The Politics of Sleep

Also by Simon J. Williams

SLEEP AND SOCIETY: Sociological Ventures into the (Un)known

DEBATING BIOLOGY: Sociology Reflections on Health, Medicine and Society (*co-edited*)

EMOTIONS AND SOCIAL LIFE (*co-edited*)

EMOTION AND SOCIAL THEORY

GENDER, HEALTH AND HEALING: The Public/Private Divide (*co-edited*)

MEDICINE AND THE BODY

HEALTH, MEDICINE AND SOCIETY: Key Theories, Future Agendas (*co-edited*)

MODERN MEDICINE: Lay Perspectives and Experiences (*co-edited*)

PHARMACEUTICALS AND SOCIETY: Critical Discourses and Debates (*co-edited*)

THE LIVED BODY: Sociological Themes, Embodied Agendas

CHRONIC RESPIRATORY ILLNESS

The Politics of Sleep

Governing (Un)consciousness in the Late Modern Age

Simon J. Williams
University of Warwick, UK

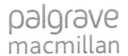

© Simon J. Williams 2011

All rights reserved. No reproduction, copy or transmission of this
publication may be made without written permission.

No portion of this publication may be reproduced, copied or
transmitted save with written permission or in accordance with the
provisions of the Copyright, Designs and Patents Act 1988, or under
the terms of any licence permitting limited copying issued by the
Copyright Licensing Agency, Saffron House, 6-10 Kirby Street,
London EC1N 8TS.

Any person who does any unauthorized act in relation to this publication
may be liable to criminal prosecution and civil claims for damages.

The author has asserted his right to be identified as the author of this
work in accordance with the Copyright, Designs and Patents Act 1988.

First published 2011 by
PALGRAVE MACMILLAN

Palgrave Macmillan in the UK is an imprint of Macmillan Publishers
Limited,registered in England, company number 785998, of
Houndmills, Basingstoke, Hampshire RG21 6XS.

Palgrave Macmillan in the US is a division of St Martin's Press LLC,
175 Fifth Avenue, New York, NY 10010.

Palgrave Macmillan is the global academic imprint of the above
companies and has companies and representatives throughout the world.

Palgrave® and Macmillan® are registered trademarks in the United
States,the United Kingdom, Europe and other countries.

ISBN: 978–0–230–22366–0 hardback
ISBN: 978–0–230–22367–7 paperback

This book is printed on paper suitable for recycling and made from fully
managed and sustained forest sources. Logging, pulping and
manufacturing processes are expected to conform to the environmental
regulations of the country of origin.

A catalogue record for this book is available from the British Library.

A catalog record for this book is available from the Library of Congress.

10 9 8 7 6 5 4 3 2 1
20 19 18 17 16 15 14 13 12 11

Printed and bound in Great Britain by
CPI Antony Rowe, Chippenham and Eastbourne

To the memory of my Dad, Alan George Williams
(17 October 1920–31 January 2008), who lives
on through me and my boys Jacob and Adam

Contents

Acknowledgements

Thanks to Philippa Grand at Palgrave Macmillan for encouraging me to write this book and to the University of Warwick for the study leave granted to do so. Thanks too to various friends, colleagues and acquaintances over the years who have shaped in innumerable ways the arguments and ideas, still in progress, that follow in the pages of this book, particularly Jon Gabe, Nick Crossley, Peter Conrad, Kenton Kroker, Philip Hancock, Mathew Thomson, Tom Crook, Steve Kroll-Smith, Brigitte Steger, Lodewijk Brunt, Sara Arber, Rob Meadows, Jenny Hislop, Sharon Boden, Clive Seale, Pam Lowe, Cathy Humphreys, Gill Bendelow, Paul Martin, John Abraham, Nigel Thrift, Nick Lee, Steve Fuller, Paul Higgs, Stephen Katz, Wendy Martin and Deborah Steinberg – apologies to anyone I've missed out here! Thanks also to Jon Gabe and Gill Shreir for comments on various bits of this book, to Angela Munro for her professional guidance, good humour and support and to Ruth Charity (as always) for putting up with me both during the writing of this book and in general!

At a rough guesstimate, I have consumed around about 840 cups of coffee and 560 cups of tea during this writing project, many in cafes I frequented if not colonised or squatted in during my sabbatical, so thanks are also probably due on this count to those friendly folks, particularly Monia Smielewska, who have fuelled and indeed benefited from my caffeine consumption and, in so doing, kept me alert/awake or wired enough courtesy of this popular drug of ours to complete this book project more or less on schedule, give or take a few months!

Last but not least, a nod in the direction of my two young boys and aspiring superheroes, Jacob and Adam (aka Batman and Robin), those saboteurs of my sleep and regular intruders into my office space, whom I love to bits but without whose 'help' this book would undoubtedly have been finished oh so much sooner! Thanks a bunch, boys. I owe you ...

Introduction: The Politics of Sleep?

To speak, let alone to write, about the 'politics of sleep' may appear strange if not absurd. Is there indeed, one might justifiably ask, by any stretch of the imagination, a 'politics of sleep' we can meaningfully point to, or even expect, in the near future?

The central argument of this book is that a politics of sleep is indeed not simply possible but evident in a variety of ways. Sleep, I will argue and demonstrate, is *political through and through*. Political, that is to say, in the sense that sleep is clearly implicated and imbricated in relations of power, authority and expertise as a site and source of claims-making, if not crisis, contestation, controversy and critique. We may in this respect, as with other aspects of the body, speak of the *regulation* or *governance* of sleep and associated socio-political issues regarding the problems, promises and prospects of sleep. This, for example, includes the rights, risks and responsibilities associated with sleepy, sleeping and sleepless bodies and, in a more critical if not radical vein perhaps, the ways in which sleep, qua unconscious somatic state, constitutes not simply a vital albeit temporary corporeal release but a potentially potent site or source of corporeal protest, refusal or resistance in an increasingly relentless if not restless or ravenous age: a 'wired awake' world indeed we might say. In our fast, flexible, work-dominated, efficiency-driven societies, moreover, as Hoffman comments, sleep problems are no longer 'a purely personal idiosyncrasy – a symptom, say, of exceptional vitality or an exquisitely fine-tuned sensibility'. Sleep (disturbance) instead has become a 'widely discussed public issue, with its own institutions, statistics, ideologies and improving ideas' (2009: 29–30): a 'matter of concern' or a 'problem in the making', in short.[1]

To consider sleep in this way, then, invites or encourages us to reflect upon the complex regulatory fields that govern not simply our waking but our sleeping lives as another problem or facet of power, politics and personhood, both past and present. My use of the term 'politics', as this suggests, is intentionally broad and wide-ranging, extending far beyond the formal political sphere or familiar references to the sleep-deprived lives of those weary or bleary-eyed politicians, to encompass many issues which, on closer inspection, turn out to be not simply political but *bio*political in character: *vital* political matters, that is to say, to do with the governance of *bodies* and hence the politics of *life itself* (cf. Rose 2007; Rabinow and Rose 2006; Foucault 1991). If sleep after all is another vital part of life, then its governance unsurprisingly perhaps is biopolitical through and through, particularly in the neo-liberal if not bio-liberal era where life itself is subsumed and capitalised upon in a multitude of ways as yet another asset or value.[2] At once a material or (neuro-) physiological matter, an arena of social, scientific and medical management, a locus of affective/emotional and inter-subjective power relations, and a powerful and potent cultural metaphor (Steinberg 2008), sleep, as we shall see in the pages that follow, is an amorphous, ambiguous, mutating phenomenon that is dispersed, deployed, deciphered, discussed, detailed, documented and debated in multiple ways, in multiple sites and settings, for multiple political ends and purposes. Sleep, moreover, doubles as both a *problem* and *prism*, a *site* and *source*, of political power relations and investments in the late modern age: a matter of growing concern today, that is to say, both personally and publicly, but also a frame of reference or point of articulation and amplification for the mobilisation of a variety of other concerns and anxieties about life and living in contemporary society, including issues of risk, stress, insecurity, injustice, time paucity or time poverty.[3]

A politics of sleep nonetheless, at one and the same time, throws up some intriguing tensions, paradoxes or contradictions. For all its ubiquity and universality, for instance, or maybe by virtue of this ubiquity and banality, sleep has no obvious political constituency beyond perhaps various patient or professional causes or campaigns of a concerted or collective kind. Rather it tends, rightly or wrongly, to be regarded as a largely 'private', 'personal' or 'individual' matter – themselves of course socio-historically constructed and contested terms of reference – and hence of little or no obvious political significance. Something we all do, in other words, but that is about all given that we tend to be asleep at the time! Consciousness-raising about an explicit lack of consciousness, moreover, as Summers-Bremner (2008) wryly notes, is not without its own ironies or contradictions.

At stake here then, we might say, are a variety of structural and ideological forces, which at first glance *conspire against* any explicit, obvious or full-blown politicisation of sleep, not least the *devaluation* and *privatisation* of sleep. Yet these very processes, I shall argue, are themselves of course deeply political and hence open to critical reflection, if not reversal or resistance. To the extent, moreover, recalling the previous notion that many sleep problems or concerns regarding sleep are not simply a *product* of society, but a *prism* or point of articulation and *amplification* for a range of other fears, worries, frustrations and anxieties regarding contemporary life and living, then talk of the politics or politicisation of sleep may not seem quite so absurd, fanciful or far-fetched after all.

To date it seems this bio- or socio-political landscape can be traced along two main axes or dimensions and characterised in terms of two main agendas, themselves of course comprising many different strands or variants on these themes. First, what might be termed the *dominant: sleep-negative* agenda (or *negative* agenda for short), expressed through numerous *sleep-negating* or *sleep-neglecting* ideas and ideologies, discourses and debates, policies and practices. This, for example, includes both the *absence* of any sustained or serious attention to sleep matters – the power evident in what is *not* said and done about sleep matters, in other words – and the multitude of ways in which sleep, as another vital aspect of the disciplinary matrix of bodies, is more explicitly denounced, dismissed, devalued and/or downsized. In both cases it is the conscious rational waking dimensions of life, and associated mandates or motifs of (self-) mastery, containment and control, which prevail or predominate over corporeal matters such as sleep. Sleep in effect, like other aspects of the body such as emotion and desire, provides yet another powerful and potentially troublesome or problematic corporeal reminder of the limits of rational modernity, which in turn, paradoxically, further fuels or redoubles attempts to 'discipline', 'contain', 'control' or 'rationalise' it. To the extent moreover, that these dominant sleep-negative or sleep-neglecting discourses and practices also serve, in the late modern age at least, to individualise and privatise sleep, or to otherwise render it a matter of little or no significance or importance, then they may also be regarded, to repeat the point made earlier, as political attempts to depoliticise sleep.

In response to this dominant or sleep-negative agenda, however, we may also now point to a second growing and altogether more *concerned: sleep-positive* agenda (or *positive* agenda for short), in which sleep is both *problematised* as matter of concern on the one hand given the costs and consequences of poor sleep for society, and *championed* on the other hand through a variety of *sleep-positive, sleep-promoting* or *sleep-friendly* ideas and ideologies, discourses and debates, policies and practices. This, for example, encompasses a variety of expert agendas, including those found in contemporary sleep science and sleep medicine today and popularised through the media and the proliferation of self-help literature, which serve to transform or translate sleep in one way or another into both a personal and public matter of concern and a prime opportunity for intervention or improvement of various kinds, if not something to be colonised, commercialised or capitalised upon through a burgeoning sleep industry which now includes everything from sleep clinics to mattresses, bedding and soporific CDs for that 'perfect night's sleep'.

The contemporary politics of sleep then, as this suggests, may in part at least be envisaged as a series of ongoing struggles, tensions and attempted resolutions or reconciliations between these two main sleep-negative and sleep-positive agendas; struggles, tensions and attempted reconciliations, that is to say, at both the micro level of individual bodies and the macro level of the body politic, and between corporeal needs on the one hand and corporate or late capitalist imperatives on the other.

To this, however, we may add a series of other newly emergent agendas more *independent: critical-reflexive* agendas, in which the social sciences and humanities now constitute a leading edge.[4] This of course is not to imply these previous two agendas are devoid of any critical edge or element. The 'sleep-positive' agenda, for example, may in part be read as a critical response to the 'sleep-negative' agenda. I term these more recent agendas 'independent' and 'critical' nonetheless in the sense that they do not simply bring other important concepts and perspectives within the social sciences and humanities to bear on the sleep/society nexus, but do so in ways which, at one and the same time, critically engage with yet go far beyond these previous two agendas. A case, in other words, of opening up other important perspectives, values, viewpoints, vistas, voices regarding the sleep and society nexus and the problems, prospects and possibilities of sleep as a socio-political matter. This for example, as my opening remarks on the politics or biopolitics of sleep suggest, includes critical explorations and interrogations of the contested nature and status of sleep today in late capitalism and contemporary risk society; the multiple ways in which sleep is governed in the neo-liberal age or era; questions of sleep, power, inequality and injustice; the social shaping/ implications of science and sleep medicine; the biomedicalisation of sleep and colonisation of everyday/night life; and the charting if not the championing of 'resistance' of various kinds to these contemporary forms of governance and control as a further important dimension, if not an altogether more radical or rival expression of the (corporeal) politics of sleep in the present or near future.

To the extent furthermore that some of these more recent engagements with sleep and society have also sought to position themselves in more or less explicit ways through critical commentaries and debates on the past and present neglect of sleep matters within the social sciences and humanities to date, then they too involve varying degrees of *reflexivity* – hence the term 'critical-reflexive' agendas above. This in turn, however, alerts us to another important fact regarding the role of the social sciences and humanities in these socio-political agendas on sleep and society, both past and present. It is not solely or simply a case in other words, as this more reflexive stance suggests, of these latter day more independent 'critical' and/or 'reflexive' engagements with sleep and society on the part of the social sciences and humanities, important and welcome as they are. A critical-reflexive stance also brings to light the ways in which the social sciences and humanities, through their past and present neglect, dismissal or devaluation of sleep matters and their privileging or prioritisation of the conscious waking if not rational dimensions of social and cultural life, are themselves to all intents and purposes silent partners, if not active participants or accomplices in the dominant sleep-negative agendas described above. To the extent furthermore, continuing in this reflexive vein, that certain strands of work on sleep and society within the social sciences and humanities, either now or in the future, share common assumptions or problematics with other expert agendas on sleep matters, or seek to ally or align themselves in some way or other with sleep science or sleep medicine through forms of collaborative or complementary research, then they too perhaps may best be regarded as part and parcel of the more 'concerned: sleep-positive' expert agendas described above.

The upshot of this therefore is clear. The social sciences and humanities do not, unsurprisingly perhaps, stand outside these relations of power, authority or expertise regarding sleep and society, even in their neglect or dismissal of sleep matters. They are instead we might say an essential part of the very production, or co-production to borrow a much favoured term in science and technology studies

(STS) today (Hackett et al. 2007), of the field in question, including of course *this very book itself on the 'politics of sleep'*: a reflexive point of no small significance and one I intend to exploit to good effect in the pages that follow as a further contribution to these debates – see also Smith (2007) on the role of reflexivity in the human sciences and the 'creation of human nature'.

These different socio-political agendas or problem spaces regarding sleep and society are schematically represented in Table 1.

The politics of sleep then, to repeat, is complex, contested and multifaceted, including as this suggests the dynamic role of the social sciences and humanities themselves in these very problems, prospects and possibilities.

My strategy in this respect, drawing on a range of arguments and evidence throughout the book, will be to trace and track, document and decipher, those actual and potential, explicit and implicit, direct and indirect ways in which sleep is being or has become increasingly politicised in the late modern age. In doing so, I seek to put further flesh on the bones of my argument that sleep is a thoroughly political and politicised matter. This moreover, I shall argue, in keeping with the foregoing reflexive point, includes the multiple roles of the social sciences and humanities in these very processes, discourses and debates and the pasts, presents and futures to which they speak.

Some caveats or disclaimers are in order perhaps at the outset. If the foregoing sketch of sleep as another important site and source of political mobilisation and investment is correct, then this of course begs important questions of the historical past as much as the present, if not of presents or futures yet to come. My focus in this respect on the *contemporary* politics of sleep in the late modernity, and associated

Table 1 The politics of sleep: a schematic outline or problem space

Position	Agendas	Examples
1. *Dominant: sleep-negative*	Neglect/dismissal/ devaluation of sleep; privileging/prioritisation of conscious, rational waking life; commitment to dominant (Western) ideals/values of corporeal discipline, self-mastery, containment/control. Emblematic expressions (and embodiments): 'No time to sleep'; 'sleep is for wimps' (Margaret Thatcher/Thomas Edison).	Contemporary work-time, work-culture, work-ethics; advent of the '24/7 society'/'wired awake' world; globalisation.
2. *Concerned: sleep-positive*	The costs and consequences of poor sleep for society; championing of sleep (in response to dominant: sleep-negative agendas); management of sleep problems; promotion of sleep-friendly policies and practices within society. Emblematic expressions (and embodiments): 'The sleep deprived/ sleep sick society'; 'the promise/pleasure of sleep'; 'Adopt a sleep-smart lifestyle' (William Dement).	Sleep experts; sleep alerts, polls, surveys, campaigns (e.g. NSF); sleep labs/clinics; (workplace) napping facilities; 'tiredness kills – take a break' motorway signs/ prosecution of (recklessly) drowsy drivers; self-help literature on sleep/ burgeoning sleep 'industry'.

Continued

Table 1 Continued

Position	Agendas	Examples
3. *Independent: critical-reflexive*	*Critical* engagements with past/present trends and transformations, discourses and debates on sleep and society (including agendas 1 and 2 above) – may or may not involve a *normative* stance on these matters. *Reflexive* awareness/ analysis of own role in these emerging discourses and debates on sleep and society and their socio-political and ethical implications.	Recent scholarship within the social sciences and humanities on sleep and society. For example: The governance of sleep(iness) (Kroll-Smith and Gunter 2005; Brown 2004) Sleep rights, roles, power relations and (gender) inequalities (Arber et al. 2007a, b) Socio-cultural and historical dimensions of on sleep (e.g. Brunt and Steger 2008; Ekirch 2005). Social shaping/implications of sleep science/medicine; biomedicalisation of sleep and the colonisation of the everyday/night life (Williams et al 2009; Wolf-Meyer 2008; Kroker 2007; Moreira 2006; Williams 2005).

issues to do with the politics of the future, is largely pragmatic given my own particular interests, preoccupations and disciplinary spheres of expertise. It also, however, rests upon and reflects what I take to be a *growing* or *increasing politicisation* of sleep, both directly and indirectly, in recent decades, or at the very least a significant *reconfigu-ration*, *refashioning* or *reformulation* of political discourses and debates regarding sleep in these contemporary times of ours, involving important elements of both *continuity* and *change* with the past.

The predominant focus of the book, for similar reasons, is also, though not exclusively, Western. To speak of sleep in the so-called 24/7 era or wired awake world, nonetheless, begs important questions regarding *global* trends and trans-formations, which alongside some comparative materials on sleep in the Asia and the West, are taken up and addressed throughout the book in the chapters that follow.

A third point concerns the eclectic theoretical stance or theoretical eclecticism of the book. To the extent, for exam-ple, that the issues to be discussed in the pages that follow revolve around the governance of sleepy/alert bodies in the neo-liberal age or era, and the broader questions and issues this raises about the contemporary politics or biopolitics of sleep, then a Foucauldian analysis or stance clearly has its merit. This, for instance, beyond a general emphasis on the productive nature of power relations, includes attention to the role of expertise in regulating subjectivity; analysis of risk as a socio-political technology in the production of the 'at-risk' self; the manner in which subjects are not simply subject to various policies and programmes but required to actively participate in them as good citizens and enterpris-ing selves (cf. Rose 1996, 1992, 1990; Miller and Rose 1990); and finally a recognition of the complexities, negotiations, subtleties and micro relations of power, spanning both rational and non-rational elements, which in turn serve to remind us, as Petersen puts it, that 'any project of gov-ernance is always incomplete and partial in respect of the objects and practices it governs' (1997: 203). Power relations then, from this perspective, involve diffuse, diverse, dispersed and dynamic investment strategies, including the ability of subjects not simply to know or come to think of themselves in particular ways, but to manage or self-regulate themselves and their conduct, including their own risks and behaviours, in new, novel or enterprising ways (Rose 2007, 1992, 1990; Rabinow and Rose 2006).[5]

I also nonetheless, given the challenges, complexities and multiplicities involved in charting or tracing the politics of sleep and the limits of any one perspective in fully or adequately doing so, draw on a variety of other perspectives and approaches throughout the book, including phenomenological approaches to the lived body; recent sociological work on the negotiation of sleep rights across the life course; elements of social and political thought on questions of rights, vulnerability, (in)equality and (in)justice; strands of work at the interface between science and technology studies (STS) and medical sociology on the social shaping/ social implications of sleep science and the biomedicalisation of society; and finally, at the broadest and most general level, various other contemporary sociological theories and debates on the contours and dynamics of contemporary capitalism, risk society and late or liquid modernity. This, to be sure, leaves me open to potential criticism on various counts, not least regarding the undoubted philosophical (i.e. ontological and epistemological) tensions or problems involved in any such theoretical eclecticism.[6] To the extent nonetheless that a strategy of this kind opens up different avenues or entry points on these complex multifaceted issues concerning the politics of sleep, then it clearly has its merits. To the extent, moreover, that we are at a relatively early stage in theorising these sleep and society relations, including the politics of sleep, and to the extent that my intent, in this book at least, is precisely to chart or explore these issues from a variety of different angles, perspectives or viewpoints, rather than attempt some sort of grand and premature theoretical synthesis or integration of these different approaches and perspectives, then a pragmatic or plural theoretical stance of this kind undoubtedly has its merits as well as its drawbacks. Given the limited work on sleep, let alone the 'politics' of sleep, within the social sciences and humanities to date, in short, and given the complex if not contested or contradictory nature of sleep itself, keeping our theoretical options open may well be a wise move, or to put it the other way around, foreclosing them may well be unwise at this particular juncture or point in time.

A final point concerns the role of sleep science and sleep medicine within all this. There is to be sure, as we shall see, a powerful argument to be made here that sleep, as a bio- or socio-political matter, is 'everywhere' today because 'knowledge' of it has increased courtesy of sleep science and sleep medicine, particularly in the information age or era where expertise of all kinds 'travels', so to speak, far beyond its original anchor points or institutional confines. On this, of course, I wholly concur and do not dissent. Rather than start with the sleep laboratory or sleep clinic, however, and then move 'outwards' into the broader realms and vistas of society, I have chosen instead to spell out where sleep science/ medicine fits into the unfolding political or biopolitical storyline towards the end of the book as a further commentary, or series of critical reflections, if you will, on what has gone before and what indeed may be around the corner in the near or not-too-distant future. To the extent, moreover, to repeat, that the politics of sleep is rich, complex, multisited and multifaceted, extending far beyond the reach or remit of sleep science or sleep medicine, even in the information age, then approaching or framing things in this way undoubtedly has its merits as well as its drawbacks.[7]

Five chapters follow in taking these issues forward and charting these many facets and features of the contemporary politics of sleep in all its richness and complexity.

Chapter 1 sets the scene for the book as a whole by placing or locating sleep within the context and contours of late or 'fast' capitalism. Attention is paid, in doing so, to charting and exploring the changing nature, pace, tempo and dynamics of life and living in contemporary society in general, and associated discourses and debates about its costs and consequences for sleep, or lack of it, in particular. The chapter, as such, provides a preliminary or provisional sketch of the problematisation and politicisation of sleep 'loss', 'debt' or 'deprivation' in contemporary society, including relations between sleep, work time, work culture and work ethics; the location of sleep within contemporary risk culture; and related socio-political matters to do with the multiple associations between sleep, risk and the politics of anxiety. This therefore, at an early stage in the proceedings, enables me to put further flesh on the bones of my argument, as outlined above, that the politics of sleep, however nascent or embryonic, involves or entails a dual point of reference in which sleep doubles or redoubles as both a problem in its own right and a prism or point of articulation/amplification for the mobilisation of a wide variety of other concerns and anxieties about life and living in the contemporary late modern era, if not the 'go faster' or 'non-stop' world of global capitalism.

Chapter 2, following directly on from these previous concerns and considerations, moves us to closely associated moral and political issues to do with the governance of alert/sleep(y) bodies in contemporary society, particularly questions of citizenship, vigilance, virtue and the politics of culpability or blame. At stake here, I argue, is not simply the remaking or refashioning of sleepiness as a culpable corporeal condition or blameworthy soporific state, but the associated recasting or revaluation of sleep itself in altogether more positive or productive terms as the aid or ally rather than the enemy of contemporary corporate capitalism. Sleep as such, recast or reconfigured in this fashion, becomes the duty, ethic and responsibility of each and every one of us in the service of both personal and public goals or goods, values or ideals, including hopes, dreams or visions of the 'well-slept' citizen and the 'well-slept' society. The chapter in this respect casts further critical light on the multiple relays and relations between the aforementioned 'concerned' political agendas regarding sleep and predominant/prized neo-liberal values and corporate ideologies of enterprise and efficiency if not enhancement or (self-) improvement in all walks of life, both inside and outside the workplace.

Further critical moral and political questions come sharply into view in Chapter 3, which takes a closer look at the *rights and wrongs of sleep*, both locally and globally. Key issues here, for example, include the contested nature and status of sleep rights across the life course, relations between autonomy, sleep and the 'just' society, the 'dark face' or 'dark side' of sleep deprivation in the guise of interrogation or torture, and related matters to do with sleep, vulnerability and *bare life*. Sleep, as this chapter clearly attests, may very well be a great 'leveller' to which we all sooner or later succumb, regardless of status, rank or position, but it also constitutes another profoundly important, yet neglected or invisible, dimension of social inequality, insecurity and injustice: something, qua basic human need and basic human right, which at once unites and divides us, both publicly and privately, locally and globally.

Chapter 4 in contrast focuses on another vital dimension to the politics of sleep in which corporeal questions of unconsciousness and unruliness, transgression and taboo, dormativity and normativity loom large. These issues are explored from a variety of angles, including phenomenological explorations of sleep and other liminal or partial states of consciousness, the policing of dreams, the spatialisation and co-mingling of dormant/deviant bodies and the politics of the night. Sleep from this viewpoint, I argue, provides something of a double corporeal point of reference as both 'limit' and 'excess'. A corporeal 'limit', that is to say, in relation to conscious waking life in general and the rapidly escalating if not excessive demand and dictates of contemporary life and living in particular; and a corporeal state of unconsciousness if not unruliness which, by virtue of this very fact, exists beyond and hence 'exceeds' the bounds or 'limits' of conscious waking life and the dreams, desire or delusions of rational modernity. The chapter as such may be read as a further corporeal exploration of the powers of sleep and hence the complexities of contemporary forms of governance, including the prospects or possibilities of corporeal protest or resistance of various kinds, both past and present, public and private.

The final chapter, as already noted, completes the storyline and fills in the missing pieces through a focus on the role of sleep science and sleep medicine within all this. Key issues covered here, for example, drawing on strands of both science and technology studies and medical sociology, include the *transformation* of sleep into an 'object' of scientific or technoscientific inquiry during the course of the twentieth century, its *translation* into a 'problem' within the modern-day sleep clinic, the shifting or blurred boundaries between *therapy* and *enhancement,* and the multiple relays or relations between medical, corporate and popular culture in the governance of sleepy/alert bodies today in the name of public health and safety, productivity and performance, wisdom and well-being, diligence and virtue. The chapter in this respect, to repeat, brings to the fore and spells out in explicit fashion themes largely implicit in previous chapters concerning the critical roles and relations between *biomedicine, bioscience* and *biotechnology* in the politics or *biopolitics* of sleep in contemporary society, and related questions to do with the very nature and status of sleep itself as an ambiguous, morphing, mutating phenomenon which is endlessly reworked or reconfigured as a problem or matter of concern within the diverse circuits and settings of the sleep laboratory, the sleep clinic and the shifting or blurred boundaries between public and private life. It also, in closing, rehearses various alternative possible futures regarding sleep, taking the military as a case study or exemplar, including both futures present and futures yet to come, in which sleep may, or may not, become a relic of the evolutionary past.

A brief Afterword follows in which I revisit and restate the central arguments of the book concerning the problems, prospects and possibilities of a politics of sleep, both now and in the near future, including the role of the social sciences and humanities within these discourses and debates. Sleep, it is argued, in its manifold guises, is a prime site and source of controversy and concern, contestation and critique: both a *problem* and a *prism,* to repeat, regarding life and living in these late modern times of ours. In these and countless other ways, I conclude, sleep is not simply political through and through, but likely to become *increasingly politicised* in the (near) future, as interest in sleep matters continues to grow both inside and outside the bedroom, the workplace, the clinic, the laboratory and the academy, and attempts to hold on to or reclaim sleep in some way or other converge, compete or clash with attempts to render it ever more 'optional' if not 'obsolete' in an era seduced by a renewed ethic of enterprise, cultural imperatives towards wakefulness and the lure or temptation of (biomedical) enhancement.

Notes

1. My use of the term 'matter of concern' here is first intended in a commonsensical, simple or straightforward fashion, to denote the multiple ways in which sleep is coming to matter today, or better still being made to matter today, in all walks of life both inside and outside the laboratory or clinic: a problem in the making, to repeat. It also of course recalls Latour's (2008, 2004) own more 'technical' rendition, as he himself puts it, of these matters in terms of the distinction he draws (as a shorthand for 'the huge sea change between two empiricisms – the first and the second') between 'matters of fact' and 'matters of concern'. 'A matter of concern', in this latter sense, 'is what happens to a matter of fact when you add to its whole scenography, much like you would do by shifting your attention from the stage to the whole machinery of the theatre' (2008: 38). See Wolf-Meyer (2008), for example, for a recent Latourian rendition of these 'matters' in relation to 'sleep, signification and the abstract body of allopathic medicine'. See also Chapters 1, 2 and 5 of this book in particular for further elaborations of these matters of concern.
2. See Rabinow and Rose (2006), for example, for a useful recent discussion of biopower today, including their own Foucauldian stance vis-à-vis the likes of Hardt and Negri (2000) and Agamben (1998). Biopower, Rabinow and Rose conclude, focuses attention on three key elements, namely: 'knowledge of vital life processes, power relations that take humans as living beings as their object, and the modes of subjectification through which subjects work on themselves qua living beings – as well as their multiple combinations' (2006: 215). See also Bull (2007)

on vectors of the biopolitical and Massumi (2002) on the 'subsumption of life under capitalism' – a term which Dickens (2000) also deploys to good effect, albeit from a somewhat different angle or vantage point.

3. This of course is not to dismiss or discount the sleep 'problems' people experience and articulate in their everyday lives, or the broader discourses and debates on sleep as a matter of concern in contemporary society. It does, however, alert us to the way in which these very articulations of sleep 'problems' may also serve, at one and the same time, as vectors or vehicles for the mobilisation of a variety of other concerns and anxieties that may or may not have much to do with sleep 'problems' as such, but which are nonetheless framed in this way through the discursive rendering of sleep 'problems' as a matter of personal and/or public 'concern'. See Chapter 1 for a further elaboration of this point.

4. See Williams (2008, 2005), for example, for recent reviews of progress, problems and prospects regarding the sleep and society nexus within the social sciences and humanities.

5. A case, in other words, as Massumi (2002) appositely puts it, not so much of an extrinsic relation of power from outside and over us but of a power which 'in-forms' us, such that in learning to follow its contours and its constraints we are, in effect, 'following ourselves' – the corollary being that we cannot easily or readily 'run away' from it either.

6. Shilling (2003), for example, takes Turner (1992) to task on precisely these sorts of counts regarding attempts to theorise body–society relations from a range of different perspectives or viewpoints.

7. My aim here, in other words, is to steer a cautious and considered path between the Scylla of underplaying the sleep science/sleep medicine story and the Charybdis of over-stretching its explanatory reach or frame of reference. See, for example, on this latter count, Smith's (2009) recent review of Kroker's (2007) book *The Sleep of Others and the Transformations of Sleep Research*. While Kroker, Smith notes, undoubtedly writes a convincing 'biography' of the sleep laboratory and the socio-historical transformations contained therein, in moving 'outwards' from these specific claims about transformations of sleep *research*, to claims about 'the *being* of sleep' – claims, that is to say, about wider transformation in the meanings of sleep and dreams in the 'centuries before and the social places beyond' – his 'conceptual framework does not serve' (Smith 2009: 110).

1
Restless Times: Wired Awake in *Fast* Capitalism?

Introduction

Any attempt to grasp or grapple with the politics of sleep in the contemporary developed world today needs to place these issues in the context of broader social, cultural, economic and political trends and transformations during the closing decades of the twentieth century and the opening decade of the twenty-first century.

In this opening chapter, therefore, we take a critical look at the contested nature and status of sleep, or lack of it, within contemporary society, with particular reference to issues of *continuity* and *change* in the *temporal regimes* of working life and living in the so-called era of *fast* or *flexible* capitalism and associated issues concerning relations between the politics of sleep, risk and anxiety in the late modern age.

At stake here, in other words, is a series of key questions, the answers to which set the scene or context for the book as a whole and themes and issues that follow. What are the implications of contemporary forms of work and leisure for our sleeping as well as our waking lives, for example? Are we all trading on 'dangerous' levels of sleep 'debt' or 'deprivation', for instance, as some claim? Is sleepiness, moreover, now being reconfigured or refashioned as an 'adverse', 'dangerous', 'problematic' or 'at-risk' state, and if so with what consequences? And what finally does all this tell us, as a first or preliminary pass, if you will, about the problematisation or politicisation of sleep in the late modern age?

Sleep, as we shall see, is indeed a contested or controversial matter in these 'restless' if not 'relentless' times of ours, at once both a *problem* or matter of concern in its own right, and a *prism* or point of articulation for the mobilisation of a range of other concerns and anxieties about contemporary life and living in the late modern age. It is to these changing contours and contexts of life and living in late or fast capitalism, therefore, that we now turn in search of sleep, so to speak.

Acceleration: a 'time-squeezed/go-faster' world?

Life, it seems, is speeding up. Everything apparently is accelerating in this time-squeezed, go-faster world of ours, so we are told. This is an era that goes by or trades under various names such as 'late', 'light', 'liquid', 'flexible' or 'post-Fordist' capitalism (see, for example, Bauman 2000; Giddens 1991; Harvey 1989; Martin 2000, 1994), but one characterised, among other things, by *speed* and the associated reworking or *reconfiguration of time/space boundaries.*

On this perhaps we may all more or less readily concur. Life for many if not most of us does indeed seem to be accelerating these days. We seem to be busier than ever before, with more to do in less time, in an increasingly restless if not relentless, frantic if not frenetic era, which leaves us feeling more or less tired, wired or just plain worn out. Even social and cultural commentators and critics concerned with the analysis of these trends and transformations struggle, it seems, to keep up with them. Agger's

(2004) book *Speeding Up Fast Capitalism*, for example, as he readily acknowledges, was written as a sequel to his previous book *Fast Capitalism* (1989), given capitalism by his reckoning had become *even 'faster'* since the 1980s, particularly in light of the rapid pace and development of new (faster and faster) information technologies in the Internet age and global era.[1]

To speak of 'fast' capitalism in this respect, Agger (2004) argues, is to highlight at least two important interconnected or interrelated ways in which capitalism has been modified, particularly over the past two decades or so and into present-day or early twenty-first-century capitalism. The first involves the *compression of time and the quickening pace of everyday life* in the face of new economic imperatives and forms of social control. The second pertains to the *erosion of boundaries* which are 'effaced by a social order bent on *denying people private space and time'* (Ibid.: 4, my emphasis). The key factor underpinning these two senses of the adjective 'fast' (i.e. acceleration and erosion of boundaries), Agger suggests, is *instanteity*; we expect things ever more quickly, instantly even, at the snap of our fingers or the click of a mouse, including 'fast food, fast cars, fast bodies, fast work, fast reading and fast writing' (Ibid.: 5).[2] This instanteity in turn engenders potentially new *global dimensions* to *contemporary experience* in the 'wired' world, thereby further contributing to these 'disembedding' processes and 'de-boundarying' effects through the compression of time and space as communication and information accelerates, and our sense and sensibilities are further rewired or reconfigured in the global age or era (cf. Giddens 1991; Harvey 1989): an 'invasion of home and head', in effect, 'by cultural imperatives delivered by advertising and the media' (Agger 2004: 9).

It is certainly true that a new *intensity* seems to character-ise or accompany this instanteity of contemporary life and living both inside and outside the workplace, an intensity at once both *structural and ideological*, based on transforma-tions in the *globalised* capitalist economy which themselves are understood and experienced if not justified through appeals to neo-liberal notions of 'enterprise', 'freedom', 'flexibility', 'freewill' and so on in which we are all some-how expected to be '(more) available', to work 'faster' and/ or 'longer', and generally to 'do more in less time'. A world, in short, characterised or predicated on a new air or ethos of 'busyness' as a badge of honour, pride or a sign of value (Gershuny 2005), and new norms of 'having too much to do', especially among the professional and managerial sec-tors of the economy (Widerberg 2006: 115).

Hopes or dreams of a 'leisure revolution' or 'surplus of free time' tied to economic progress and technological change have, in this respect, failed to materialise or all but disappeared. Instead, transformations in work-time rela-tions – such as the shifting boundaries of work and social life, the drive toward greater efficiency and competition in the global economy, neo-liberal shifts in governmental policies, and associated trends such as the deregulation of working time and the weakening of trade unions – appear to have 'halted the long-term trend of reduction in full-time working hours' (Chatzitheochari and Arber 2009: 31; see also Wainwright and Calnan 2002; Green 2001; Kodz et al. 1998).

These trends and transformations, for example, are clearly evident in the United Kingdom, which at the time of writ-ing still has the dubious honour of being the only EU mem-ber state to retain the right for exemption (via an opt-out agreement, first won by John Major in 1993) from the 1993

European Working Time Directive (EWTD) which set the upper weekly limit for full-time paid work at 48 hours. This is a position the British government continues to defend despite various EU challenges to or rulings regarding this exemption (see also Chapter 2). Britain indeed is renowned for its 'long hours culture', with over a quarter of employees working over 48 hours a week, especially among men at *both ends* of the occupational spectrum (Chatzitheochari and Arber 2009: 31; see also Warren 2002). A large proportion of the British population, moreover, according to Kreitzman, believe they are 'overworked, and that life is out of control' (1999: 25).

It is not, however, as already noted, just working *time* which is at stake here but the concentration and *intensification* of work – a broad trend it seems across most sectors of the economy or workforce since the mid-1980s (Wainwright and Calnan 2002; Green 2001) – and associated trends such as the decline in job tenure or increase in *job insecurity*, particularly in the wake of the recent economic downturn. A recent UK survey commissioned by the mental health charity Mind (2010), for example, found that one in four employees dreaded going back to work the next day due to the pressures people are under in the current economic climate, with high rates of unpaid overtime, and almost all the people surveyed saying they were unhappy with their work/life balance (McVeigh 2010).[3]

Unpaid workloads associated with domestic and child-care activities also, of course, weigh heavily in the balance sheet here, leaving employed individuals, particularly working mothers, less time for other pursuits and pastimes – a 'second shift' (cf. Hochschild 1990) in effect, resulting in a further 'time-squeeze' or 'time-bind' (Hochschild 1997) from paid work and family responsibilities that is clearly gendered (Chatzitheochari and Arber 2009; Venn et al. 2008). 'Time paucity', 'time poverty' or a lack of 'discretionary time', as a consequence, appears to be a growing problem for many people today in advanced countries across the globe (see, for example, Goodin et al. 2008);[4] the implication being that 'temporal autonomy' is a basic measure of individual freedom and that for some, as Hoffman notes, 'time has become a more valuable and less attainable commodity than money' (2009: 11–12).

These trends, to be sure, are important. The pace or tempo of life does indeed, to repeat, appear to be accelerating, quickening or speeding up for many if not most of us today in the advanced minority world. Caution nonetheless is clearly needed with respect to any such broad brush or unqualified portrayal of this global 'go-faster', 'speeded-up' or 'runaway' world. This, for example, as Thrift (2008, 2000, 1997, 1996, 1995) rightly notes, includes the danger or risk of a crude, overly simplistic technological determinism, or the lack of other important points of *continuity* or *challenge* to any such trends (see also Wajcman 2008).[5] To the extent, moreover, that speed itself is in part a 'cultural creation' if not a rhetorical resource (i.e. a 'rhetoric of "speedy" things'), then this itself depends upon the 'depiction of certain places, things and people as slow-moving' (Thrift 2008: 63). In particular, it may be argued that this greater awareness of movement has in turn produced a set of resources that enable us to separate out a 'present-oriented stillness, thus promoting a *"politics" based on intensified attention to the present*' (Ibid.: 64, my emphasis). This, for example, includes a host of cultural practices associated with quiet contemplation, which 'distil or concentrate time', and other technologies and body techniques or practices which 'stretch out the moment' and 'expand the size of consciousness', thereby allowing each moment to be 'more carefully attended to' and which, taken together, may be viewed as constructing a 'slow-down perception, as much as a speed-up' (Ibid.: 65). Boredom furthermore, qua discourse and experience, remains a distinct possibility if not a characteristic feature of modernity to the present day. In a time, in other words, where the:

> drive to novelty and innovation, speed and progress that have always defined modernity become the foundation of a process of continuously accelerating transformation, *boredom haunts the Western world*... as both cause and effect of this universal process – both as the disaffection with the old that drives the search for change and as the *malaise produced by living under a permanent speed-up*. A symptom, then, of modernity, this experience without qualities, an adaptation at once visceral and intellectual to life in a world where nothing stays put, to an era in which the idea of transcendent meaning seems hopelessly old-fashioned. (Goodstein 2005: 1–2, my emphasis)

Contemporary culture then, as this suggests, involves important elements of *continuity* as well as *change* in relation to any such trends and transformations in the pace or tempo of life in late or fast capitalism. This, moreover, includes multiple acts of 'slowness', both individual and collective in kind, which are not so much, Honoré comments, about a 'backlash' as about finding the right sort of 'balance' in a fast-paced world, and might even embrace or encompass the possibility of doing things quickly while maintaining a 'slow frame of mind' (2004: 15), of which more in the next chapter of this book.[6]

Debt: no time to sleep?

It is in this context of continuity and change in the temporal rhythms, routines and regimes of contemporary capitalism and its global reach that sleep in general, and sleep 'debt', sleep 'deprivation' or sleep 'loss' in particular, comes to the fore as a critical yet neglected issue or matter of concern which itself provides a further vantage point and embodied expression, if not critique, of prevailing sociocultural, political and economic imperatives that privilege or prioritise alert wakefulness and valorise vigilance. 'Wakefulness and the wired world go together', in other words, as Summers-Bremner comments, with the 'expansion of the 24-7 economy into more and more lives, and more of each life' (2008: 131).

Sleep-deprivation, therefore, according to various experts, commentators and campaigners, is a widespread and growing problem in contemporary society; a casualty, symptom or victim of the wired world, that is to say, the costs and consequences of which have yet to be fully counted. A number of sources may be pointed to in this respect, some more credible than others. Dement (1999) for example, an eminent American sleep expert, claims that: (i) people now sleep on average 1½ hours less each night than they would have a century ago; (ii) there is an 'epidemic' of sleep deprivation in our midst; and (iii) most people in advanced industrialised countries, as a consequence, are walking around with an accumulated 'sleep deficit' of between 25 and 30 hours.

A litany of supposedly 'sleepy' people are pointed to or singled out for attention in this regard, including sleepy drivers, pilots, doctors, parents, children, teachers and politicians, all of which it is claimed represent a risk or danger not simply to themselves but to others and to society at large through this lamentable soporific state of affairs.

Politicians, in particular, are frequently criticised on this count as 'poor role models' given a macho political culture where sleep is seen as for 'wimps' (epitomised in the Thatcher era) and sleep-deprivation treated as a sign of dedication, drive or devotion to the cause (see Table 1). When it comes to the list of famous insomniacs, indeed, then 'care-worn politicians loom large', as Summer-Bremner (2008: 129) wryly remarks. Awakeness 'beyond the degree expected from the general population', she continues, 'is endemic to contemporary governance' (Ibid.), albeit with the important rider that greater alertness or vigilance is required on the part of us all these days of course in contemporary *risk* culture or risk society (cf. Beck 1992; Giddens 1991), of which more shortly. Consider, for example, a recent article in the *Guardian* newspaper (Barkman 2008), in the midst of the financial crisis/credit crunch, entitled 'Sleepless in SW1'. 'The financial crisis', it is noted, 'is keeping politicians', such as Alistair Darling and Gordon Brown, 'from their beds with rounds of all-night meetings'. But 'Is this wise?' it then proceeds to ask. 'How much sleep deprivation can anyone take before their judgement takes a fall?' (Ibid.).

The recent British election campaign was also something of an eye opener on this count, quite literally. This, for example, included desperate last-ditch attempts on the part of the main party leaders to drum up potential votes in the last 36 hours prior to polling day. Cameron, for example, the Conservative Party leader and subsequent Prime Minister in the new coalition government, undertook a punishing 36-hour schedule, including visits to night-workers at an engineering plant in Lancaster, fishermen on the night-shift in Grimsby and supermarket staff, bakers and paramedics in Bristol, while also apparently 'grabbing some sleep' in the back of the campaign bus between visits 'in a bid to stay fresh in the run up to polling day' (*Channel 4 News* 2010).

As for the costs and consequences of this stinting on or selling ourselves 'short' of sleep, these it is claimed are borne both individually and collectively, including various large-scale accidents, catastrophes or national disasters such as the Exxon Valdez oil spill, the Challenger space shuttle disaster, and the Chernobyl nuclear meltdown (see Moore-Ede 1993, for example).[7] Sleep-related accidents, as this suggests, are costly on many counts. Even when expressed in purely financial terms indeed, these costs and consequences quickly escalate or multiply. Mitler et al. (2000), for example, estimate these costs to be in the region of $56 billion each year in the United States alone, excluding lost productivity, medical illness or shortened life span.

Many of these discourses and debates, however, are North American in origin. Is this then, we may justifiably ask, a distinctly American crisis, or problem 'in the making', so to speak? Certainly, there is plenty of campaigning or lobbying about sleep-related matters in North America, through bodies such as the National Sleep Foundation (www. sleepfoundation.org), which conducts an annual 'Sleep in America' poll to help both document the extent of sleep problems among the American public and raise the profile of sleep as a matter of public concern. The executive summary of the NSF 2005 Adult Sleep Habits and Styles Poll (NSF 2005), for example, informs us inter alia that:

- on average, adults in America are sleeping 6.8 hours a night on weekdays and 7.4 hours a night on weekends. Overall, adults in America report sleeping an average of 6.9 hours a night when considering both weekday and weekend sleep.

- a significant proportion of the respondents (40%) report getting less than 7 hours of sleep a night on weekdays. About seven in ten adults (71%) are getting less than 8 hours of sleep a night on weekdays.
- over the past several years, there has been a downward trend in the proportion of respondents who report sleeping 8 or more hours a night on weekdays (from 38% in 2001 to 30% in 2002 and 26% in 2005).[8]

North America has also, of course, as will be more fully discussed in Chapter 5, been at the forefront of sleep science and sleep medicine over the past half-century, thereby helping raise the profile of sleep as a matter of concern in contemporary society still further. Sleep-deprivation nonetheless, according to a variety of studies and sources, is a widespread and growing problem in many if not all advanced industrial societies and 24-hour economies in the global age or 'wired' world. Martin (2002), for example, drawing on studies in countries as diverse as Australia, Sweden, Poland, Finland, France and Japan, concludes that 'overall' it is safe to say at least 'one in ten adults in the general population (you, me and the people next door) are currently affected by moderate or severe daytime sleepiness. Some scientists believe the situation is much worse, with up to one in three adults suffering from significant sleepiness' (Ibid.: 20).

These findings in turn are echoed and amplified in other specially commissioned public surveys and popular opinion polls. A recent Demos report, for example – tellingly entitled *Dream On – Sleep in the 24/7 Society* (Leadbeater 2004) – finds (on the basis of a specially commissioned MORI poll[9]) that:

- 39 per cent of British adults say they 'do not get enough sleep'
- sleep deficit/deprivation is most concentrated in the 25–54 age bracket (i.e. those of working age who are likely to have family

responsibilities); among managers and white-collar workers (51%) and full-time workers (49%)

- self-reported consequences of sleep deprivation included irritability and shouting, mistakes at work and behind the wheel, and falling asleep at work
- key sleep disrupters identified were children (reported by 41% of parents), worry at work (15% of managers) and noise (Leadbeater 2004).

Similarly, *Insomniac Britain – Does Anybody Sleep Here Anymore?* – a report by the British Association of Counselling and Psychotherapy (BACP 2005)[10] – claims that 'the nation is "sleep deprived"', based on further survey findings that:

- people report they only get on average 6 hours 53 minutes of sleep per night
- 12+ million people in Britain (27% of the adult population) experience at least three bad nights' sleep in an average week
- there is a 'night-time gender divide' – women are significantly worse sleepers than men.

Caution nonetheless is once again required here regarding many of these claims about sleep and society. Horne (2006), for example, highlights a number of important points in response to both current evidence and assumptions of a '(chronically) sleep-deprived society', including: (i) the limits of historical comparative data regarding the quality and quantity of sleep; (ii) the problem of asking people about their sleep; and (iii) the costs versus benefits of encouraging people to get more sleep.

With respect to the first of these issues, for example, the partial or patchy historical data available make firm claims about either the quantity or quality of our sleep relative to our ancestors at best difficult and at worst impossible in anything other than the most general or broad terms. It may very well be indeed, as Ekirch (2005) rightly notes, that the *quality* of our sleep has improved over time – through, for example, better housing, heating, bedding, pain relief and the like – even if, and it is still a big 'if', its *quantity* has declined. Many people today indeed, as Klug posits, 'can hardly imagine the various threats our medieval ancestors were exposed to in the dormant part of their lives, given the warmth and security of modern day centrally heated bedrooms and our safely locked if not gated houses or apartments' (2008: 33). (See also Cox (2008) on the perils and potential of sleep in the eighteenth century.)

Caution too is clearly needed on this historical count in relation to current claims about our so-called long work-hours culture. The picture indeed, unsurprisingly perhaps, is more complex than this on closer inspection, depending on sector or occupation, and the time period in question. Generally, nonetheless, working hours have declined over time, even if work intensification, as noted above, has increased since the mid-1980s (Wainwright and Calnan 2002; Green 2001).

As for self-reports of sleep-deprivation, these too of course are potentially problematic on a number of counts. While 'tiredness' and 'sleepiness', for instance, are clearly separate states, they are frequently equated or conflated in everyday life (see, for example, Widerberg 2006). These meanings in turn are likely to be gendered and to differ according to other sociological or socio-demographic factors such as class, occupation, education and age (Williams et al. 2010; Meadows et al. 2008a; Arber et al. 2007a, b; Meadows 2005). Just because people say they are 'tired' or 'sleepy' or not getting 'enough' sleep, moreover, does not necessarily mean they need 'more' sleep or therefore, as a corollary, that more sleep would be a worthwhile investment of their time compared to other possible investments such as more exercise, for example (Horne 2006). Individual sleep 'needs', furthermore, are known to vary considerably, while any such self-defined sleep 'shortage' or 'deficit' may be as much a *product of perception* as it is of actual time spent asleep (Williams 2005).

Most available evidence anyway, Horne (2006) notes, seems to show that people actually get 7 to 7½ hours per night which, depending on quality, the majority of sleep experts would probably deem to be adequate for most healthy adults.[11] The UK 2000 Time Use Survey (ONS 2003) indeed points to a fairly constant 8 hours per night for adults until people get into their 60s, when it begins to rise to an average of 9 hours, with women on the whole appearing to sleep longer than men, particularly in the 30–60 age range[12] (see also ONS 2006).[13] Similarly, a recent international OECD survey recorded an average sleep time across all OECD countries surveyed of 502 minutes per night, or 8 hours 22 minutes, with France topping the table at 530 minutes per night compared to Korea with the lowest average sleep time of 469 minutes per night, just 11 minutes short of 8 hours (Cartwright 2009; OECD 2009).

Sleep then, as this preliminary discussion suggests, is indeed a contested issue or matter within contemporary society. Something, that is to say, which is becoming increasingly problematised if not politicised through discourses and debates regarding sleep loss, debt or deprivation as an 'adverse' or 'at-risk' state, for self and society, and hence a matter of concern.

Anxiety: sleep as problem and/or prism?

It is precisely at this juncture that further pertinent questions come to the fore concerning relations between the politics of sleep, risk and anxiety in contemporary culture and society. To what extent, for example, as a consequence or corollary of these discourses and debates, are people becoming or made to feel increasingly anxious about their sleep? To what extent, moreover, are sleep problems themselves a symptom or expression of broader cultural concerns and anxieties about life and living in contemporary society? And perhaps most importantly of all for our purposes, what does this tell us about discourses regarding sleep 'problems' themselves?

As to the first of these questions, the aforementioned discourses and debates on the costs and consequences of sleep (debt/deprivation) for both self and society, certainly runs the risk of *anxiety inflation*. Consciousness-raising campaigns or public alerts, for example, may not only sound like a contradiction in terms when it comes to sleep, they may also, paradoxically or unintentionally, *promote or fuel the very sleep problems they are designed to alleviate* through the concerns and anxieties they engender regarding sleep (Horne 2006). The last thing an insomniac needs, for example, is a further reason to worry about their sleep! This, of course, is not to belittle, discount or devalue the possibility that calls or campaigns of this kind may result in a better-rested if not well-slept public, populace or citizenry. It does nonetheless introduce an important note of caution with respect to any such campaigns or public alerts of this kind, however well intentioned.

The aforementioned construction of sleep loss, debt or deprivation as an 'adverse', 'at-risk' or otherwise problematic state, nonetheless, is itself of course part and parcel of a broader landscape or proliferation of risks in contemporary society (Beck 1992; Giddens 1991),[14] which not only compete or clamour for attention but *engender their own particular or peculiar anxieties, fears, uncertainties*, if not outright states of panics or paranoia, with potentially important implications once again for our sleep (or lack of it). Fear and anxiety, indeed, appear to be characteristic if not predominant affective states in contemporary society. We have long since, for example, according to writers such as Furedi (2005), been 'enveloped' in a 'culture of fear' as an 'ever expanding part of life' tied to the multitude or explosion of risks we now face – from GM food, BSE, prospective flu pandemics or the health dangers of mobile phones, to 'stranger danger', potential acts of terrorism, energy security, climate change or global warming and other environmental disasters – with 'scaremongering' increasingly represented as the act of a 'concerned and responsible citizen' (Ibid.: vii–viii) – see also Booker and North (2007).

Scare stories, however, Furedi (2005: ix) argues, do not simply make people more anxious or fearful, they also 'reinforce existing apprehensions and help to shape and even alter the way that people conduct their lives', including the parenting or 'paranoid parenting' of their children (Furedi 2002). Once the mindset of fear prevails, in other words, 'it creates a world where problems and difficulties are inflated' and fear, panic or paranoia are driven by a 'self-fulfilling dynamic' (Furedi 2005: xi).[15] This, moreover, as we shall see in the next chapter, contributes in no small part to ever-renewed efforts at *vigilance* which in turn are based upon and underwrite a heightened alertness in all walks of life as the active duty and responsibility of all good citizens.

While a distinction is frequently drawn in this respect, for psychological or psychiatric purposes, between fear and anxiety – the former considered a more specific or immediate state and the latter a more generalised, free-floating or diffuse state – it is clear nonetheless, as Bourke (2005: 191) rightly notes, that any such differences 'oscillate wildly' in socio-historical time, with 'anxiety easily converted into fear' and vice versa. The uncertainty of anxiety, for example, can quickly be converted into more focused fears through the cultural and political process of naming an enemy or scapegoating (Ibid.). The conversion of fear into more diffuse anxiety states may also serve social and political ends or purposes given that anxiety states tend to promote withdrawal and tighter forms of individual bodily control (cf. Douglas 1992, 1970), unlike fear states which are more likely or liable to draw people together (Bourke 2005: 191). It is no coincidence, moreover, Bourke astutely comments, that the very word 'anxiety' became more popular as the twentieth century progressed, given the 'modern construction of the unique self residing "within" the body and accessible to psychotherapeutic confession' which 'prioritises the language of anxiety' (2005: 191).

Viewed in this latter light then, it is not simply a question of the anxieties associated with sleep, including potential anxiety inflation through sleep awareness or sleep promotion campaigns, but of *sleep problems themselves as symptoms or expressions, products or reflections of the age of anxiety*, and all that this implies. Consider, for example, the aforementioned BACP *Insomniac Britain* report, which concludes that:

We are prosperous but live in an *anxiety society*. General anxiety and the *excessive pace of modern life* are felt by the highest proportion of the population to affect the quality of their sleep. We view this as evidence that the broader trend toward 'Anxiety Society' is *penetrating our sleeping life* and acts as a *barrier to peaceful sleep* for many. (2005: 1, my emphasis)

This in turn, however, returns us to the final critical question raised above regarding the cultural *framing* of sleep in this way. Sleep problems, to be sure, may well be very real for those who experience them, of that there is no doubt, but the sleep 'discourse' nevertheless, if we may call it that, may itself be partial, problematic or at the very least far from adequate. Are we talking about sleep, for example, because it is a convenient cipher, metaphor, *surrogate* or *substitute* way of talking about or framing other things such as anxiety, fear, stress, worry, frustration, pessimism, insecurity, inequality or injustice (Williams 2005), and associated issues to do with the changing dimensions and dynamics of lived time? Like the stress discourse, moreover, these discursive articulations or configurations of sleep may themselves in part reflect and reinforce other socio-cultural changes prevalent in contemporary times such as the heightened awareness of vulnerability if not victimhood and the rise of a therapeutic culture or state (Wainwright and Calnan 2002).[16] Sleep, in this respect, as both discourse and experience, becomes yet another critical *point of reference or articulation for the mobilisation of a variety of other concerns and anxieties about life and living in contemporary times*, including the stresses and strains of work and family life (Hinsliff 2004), associated feelings of time paucity or time poverty, and the multiple risks and uncertainties which clamour for attention if not beset us on all sides.

Conclusions

Sleep, we may safely conclude, is indeed a contested matter in the global age and the 'wired awake' era of go-faster or turbo-capitalism. This, for example, as we have seen, includes ongoing discourses and debates as to the extent of sleep debt or deprivation in society and associated concerns over the personal and public costs and consequences of poor sleep as an 'adverse' or 'at-risk' state. Sleep, moreover, I have argued, may be viewed as both a problem in its own right and a prism or point of articulation for the mobilisation of a variety of other concerns and anxieties about life and living in the late modern age, not least the changing character and dynamics of (lived) time and the multiplication of risks and uncertainties. Sleep indeed one might say is very much a 'problem in the making' today, around which a variety of claims and concerns converge, compete, clash or clamour for attention.

We may in this regard, returning to the differing sociopolitical agendas sketched in the introduction to this book, view these issues in terms of an ongoing tension between the dominant ideologies and imperatives of late or fast capitalism and the global economy on the one hand, which continue to neglect or negate sleep, and other recent discourses and debates which, at one and same time, render sleep a matter of growing 'concern' if not a 'crisis' today and therefore 'champion' sleep through a variety of sleep-positive or sleep-promoting discourses and debates, policies and practices: what I termed the 'concerned' or 'sleep-positive' agenda.

To the extent, however, that states such as 'busyness' or having 'too much to do', if not feeling 'tired', 'exhausted', 'sleepy' or just plain 'wasted', are normal if not banal features of contemporary life in the global economy or wired awake world, and to the extent that the 'hectic' nature and pace of modern-day life and living is described as 'exciting' or 'positive' (Widerberg 2006: 109), or justified in the name of 'freedom', 'flexibility' or 'freewill' (cf. Maasen and Sutter 2007; Martin 2000, 1994; Rose 1990), then this at once confirms both the warrant or mandate for these latter day 'concerned' or 'sleep-positive' agendas and the problems and difficulties any such agendas face given the continuing power of these dominant sleep-neglecting or sleep-negating ideologies and imperatives. It tends to be assumed, as Summers-Bremner astutely comments, that 'our desire is of the same order as that of the global economy, which is voracious and can turn itself to any object', the net result being a *'vexed wakefulness and a volatile ambivalence'* (2008: 138, my emphasis). To the extent, furthermore, that we remain reluctant or unwilling to acknowledge let alone embrace the *corporeal limits* to which sleep speaks,[17] and to the extent that the causal chain or link between personal sleep problems and these broader public, structural and ideological factors remains obscure or at least difficult to articulate (Ibid.: 137–8), then any attempt to challenge or problematise these dominant late capitalist values and ideologies through other more sleep-positive, sleep-friendly, sleep-smart or sleep-wise agendas are likely to have only partial or limited success.

These struggles or tensions nonetheless, at one and the same time, should clearly not be overplayed. To the extent, for example, that these latter more concerned or sleep-positive agendas seek to emphasise the power and promise of sleep as a boost to productivity and performance, both inside and outside the workplace, and to the extent that in so doing they subordinate sleep to the very same logic, ethos or ethic of essential if not enhanced efficiency and productivity from which sleep problems themselves arise in the first place (Hoffman 2009), then this suggests important points of convergence or compatibility rather than contestation or conflict between these agendas, as corporeal needs are reconciled or realigned with corporate values and neo-liberal imperatives in the governance of sleepy/ alert bodies – of which more in the next chapter. It is surely no coincidence moreover that lack of sleep itself is now commonly described through terms with distinctly capitalist overtones, as notions such as sleep 'debt' or sleep 'loss' suggest.

Here then we return once again to other more critical and reflexive agendas regarding the contemporary politics of sleep in which the social sciences and humanities themselves play a leading role. To the extent moreover that sleep constitutes not simply a temporary release or remission from our everyday roles and a vital opportunity to recharge, rejuvenate or revitalise ourselves ready for the day ahead (i.e. sleep as preparation), but a potential source of corporeal refusal, renunciation or resistance in a world of rapidly escalating demands and dictates (i.e. sleep as corporeal protest),[18] then we glimpse here in principle if not practice the outlines of an altogether more radical if not romantic or utopian politics of sleep: a resistant or reclaimed politics of sleep in short, as a final frontier of sorts, given the corporeal 'limits' to which sleep speaks in an increasingly restless or relentless if not ravenous or voracious, time-hungry, 'go-faster' world.

These are issues I shall return to and elaborate upon more fully throughout the book. The chapter in this respect, to repeat, is best read perhaps as a first pass or preliminary exploration of the politics of sleep today in all its complexity and contradictions, the multiple facets and features of which form the subject matter of the chapters that follow.

Notes

1. See Castells' (2000/1996), for example, for a sustained sociological analysis of the 'information age' and the 'network society' – a new 'techno-economic system' of 'informational capitalism', in his view, including new forms of 'timeless time', facilitated by new information technologies and 'embedded in the structure of network society' (Ibid.: 464). Thrift (2005) also usefully refers here to a new phase of 'knowing capitalism' in which 'capitalism has begun to consider its own practices on a continuous basis' and hence started to 'make business out of, thinking the everyday' (Ibid.: 1). See also Massumi (2002) on this new phase of capitalism and the associated transformations of power and control which he succinctly summarises in terms of power no longer embodied in the 'billy club of the policeman but the bar code or the PIN number' as 'checkpoints' rapidly multiply and society becomes an 'open field' of 'thresholds' and 'gateways'; a continuous space of 'passage' and 'flows'.

2. See also Tomlinson (2007) on 'the condition of immediacy', which, he argues, has become a 'core feature of control' in the twenty-first century, given the combination of fast capitalism and media technologies which saturate everyday life. Like Agger (2004, 1989), therefore Tomlinson takes seriously the notion that: (i) 'acceleration rather than deceleration has been the constant leitmotiv of cultural modernity', and; (ii) 'the sense of living a "faster life" is not a sort of anthropological constant of generational succession, but a contingent state of affairs: a genuine and significant shift in temporality that occurs and accelerates specifically in modern societies' (2007: 1). Virilio's (2000, 1991, 1986/1977) hypermodern writings on *perpetually increasing speed* or *dromology* – defined by Virilio as the 'science (or logic) of speed' derived from the Greek term *dromos* meaning to race (1986/1977: 47) – are also of course relevant here, though I do not seek to elaborate on them at length in this book. See Armitage (2000), for instance, for a critical appraisal of Virilio's work.

3. Of the 2000 people surveyed in the Mind study, 70 per cent also said that they felt 'dread and apprehension' the day before going back to work following time off. Mind therefore is calling on employers to improve working conditions, including a 'reclaiming' of staff lunch breaks. See also Campbell (2010), for example, for other recent coverage in the news of how Britain's 'binge working culture is taking its toll', particularly in the new economic climate where jobs are at risk and demands in the downsized workplace are rapidly escalating.

4. Goodin and colleagues' (2008) study usefully explores comparative time use data from the United States, Australia, France, Germany, Finland and Sweden. In doing so they show how well-being depends as much on the amount of time as the amount of money people have at their disposal or discretion, and how this 'temporal autonomy' or control varies significantly between different countries and according to differing living conditions within countries.

5. Time compression, Wajcman (2008) reminds us, has multiple dimensions and the effect of technological devices is not simply one of acceleration. These relations between technological innovation and changing time processes moreover are reciprocal and merit far greater empirical specification, in Wajcman's view, in order to distinguish social science from science fiction.

6. For other contemporary writings in praise of slowness see, for example, Kundera and Asher (1996), and much further back in time Russell's (2004/1933) *In Praise of Idleness*. See also Hoffman (2009) for a recent critique of any such incipient 'worldwide movement' or 'challenge' to the 'cult of speed' (cf. Honoré 2004). In the context of contemporary acceleration, Hoffman states, citing Connolly's (2002) *Neuropolitics: Thinking, Culture, Speed* approvingly, projects aiming for:

   > a return to earlier forms of temporality become even more untenable, calling for a sort of collective equivalent of psychic regression, or at least living in the past. Moreover, the costs of reactive slowness in productivity and economic competitiveness are too high…In a world riven by 'asymmetries of pace', fast time trumps slow time every time. (2009: 167–8)

7. Ongoing federal investigations into the recent Deepwater Horizon oil rig disaster on 20 April 2010 which killed 11 people are also instructive on this count, given recent evidence which seems to suggest that the sleep of workers for once was prioritised over other safety concerns or considerations as vital warning systems on the rig were apparently switched off 'to help workers sleep' (Pilkington 2010).

8. See also other NSF Sleep in America Polls on: *Sleep and Ageing* (2003); *Children and Sleep* (2004); *Teens and Sleep* (2006); *Women and Sleep* (2007); *Sleep, Performance and the Workplace* (2008); *Health and Safety* (2009) at: www.sleepfoundation.org/article/sleep-america-polls/.

9. The Demos study involved a MORI poll of a representative sample of 1006 British adults interviewed by telephone in June 2004.

10. The BACP (2005) survey involved a nationally representative sample carried out by ICM Research of 1008 British adults interviewed on

26 and 27 January 2005. See also the previously mentioned MIND (2010) study findings regarding the effects of recession on sleep patterns.

11. A recent systematic review and meta-analysis of sleep duration and all-cause mortality, for example, concludes that both short- and long-sleep duration are significant predictors of death in prospective population studies. For those sleeping 6–8 hours per day, however, no adverse effects were found (Cappuccio et al. 2010).

12. The UK Time Use Survey (ONS 2003), admittedly, is far from unproblematic in terms of sleep duration estimates and is liable to *overestimate* sleep duration, recording as it does 'sleep' from duration of 'time in bed', which therefore includes 'trying to sleep' and 'lying awake' (Chatzitheochari and Arber 2009). Once again, however, this simply underlines the need for caution regarding much of the evidence both for and against sleep-deprivation at present.

13. A smaller-scale Time Use Survey in 2005 (ONS 2006), conducted as part of the National Statistics Omnibus Survey, records an average of 527 minutes (8.78 hours) of sleep per day for men, and 546 (9.1 hours) for women. Overall, the survey reports, three main activities (sleeping, working and watching television and videos/DVDs or listening to music) account for more than half the day (13 hours and 38 minutes out of 24 hours), with about one-third of the day spent on sleeping. At the weekends, moreover, time not spent at work or in school is taken up by an increase in sleep and an increase in domestic work and leisure activities (ONS 2006).

14. Risk, according to these authors, becomes a pervasive feature of life and living in late modern or reflexive modernity. Not only does modernity create risks through our current ways of living, working, systems of production, consumption, transport and so forth, it also seeks to compensate for them by means of calculation and political regulation (Beck 1992). The profiling of risks, in this respect, becomes an important means of 'colonising the future' (Giddens 1991). Risk nonetheless involves many imponderables and uncertainties given that its locus lies in the future. It also, therefore, at one and the same time, exposes the limits of modern systems of authority and expertise: a 'dialectical relationship', in Beck's (1992) terms, of 'expertise and 'counter expertise'. See also Douglas (1992) for a cultural theory of risk and blame, and the next chapter (Chapter 2) of this book on sleep, virtue and the politics of blame.

15. Instructive comparisons and contrasts may be drawn here, in this respect, with other work on moral panics (Cohen 2002/1972); epidemic psychology (Strong 1990); panic bodies (Lupton et al. 1995;

Lupton 1994; Kroker et al. 1990; Kroker and Kroker 1988); and the 'shock doctrine' (Klein 2007).

16. Relations between sleep and stress are themselves, of course, complex if not contradictory. Sleep problems, for example, are a commonly reported symptom of (work) stress (Hinsliff 2004). Sleep loss or sleep-deprivation itself, however, also seems to manifest or mimic the same physiological changes as stress such as raised cortisol levels in the body (Åckerstedt 2004, 1995; World Health Organization 2004). While stress, moreover, is something we can all more or less readily identify with in contemporary times, it is also (like the sleep discourse) the subject of much controversy and debate. (See, for example, Wainwright and Calnan 2002; Williams 2005.)

17. We cannot after all, as Summers-Bremner (2008: 138) states, have sleep 'restore our energies if we are unwilling to embrace the original limit to capability to which its restorative power belongs'. Sleep moreover has its 'own phases and its own temporality. Its relation to our world is *one we cannot fully master*' (Ibid., my emphasis).

18. Hoffman's remarks are also once again instructive here. 'No matter how severed from the natural cycles of day and night we have become,' she notes, 'sleep continues to be stubbornly attuned to them' (2009: 31). The struggles and problems associated with shift-work and jetlag, for instance, suggest that 'we try to prise ourselves out or our natural diurnal cycles at our peril' (Ibid.: 32).

2

Vigilance and Virtue: Sleep, Citizenship and the Politics of Blame

Introduction

If sleep, as the last chapter suggests, is now becoming a matter of concern in late or fast capitalism, and if sleep debt or deprivation is now being recast or refashioned as an adverse or 'at-risk' state, then further important questions arise here of course to do with associated matters of accountability, responsibility and blame in the governance of sleep today. To what extent and in what ways, for example, are we rendered increasingly accountable, responsible or culpable for our sleep as well as our waking lives today, and how precisely, if so, does this relate to broader socio-political and moral questions of vigilance and virtue, citizenship and the public good?

It is to these very matters therefore that we now turn. The chapter in this respect, taking a broadly Foucauldian and Deleuzian line on these matters, sheds further important light on the governance of alert/sleepy bodies and the complex relations between these contemporary modes of governance and the dominant values and ideologies of our times, particularly those associated with corporate or enterprise culture and neo-liberal values and imperatives.

The wise or prudent management of sleep in 'good' or 'due measure', I will argue, is now becoming the active duty and civic responsibility of each and every one of us qua responsible citizens given the costs and consequences of poor sleep for society. Another vital aspect of the governance of bodies, that is to say, through a more or less continuous processes of self-inspection and control, such that the wilful or wanton neglect of sleep is now equally worthy, like the corporeal excesses and self-indulgent pleasures of 'too much' sleep, of outright condemnation, correction and control. To the extent, moreover, that sleep is now increasingly valued through practices such as (workplace) napping as an aid or boost to productivity and performance and a smart low-cost route to success, particularly in those cognitively rich sectors of the economy, it resonates with prized neo-liberal values in which corporeal needs and corporate imperatives are once again ever more closely aligned in the management of life both inside and outside the workplace.

Sacrifice and salvation: 'Early to bed, early to rise, makes a man healthy, wealthy and wise'

Our starting point here, returning albeit briefly to the historical past, concerns the multiple associations, in words and deeds, between sleep, time, wealth, wisdom and moral virtue. The above well-known proverb, 'Early to bed, early to rise, makes a man healthy, wealthy and wise',[1] for instance, captures and conveys many of these material and moral issues and associations, both past and present, which converge and coalesce around the disciplines of the body in one way or another as a sign or source of both secular and spiritual salvation.

These disciplines of the body, of course, pre-date the modern period and have long been in existence in monasteries, armies and workshops, for instance. The seventeenth and eighteenth centuries nonetheless, as Foucault (1979) reminds us, were a significant turning point in European societies as far as the history of such methods are concerned. At stake here in effect was a transition from the disciplinary use of time in its traditional (monastic) form based on principles of 'non-idleness' (in which wasting time was 'counted by God and paid for by men'), to a far more positive economy concerned with how one could 'capitalise' on the time of individuals and organise 'profitable durations' in terms of the 'maximum speed and efficiency' (Ibid.: 154).[2]

Protestant writings at this time, as Weber (1974/1930) emphasises, were dominated by continual, passionately preached virtues of hard work and unrelenting physical and mental toil in one's 'calling' as the surest proof of genuine faith and spiritual salvation: the most powerful conceivable lever, in Weber's view, for the expansion of that attitude in life which he termed the 'spirit of Capitalism'.[3] Implicated in puritan doctrines in which time-wasting was the first and, in principle, the worst or deadliest sin, and embodied in a new form of 'possessive individualism' which created a culture dedicated to hard work, bodily asceticism and the transformation of the human environment (Turner 1993a), sleep was now part of a new economy in which time, recalling Franklin, was money and 'loss of time through sociability, idle talk, luxury ... even more sleep than is necessary ... six to eight hours, is worthy of absolute moral condemnation' (Weber 1974/1930: 157–8). While time in this respect, as noted in Chapter 1, may now for some have become more valuable than money (Hoffman 2009), this itself perhaps is expressive or symptomatic of a culture in which these older values and ideologies are not so much replaced as *reworked* in the newly configured contexts and circumstances of late or fast capitalism where the character of lived time is changing dramatically.

The disciplining of sleep nevertheless, as already noted, is clearly bound up with more than simply economic value – in which time is money and less time for sleep equals more time to be productive – however important an historical reference point this may be. It is also of course part and parcel of a wider moral economy of bodies, both past and present, which involve, express, embody and exemplify age-old corporeal themes or struggles between self-indulgence and self-control, self-mastery and self-sacrifice, if not salvation. These sentiments and struggles, moreover, as Steger (2008) reminds us, can be found in both Eastern and Western traditions of religious, social and political thought and practice, including both Confucianism and Buddhism, where the desire to sleep has to be suppressed in line with other bodily needs or desires such as the desire to eat, drink or have sex (see also Richter 2003; Steger and Brunt 2003).

The phenomenon of early rising is particularly instructive on this count, both individually and collectively. The demand to rise early indeed, Steger (2008) notes, has been reported throughout the course of human history in many parts of the world, including Europe, India, China and Japan. Both nationally organised early-rising movements in the first half of the twentieth century and current 'early-bird' activities in Japan, for instance, claim to provide a 'bouquet of merits', including 'health, wealth, wisdom, happiness and even beauty' (Ibid.: 233). The key reason for early rising nonetheless, Steger stresses, is to learn to *suppress* or *control one's bodily desires, feelings and inclinations.*

By 'overcoming' inclinations towards 'weakness' or 'laziness' and dealing with 'hardship', moreover, one is said to gain 'positive energy': a particularly powerful or potent method of 'cultivating the body' by means of early rising, that is to say, which has been used by religious faiths around the world for centuries (Ibid.). In Japan furthermore, from the early twentieth century:

> nation-wide government-controlled organisations such as the *hōtokukai* and *seinendan*, have worked with early-rising activities in order to *increase patriotic sentiments and achieve national goals of economic advancement and military power.* It is thus no coincidence that nation-wide initiatives to encourage early rising have re-gained momentum at a time when Japanese leaders have worked towards increasing love for their nation. (Ibid.)

The 'disciplining' of sleep, then, as this suggests, is intimately bound up not simply with issues of work time, work culture and work ethics, but also with the control, suppression or transcendence of bodily needs and desires in the service of broader moral or spiritual, individual or collective, personal or patriotic goals and values, both past and present.

Accountability and blame: drowsiness as the new drunkenness

Sleep nonetheless, however construed or constructed, remains a vital bodily need or corporal matter. Sooner or later, as we all know, we need to sleep. Without adequate sleep, moreover, our performance, let alone our well-being, will suffer.

One may point in this respect, as a further facet of the politics of sleep and risk today, not simply to a growing *recognition* or *revaluation* of sleep as vital *preparation* for the *performance* of everyday roles, routines and duties, but to a growing sense of both personal and public *duty* or *responsibility* in making sure we get 'enough' sleep, or at the very least, 'sufficient' sleep to ensure we are not 'dangerously' or 'excessively' sleepy (and hence 'a risk' to ourselves and others) in our day-to-day lives.

Sleepiness, in this way, becomes not simply a matter of individual and public concern, but a personal and moral *failure* or *failing* – a *reprobate* condition, as Kroll-Smith and Gunter (2005) appositely put it, requiring both social and individual attention and correction – which at one and the same time both *reflects* and *reinforces* the *cultural premium placed on alert wakefulness and the valorisation of vigilance in all walks of life*. We are all, in other words, *rendered increasingly accountable if not culpable for our sleep or lack of it*: a problem that is to say, cast in Foucauldian terms, of self-administration or governance, or a further postscript, borrowing from Deleuze (1995), on the pervasive nature of 'control societies' as a more fluid, flexible, fluctuating yet continuous and dynamic series of (extra-institutional) power relations regarding conduct and existence.[4]

While tiredness or sleepiness therefore, as noted in Chapter 1, may well be considered normal, commonplace, inevitable and hence unremarkable for many of us today, and while lack of sleep may continue to be worn as a badge of pride or a sign of moral fibre and commitment – as embodied and expressed in the Thatcheresque 'sleep is for wimps' or 'sleep is for losers' slogan (see Table 1) – these 'truths' are now being joined if not eclipsed by another 'truth' or series of truths which render any such stance problematic, suspect if not downright *irresponsible*. At the very least, it seems, this former (macho) sleep-denying or sleep-negating stance can *no longer be taken too far* without incurring criticism or outright moral condemnation, particularly in safety-critical occupations such as transportation and medicine, but also more generally given the aforementioned risks and dangers (and associated alerts and reminders) of poor sleep and sleepiness for both the individual and society alike.

We see this, for example, very clearly in the *moral equivalence* now increasingly drawn between *drowsiness* and *drunkenness*. Consider, for instance, as indicative of these trends, Coren's remarks back in 1996, in his popular book *Sleep Thieves*, that sleepiness is a:

> danger to the general public because of the probability that a sleepy individual might cause a catastrophic accident... Perhaps someday society will act to do something about sleepiness. It may even come to pass that someday the person who drives or goes to work sleepy will be viewed as *reprehensible*, dangerous, or even criminally negligent *like the person who drives or goes to work while drunk*. If so perhaps the rest of us can all sleep a little bit more soundly (1996: 286–7, my emphasis)

These remarks indeed are prophetic, given that cases of this kind are now on the statute books and sanctioned by the law. The US state of New Jersey, for example, is the first state in the United States to decree drowsy driving 'recklessness' under a vehicular homicide charge (the so-called Maggie's Law[5]) – a measure based on the calculus that 24 hours of sleep deprivation is equal to a blood alcohol level of 0.1 per cent which, it just so happens, is New Jersey's legal limit for drunk driving (Kroll-Smith and Gunter 2005: 366–7). The critical issue here nonetheless, as the very notion of *reckless-ness* suggests, turns on the fact that to be so charged under this new law, a driver would not simply have to be awake at least 24 hours but have *knowingly* driven while drowsy. And the merit of wisdom of such measures, it seems, is now catching on. At least eight other US states indeed, at the time of writing, are now considering similar laws with 12 bills pending that address fatigued driving in various ways. The National Sleep Foundation (NSF), meanwhile, has also now launched its own *Drowsy Driving Prevention Week* (DDPW) with an accompanying website (www.DrowsyDriving.org) where individuals can find information about drowsy driv-ing. This, moreover, includes a 'drowsy driving' memorial and testimonials site for those who have been affected by a drowsy driving accident or incident, thereby adding further moral weight and emotional force to the campaign through the power of the personal and the tragic.

The Selby rail disaster was also something of a critical test case in the United Kingdom. The incident in ques-tion involved a male motorist, Gary Neil, who confessed to 'often' going 36 hours without a break and who had spent the previous night on the phone chatting to a female friend of his. On this fatal occasion he apparently fell asleep at the wheel, causing his Land Rover to leave the M62 motorway onto the East Coast Main line – and to sub-sequently collide with a southbound GNER express train, before being deflected into the pathway of a fully laden northbound coal train – thereby resulting in ten deaths and more than 70 injuries. Neil was charged and subse-quently convicted of causing death by dangerous driving given that he *knew*, or more to the point *ought* to have known, he was *at risk* of falling asleep but nevertheless continued to drive regardless. Not only, moreover, was this case widely reported in the press, both at the time of the incident and during the subsequent trial, it also provided a further high-profile opportunity for detectives involved in the incident to roundly condemn 'sleep-deprived driving' while simultaneously warning that 'all sleep-deprived drivers should be treated as "social outcasts"' (*BBC News* 2001).

Strohl's (2008) recent remarks are also instructive on this count. The current inability to forecast sleepiness risk and therefore to legislate solutions makes the subject problematic, he notes. There is nonetheless, Strohl continues:

> a case to be made for more public education on sleep and the impact of sleep loss on driving. This would move the objective from one of punitive responses to one of prevention through recognition of risk, and prevention of sleepiness while driving would become *more like alcohol policy*, in which both an educational and legislative focus are important to make a significant impact on public health. (2008: 582, my emphasis)

At stake here then, to repeat, is not simply a moral equivalence now increasingly drawn between drowsiness and drunkenness (behind the wheel, but also more broadly or widely in society at large) as a morally reprehensible state, but the transformation of this 'risky' or 'dangerous' corporeal state into an accountable, preventable or *potentially criminal act* for which the wantonly or recklessly sleepy may be culpable and thereby prosecuted in a court of law. Making sleepiness akin to drunkenness, in other words:

> transforms this – some might say – unavoidable state of consciousness into a *morally suspect somatic condition*. Moreover, like drunkenness, it is assumed that the sleepy

person is either unable or unwilling to control this cor-
rupted somnolent state. Like drunkenness, sleepiness is
framed as a *loss of self-control*; and like drunkenness, any
untoward or unwanted consequences of being sleepy are
ultimately the responsibility of the sleepy person. (Kroll-Smith
and Gunter 2005: 366, my emphasis)

The message here is simple, then: namely that 'you' (yes,
you, me and the rest of the populace), are responsible for
your sleep, or at the very least for any *unwelcome, unfortunate* or *untoward* consequences stemming or resulting from
your dangerous, reckless or wantonly sleepy corporeal
(in)actions: a matter of self-governance, in effect, or what
Crawford (1977) long ago, albeit from a more avowedly political economy perspective, termed a 'victim blaming ideology' which deflects attention away from the broader drivers
or dynamics of these problems in late or fast capitalism.

Deprivatisation? Putting sleep to work...

Other contemporary re-workings of sleep, as further variants on these questions of risk, responsibility and blame
and another prime instance of more 'sleep-positive' agendas, seek to recast or realign corporeal needs and corporate
imperatives in newly productive ways. No longer solely or
simply construed in other words, if ever it was, as the 'antithesis' or 'enemy' of late/fast capitalism, sleep is now being
recast, reconfigured or repositioned in altogether more positive and productive terms as the 'ally' or guarantor of contemporary work time, work cultures and work ethics. To the
extent indeed, as already noted, that sleep is now increasingly recognised as vital and valuable *preparation for* (rather
than simply the unfortunate, inevitable and inescapable

by-product of) everyday waking roles and working life, and to the extent that even a short spell or bout of sleep may help 'boost' or 'enhance' the performance and productivity, if not creative flair and imagination, of the workforce (see, for example, Mednick and Alaynick 2009; Stickgold 2009), particularly in those cognitively rich sectors of the economy, then important avenues and opportunities are opened up here for the colonisation and capitalisation of sleep in the service of corporate goals and ideals.

While sleep and corporate culture then, at first glance, may make odd bedfellows, they are now it seems becoming increasingly acquainted, aligned or reconciled in ways that suggest 'profitable' relays and 'productive' fusions through the corporate colonisation or control of sleep *both inside and outside the workplace*, couched in the language or rhetoric of productivity, performance and (self-) improvement (Hancock et al. 2009). These trends, to be sure, cannot be pushed too far. Sleep indeed, as Brown (2004) rightly notes, remains a somewhat muted or marginal theme in many workplaces to date. It has nonetheless, she rightly notes, entered the corporate realm through the increasing emphasis on managing or micro-managing sleep in the service of corporate goals and busy lives, and through the inclusion of expert advice about the cultivation of 'good' sleep habits in various worker-friendly or sleep-friendly policies and practices (see also Chapter 5).

A number of examples may be pointed to on this count which each, in their different ways, seek to 'capitalise' on sleep to good effect, harnessing its promise, powers and potential in ways which reflect or reinforce corporate imperatives and resonate with broader trends towards the colonisation or management of everyday life. Sleep's changing fortunes and emerging significance within business culture and business discourse, in this respect, 'suggests just how *ubiquitous contemporary corporate training has become*; even a basic bodily need is now being deployed for the *objective of improving performance and productivity*' (Brown 2004: 178, my emphasis). Sleep, in other words, as Hoffman comments, becomes yet another *'activity* – something we must *accomplish'* (2009: 35, my emphasis).

It is in this context, for example, that various sleep-related consulting firms have begun to spring up, particularly in North America. The prime target or market here, it seems, as already noted, are those safety-critical companies, organisations and occupations where drowsiness poses particular risks and problems. Alertness Solutions, for instance, according to its website (www.alertness-solutions.com/products_sciences/products/html, accessed 16 August 2009), caters to: 'Anyone challenged by around-the-clock operations, time-zone changes, or altered shift schedules' who will 'benefit' from the 'broad range of products and services offered'. This includes a wide range of products, programmes and services, such as: (i) 'Awake at the wheel' – designed to promote safe driving and reduce risks of driving while tired; (ii) 'Alert Traveller' – to help 'corporations reduce the hidden costs of travel and optimise business outcomes'; (iii) comprehensive 'Alertness Management Programmes' (AMP), to promote alertness and performance 'on the job'; (iv) a dedicated 'AVAlert' (AMP) for corporate flight operators; (v) 'Alertness Metrics Technologies' (AMT) to monitor fatigue, alertness, safety and performance in 'real time operational settings'; and finally (vi) various other services such as scheduling guidance, scientific reviews and technical evaluations, education and training programmes related to human fatigue, specialised or tailored modules and projects, and research, legal and policy advice.

These corporate dreams or drives are also evident of course in other more popular writings, cast in a self-help vein, with business culture and business ethics firmly in mind. In books such as Maas and colleagues' (1999) *Power Sleep: The Revolutionary Program That Prepares Your Mind for Peak Performance*, for instance, the benefits of sleep in terms of enhanced *productivity* and *performance* are emphasised (see also Chapter 5, below). It is in this context, furthermore, that that the changing fate or fortunes of the (workplace) nap come sharply into view as another significant index or barometer of these corporate trends and transformations. A common feature of many safety-critical occupations, workplace naps are now, it seems, being advocated far more widely, both inside and outside the workplace, as a kind of *compromise* or newly struck bargain between *corporeal* needs and *corporate* imperatives which caters to already-busy people with over-burdened lives.

The guru figures here perhaps, with their own *Napping Company* (www.napping.com) and a host of associated mantras, motifs, messages and merchandise (from T-shirts to doorknob signs stating 'working nap in progress'), are William Anthony and Camille Anthony – the former a professor of psychology at Boston University, the latter a finance consultant. Consider, for example, William Anthony's book *The Art of Napping* (1997), in which we are told, among a barrage of nap-related terms and excruciating puns (from 'naptitute' to 'napnasium', 'napophobes' and 'no-nap-apology'), that it is time for 'napping to come out of the closet and take its rightful place in the living room, the workplace, and any other place' (Anthony 1997: 2); that scientists are 'discovering the awesome power of napping', and; that our 'future will be more supportive of napping' (Ibid.: 5), given a 'myriad of napping advantages, including increased productivity' (Ibid.: 79).

The Art of Napping at Work (2001) co-authored with Camille Anthony, is even more revealing on this count. Workplace napping, it is stated, can both *'prevent* and *cure* the effect of sleep deprivation'. Workplace napping, moreover, is 'one of the few habits that's good for you (improves your mood), good for your employer (improves productivity), good for your personal relationships (makes you more attentive) and *good for your country* (decreases accidents)' (2001: 16, my emphasis). Like so many other 'good ideas that directly oppose our prevailing culture', it is conceded, 'workplace napping is *not an easy sell'*. But it is an idea nonetheless, we are told, 'whose *time has come'* (Ibid.). Starting now then, these authors boldly proclaim or forecast:

> more and more workers will be asking their bosses the simple question 'Why can't I nap, without guilt or fear, on my break time'? And the common answer will be 'You can.' Starting now, more and more bosses and supervisors will ask themselves 'Why not use workplace napping as a no-cost way to improve worker productivity and morale?' And the common answer will be, 'We will'...The immediate workplace policy is to allow (encourage) napping during breaks. The not too distant change will be to accept napping *while* working on company time...We can hear the napophobes reacting 'Now you've gone too far! That's ridiculous!' But have we? While napping can *increase* productivity after one awakens, we believe it can also improve productivity *while* one is napping. How else could we have written this book? (2001: 116, original emphasis)

MetroNaps are also now, according to its website, a '... leading provider of fatigue management solutions to public and private sector organisations'. Since its inception in 2003 and expansion across four continents, we are told, MetroNaps 'has continued to pioneer news ways of identifying and tackling fatigue'. We are 'ideally placed', the website continues, to:

> help you understand the levels of fatigue within your organisation and suggest appropriate steps to tackle problem areas. We have designed a range of services from our online learning, fatigue assessments, seminars and events as well as workplace interventions and solutions which can help you understand and control the crucial issue of workplace fatigue ... *Act now to help prevent fatigue and improve key metrics.* (www.metronaps.co.uk/pages/view/profile accessed 29 September 2009, my emphasis)

MetroNaps clients, as listed on their website, range from PriceWaterhouseCooper and Procter and Gamble, to Google, W Hotels and the British Lawn Tennis Association. Products, moreover, range from the latest noise cancelling headphones to the Zero chair (based on NASA technology) and the Pzizz handheld unit which not only 'looks and feels amazing', but 'allows you to nap any time, any place' and is therefore 'recommended for frequent travellers, commercial drivers, mobile workforces and in combination with purchases of the Zero chair'. Pzizz, apparently, combines:

> Neuro Linguistic Programming (NLP), enchanting music, sound effects and a binaural beat to achieve a wonderfully relaxed state in the listener, similar to that experienced during the Rapid Eye Movement (REM) stage of

sleep. It's portable and pocket size and weighs less than most mobile phones. Pzizz comes complete with a built in alarm clock and in-ear headphones. (www.metronaps. co.uk/pages/view/pzizz accessed 29 September 2009)

The potential reach of these products, however, extends far and wide. If mental rather than manual skills indeed are the most highly prized today in this 'information rich' if not 'hypercognitive' age of ours,[6] then it is unsurprising or understandable perhaps that expressions of interest in the merits or promise of napping are also now evident in that bastion or intellectual powerhouse of cognitive capital, the university sector. My own university (the University of Warwick, UK), for example, has recently flirted with this idea of a nap-friendly environment through the trial installation of MetroNaps' EnergyPods (a sort of pod-like reclining chair with sleep or napping in mind)[7] in three locations on campus. 'We are the first UK University,' the website stated when first launched, 'to introduce Energy Management and EnergyPods to campus and will be investigating their use over a trial 10-week period to determine their effectiveness as a relaxation, *learning enhancement* and stress-relief tool' (www2.warwick.ac.uk/services/ tutors/counselling/sleep/, accessed 30 September 2009). EnergyPods, it is claimed:

allow for effective sleep in the day to offset fatigue brought on by conditions that are often found in the University environment, such as poor sleep hygiene, high intellectual workloads, a 24-hour, sometimes chaotic and stressful lifestyle that can lack calm routine. (www2.warwick.ac.uk/services/tutors/counselling/sleep/, accessed 30 September 2009)[8]

Whether or not of course the workplace nap is quite the positive step forward its advocates, converts or champions claim, remains a largely open question at present. One thing is clear nonetheless, as Baxter and Kroll-Smith comment, namely that the workplace nap, recalling themes discussed in the previous chapter, highlights an: '... increasingly ravenous work culture that encroaches on modern boundaries between work and home; a culture capable of transforming private non-productive acts like workplace naps into regulated time-space behaviours' (2005: 52). These trends, moreover, the authors continue, are not simply *variable in relation to economic sector and the mental-manual division of labour* (i.e. more common in those creative or cognitively rich activities and occupations), but *globally* depending on factors such as stage of economic development and the socio-cultural and political context of change (Baxter and Kroll-Smith 2005). Thus, while workplace napping may become increasingly popular in places such as the United States, Northern Europe and Japan, in other countries, such as Spain, Italy, Greece, Mexico, China and Taiwan, it may be in decline given economic pressures. Indeed, the 'more Fordist the production process', Baxter and Kroll-Smith (2005: 21) venture, the 'less likely' the traditional nap, siesta or *Xiuixi* 'will survive' – see also Li (2003) and Steger (2003a).

The changing fate or fortunes of the workplace nap then, as this suggests, cast further valuable light on the corporate colonisation or management of everyday life in general and the *deprivatisation* of sleep in particular,[9] in an era where alertness, vigilance, mental acuity and cerebral or cognitive labour is increasingly prized (Kroll-Smith 2008).

More broadly, what we see here, as a further instance or iteration of the governance of sleep – disseminated and dispersed, mobilised and popularised in a variety of forms and fashions, from self-help books and newspaper and magazine articles to websites and consultancy firms – is the way in which sleep is now increasingly tied to notions of (self-) improvement, optimisation, enhancement or success (Brown 2004). It is no longer simply the case, in other words, of growing moral and legal *accountability* or *culpability* in relation to soporific states of drowsiness or sleepiness that put both self and others at risk. Sleep is also now increasingly valued or valorised as the latest low-cost means, passport or route to 'success' in all walks of life: another huge potential *reservoir, resource* or *opportunity* to tap into, in effect, in advanced neo-liberal enterprise culture as the latest if not the ultimate performance enhancer (cf. Stickgold 2009) in an era of cerebral labour and the cult or quest for self-improvement in all walks of life. In an age or era, moreover, where there is now reputedly an 'app' for almost everything, it is perhaps unsurprising or unremarkable that you can now monitor if not micro-manage or 'optimise' your sleep, courtesy of apps such as 'Sleep Analyzer', 'Sleep Hygiene' or even a 'Snore Monitor Sleep Lab': a case in short where the question 'How do I sleep?' takes on an altogether new technosocial dimension far away from the sleep laboratory in the interstices of everyday/night life.

The well-slept society? Policy, politics and citizenship

Here we arrive at a further, more explicit set of political questions concerning the problems, policies and prospects of a 'well-slept' society. What evidence is there, for example, beyond the fragments discussed above, that sleep is now being taken up and addressed in more formal or orthodox political and policy-making arenas, and what does this tell us about relations between sleep, citizenship and the public 'good'? Is the notion of a 'well-slept' society, for example, however envisaged or sold, a utopian dream or a realistic ideal, particularly in the so-called 24/7 era?

It is certainly possible, in the light of the foregoing discussion, to suggest that discourses and debates about sleep are implicated or closely bound up with contemporary notions of citizenship given the *rights* and *responsibilities* they involve or entail on the part of us all in risk society.[10] The 'well-slept citizen' in this respect, if indeed we may meaningfully speak in these terms, is one who in principle if not in practice, actively, attentively and wisely manages their sleep in the light of these rights, risks and responsibilities. Sleep, in other words, becomes a duty or obligation of the 'good' citizen in the service of both self and society; another vital matter to remain alive and alert to, in effect, and hence vigilant about in the interests of responsible (self-) governance and the public 'good'. This, moreover, as we have also seen, takes place in a climate or culture where moral if not legal sanctions are now increasingly evident for those failings or derelictions of duty on our part to live up to such *dormative-normative* standards and somatic ideals. We may not, indeed, be morally or legally responsible for our actions while asleep (see Chapter 4), but we are now, it seems, rendered increasingly accountable if not culpable for those soporific corporeal states of sleepiness or drowsiness that befall or beset us, and their untoward effects.[11] Sleep, in short, may well be a 'right', or measure, of a 'just' society (of which more in Chapter 3), but it is also a *responsibility* to be exercised *wisely* or *prudently* in the interests of both the individual and society or the public 'good'.

As for more explicitly articulated or formulated policies, discourses and debates on the 'well-slept society', a number of recent public examples may now be pointed to. The Demos *Sleep in the 24/7 Society* (Leadbeater 2004) report mentioned in Chapter 1, for example, sets out a blueprint to address the so-called national 'sleep deficit' in a sustained and systematic fashion as a matter of public policy. On the face of it, it is noted, the case for 'the government becoming involved in how we sleep seems a ridiculous extension of the nanny state' (Ibid.: 3). Sleep, on this reading, is surely a 'private matter' of individual choice involving consenting and responsible adults, not a concern of the state or legislature. To the extent, however, that the very 'choices' we make about sleep are socially shaped or structured (see Chapter 3), and to the extent that the costs and consequences of any such 'sleep deficit' are also social, then some form of *sustained or systematic public policy on sleep*, Leadbeater argues, is clearly called for, if not long overdue. Public policies to *support* sleep indeed, we are told, would pay 'social and economic dividends' (Ibid.: 33). There are strong precedents moreover, it is noted, for government interventions to limit working hours and promote sleep for some safety-critical occupations. Finally, as market-based solutions – such as sleep and wakefulness-promoting drugs and devices (see Chapter 5) – to address the sleep deficit multiply, it will, it is claimed, become 'increasingly difficult for the government to stand on the sidelines, and it will be called in as a regulator' (2004: 33).

What then, the Demos report asks, might be 'the ingredients of a public policy on sleep'? The answer, it seems, involves a comprehensive package of measures, including: (i) further *regulation* of (the non-medical uses/abuses of) sleep and wakefulness *drugs and devices*; (ii) the provision of *sleep education in schools*; (iii) greater *employer responsibilities* to promote *sleep-friendly policies* and principles at work such as workplace naps and other flexible sleep management training programmes or packages, particularly for employees working long hours or irregular hours such as shift workers; (iv) the promotion of *public napping facilities*, including shut-eye pods at airports, libraries, railway stations, cafes and parks; and (v) the *regulation of working hours* (Leadbeater 2004: 30–40). Politicians, the report concludes, should also 'do their bit', even though they are terrible role models:

> The norm, at least since Mrs Thatcher, is for government ministers to work most evenings, returning to their homes after dinner to deal with their papers till the early hours. One can only wonder at the role that sleep deprivation plays in some of the decisions politicians take. It will be difficult to redress the wider sleep deficit if politicians, managers and other public figures don't *show some responsibility by demonstrating that getting a decent night's sleep is an indication of good sense rather than weakness.* (Ibid.: 39, my emphasis)

Even here, however, in the corridors of power, the picture is somewhat more complicated or complex than this implies or suggests. The history of modern political life indeed, as we know, includes both US presidents such as Reagan and Bush Jr, and British prime ministers such as Churchill, who valued or guarded their sleep time, or even conducted some of their political affairs from the comfort or confines of their beds. Many politicians, moreover, Thatcher included, are not (or were not) averse to napping or dozing when time allows or they can get away with it – see also Steger (2003b), in a comparative vein, on napping in Japanese parliament.

If certain politicians then are poor if not terrible role models, others perhaps may point the way to a more 'intelligently governed' country (Leadbeater 2004).

The explicit reference in the Demos report to the regulation of working hours also returns us once again to the implicit and explicit ways in which sleep and fatigue now figure or feature in political and policy-related discourses and debates on work time, work culture and work ethics. This includes ongoing wrangles regarding the European Working Time Directive (EWTD), and the regulation of working hours in safety-critical occupations in which problems of sleep and fatigue management loom large. We see this very clearly, for example, in the recent controversy over the implementation of the European Working Time Directive regarding junior doctors' working hours. The UK medical profession it seems is divided over the merits of a 48-hour working week on a number of counts, with some claiming it will have disastrous consequences for both patients and doctors, and others claiming it will benefit doctors and patients alike through reduced fatigue and hence reduced risk of errors (House 2009). While the British Medical Association's Junior Doctors Committee, in this respect, has supported the introduction of the EWTD to improve work/life balance and reduce excessive hours, other bodies, such as England's Royal College of Physicians (RCP), Royal College of Surgeons (RCS) and Royal College of Anaesthetists (RCA) have warned that the 48-hour week will stretch staffing levels to breaking point, disrupt continuity of care and substantially reduce the clinical exposure or training doctors receive (Ibid.: 2011).[12]

Another storm, at the time of writing, is brewing within the aviation industry. Pilots from 36 countries, according to the British Air Line Pilot's Association (BALPA) website, are now protesting that the European Parliament and European Commission are 'putting at risk airline passenger lives' through new standardised flight-time rules that are potentially 'unsafe' and likely to result in more pilot fatigue (BALPA 2009). 'Fatigue is a factor now in 10–15 per cent of all air accidents, and pressure on pilots is growing,' the General Secretary of BALPA, Jim McAuslan, states. The United Kingdom therefore, McAuslan concludes, 'has a choice. Bring the rest of Europe up to its standards or join a drive to the bottom. This is a defining moment in how passengers will be protected' (Ibid.).

It is to other advocacy or pressure groups such as the American National Sleep Foundation (NSF), however, that we must turn for the clearest and most sustained examples of political lobbying to date with the well-slept society in mind (www.nationalsleepfoundation.org). Established in 1990 with the motto 'Alerting the public, health care providers and policymakers to the life-and-death importance of adequate sleep', the goals of the NSF, according to its website, are to ensure that:

1. Americans are aware that sleep is an important component of their health and safety, and that they make obtaining sufficient sleep a priority;
2. Americans recognise the signs and symptoms of sleep disorders and seek effective treatment for them;
3. public and private institutions operate in a manner consistent with providing optimal sleep for human performance;
4. the incidence of drowsy driving is reduced so that it is rare and an exception;
5. new sleep-related discoveries are made that optimise public health and the detection and treatment of sleep disorders.

National Sleep Foundation programmes and activities, in this respect, include a 'National Sleep Awareness week', 'Sleep in

America Polls' (see Chapter 1) and other events such as the previously mentioned 'Drowsy Driving Prevention week'. Public health agendas, moreover, are clearly an important part or plank of these NSF agendas (of which more in Chapter 5).

The slow 'movement' too of course, as noted in Chapter 1, embraces or encompasses many implicit or explicit sleep-related themes, based on a 'shared' philosophy of *deceleration* or perhaps more correctly 'balance' in which life is lived at the right speed, pace or tempo, with a variety of pro-slow groups and spin-offs springing up around the globe – from slow food to slow cities, slow schooling, even slow sex. Inevitably, Honoré (2004) notes, the slow movement overlaps with the anti-globalisation crusade, given both are set against 'fast' or 'turbo' capitalism as bad news for both people and the planet. In common with moderate anti-globalisers, however, he stresses, slow activists are not out to destroy or dismantle capitalism but rather to give it a more 'human' if not 'humane' or 'virtuous' face by taking aim against the 'false god of speed' and fighting for the 'right to determine our tempos' or a 'better balance between work and life' (Ibid.: 16–17).

This may well be so, but therein lays the dilemma: a more 'humane' face, to be sure, but one that potentially or ultimately risks subordinating sleep to the self-same logic or ethos from which sleep problems arise or materialise in the first place (cf. Hoffman 2009). While Honoré (2004: 35–6), for example, laments the way in which 'sleep is no longer a haven from haste', he nonetheless proceeds to cite approvingly practices such as workplace naps, chill-out or meditation rooms and the like, as evidence that companies are beginning to take deceleration seriously and taking steps to help staff 'slow down' (Ibid.: 213–14). Despite acknowledging the undoubted merits of such practices in boosting energy and productivity indeed, the manner in which this serves to further *deprivatise* sleep, rendering it amenable to ever-greater corporate 'colonisation', 'capture' or 'control', both inside and outside the workplace, is significantly underplayed or overlooked here. The irony, moreover, that practices of this kind actually *embody* and *express or underline, rather than challenge or call into question* the cult of speed (i.e. ultra-short or smart-sleep, sleep-wise strategies as solutions to fast or turbo-capitalism) is largely lost in Honoré's analysis.[13] Here we return once again then to other more 'critical', 'reflexive' if not 'radical' political agendas concerning sleep in which corporeal questions of resistance, refusal or renunciation, or at the very least a politics of corporeal 'limits', themselves of course contested socio-historical matters, loom large.

Conclusion

Sleep, as this chapter clearly demonstrates, is another vital part of the governance of bodies today in the late modern age. To the extent, for example, that drowsiness or sleepiness is now being recast not simply as an 'adverse' or 'at-risk' state but a culpable corporeal condition tied to the politics of blame, and to the extent that sleep in 'good' or 'due measure' is now being repositioned and revalued as an asset or ally of neo-liberal enterprise culture, then sleep effectively becomes the duty and responsibility of each and every one us in the service of both personal goals and the public good: part and parcel, that is to say, of contemporary forms of *active* citizenship in which we are all obliged to govern ourselves through a more or less constant process of self-management and continuous 'control'.

The underlying message here it seems, to repeat, is that you are responsible for your sleep and that sleep, like all other aspects of our lives today, is something to be actively worked at or managed in the interests of all: a process it seems in which 'too little' and 'too much' sleep are both now equally culpable corporeal states, particularly when the costs and consequence for self and society are fully weighed in the balance. To the extent, moreover, that corporeal needs and corporate imperatives are now being increasingly reconciled or realigned through more sleep-friendly policies and practices, such as the not-so-humble workplace nap, and to the extent that sleep is now being transformed in and through such 'enlightened' or 'humanistic' practices into a 'productive' act and a 'regulated time-space behaviour' (cf. Baxter and Kroll-Smith 2005), then this further underlines the complexities of these contemporary modes of governance, which despite their seemingly pervasive nature nonetheless remain open to contestation, challenge or critique. The chapter, in this respect, may be read as a further 'postscript' of sorts to both Foucault's notions of self-governance and Deleuze's notion of continuous 'control' societies, this time albeit with sleep in mind.

The 'well-slept' society then, to conclude, may well be a distant dream. Sleep nonetheless, as this and the previous chapter attest, is clearly another vital aspect of the contemporary governance of bodies, and hence, to repeat the central message of this book, a political matter through and through.

Notes

1. The proverb, of course, is attributable to Benjamin Franklin (1855) in his book of the same title, although Aristotle (2002) had already long since advised that 'It is well to be up before daybreak, for such habits contribute to health, wealth, and wisdom.' Franklin also of

course equated time with money and is famously quoted as saying: 'The early morning has gold in its mouth.'

2. See also Thompson (1967) for whom, albeit in a more Marxist vein, neither industrial capitalism nor the creation of the modern state would have been possible without the imposition of synchronic forms of time and work discipline.

3. There are, as writers such as Turner (1993a) rightly note, significant points of convergence here between Foucault and Weber in terms of the *rationalisation* of life.

4. Articulated and elaborated as a 'postscript', Deleuze's (1995) notion of 'control societies' was intended to signal the multiple ways in which societies were no longer 'disciplinary' in Foucault's (1979) terms, given what Deleuze took to be the breakdown of contemporary social institutions whose authority nonetheless, he insists, becomes more continuous, intrinsic and integral to all activities and practices of everyday life and existence today. Control, in other words, becomes more pervasive and far-reaching, a lifelong task or life's work in which we are all obliged to monitor, manage, modulate, improve or optimise our capacities and conduct in a continuous fashion through a finer and finer process.

5. So-called following the death of a New Jersey citizen (Maggie), killed by a driver who admitted to falling asleep after nearly 24 hours of wakefulness. Maggie's Law in this respect, following a public outcry, made injury or death by a driver who has been shown to be awake for 24 hours before a crash a felony (State of New Jersey NJS 2C: 11-5; Strohl 2008).

6. To speak of a 'hypercognitive' age in this respect (cf Post 2000) is to highlight the premium placed on cognitive skills, performance and functioning, particularly within certain sectors of the economy but also more generally within contemporary culture. The notion of an 'information rich' era also of course meshes closely with both Agger's (2004) account of 'fast' capitalism and Thrift's (2005) analysis of 'knowing' capitalism – see Chapter 1, note 1.

7. The accompanying blurb on the MetroNaps website for the EnergyPod runs as follows: 'Raise your feet to improve circulation, set the built in timer and relax to the ambient music. At the end of your rest you will be awoken by a combination of light and vibration leaving you to return to your day with renewed energy' (www.MetroNaps.co.uk/pages/view/energypod, accessed 30 September 2009).

8. This presumably coincides with popular notions of 'around-the-clock' student lifestyles if not the advent of the '24/7 university campus'.

9. The 'privatisation' of sleep in the past of course was itself something of a socio-historical accomplishment and has never in fact been total. See Elias (1978/1939), for example, on the civilising process and the gradual privatisation of sleep, and Gleichman (1980) for a further development of these issues along Eliasian lines. See also Ekirch (2005) on sleep in pre-industrial times, and Crook (2008) on the spatialisation of sleep in Victorian Britain (discussed further in Chapter 4). Current trends towards the *deprivatisation* of sleep in this respect may themselves represent something of a *return to the past* when sleep was a more public affair, this time albeit in newly configured or reconfigured contexts and with very different implications for the late modern individual.

10. My use of the term 'citizenship', in this context, implies significant transformations since T.H. Marshall's (1950) classic formulation in which citizenship is now increasingly tied to notions of free choice and personal responsibility. At stake here, in other words, is a new form of citizenship which has less to do with social solidarity, collective rights and welfare entitlements associated with the nation state, than with individual obligations and a new ethic or civic duty of responsibility tied to the minimal state. Citizenship, in this respect, signals new forms or modes of governmentality (cf. Foucault 1991) in which we are all obliged through the language or discourse of risk and associated socio-political notions of individual freedom, personal choice and self-fulfilment, to take care or responsibility for ourselves as *active, responsible* citizens, and to engage in constant risk management through ever finer, more continuous processes of (self-) surveillance and control (cf. Deleuze 1995 – note 4 above). For useful recent commentaries and analyses of these issues, see, for example, Turner (1997, 1993b); Higgs (1998); Rose (1996); Miller and Rose (1990). See also Rose (2007); Gibbon and Novas (2008); and Petryna (2002) on related notions such as 'biological citizenship'.

11. Having a sleep disorder, in this respect, may absolve moral responsibility. Even here, however, the onus of responsibility still falls on the individual not to drive while knowingly sleepy, and indeed to seek professional help for their sleep problems should these problems persist.

12. Up until the 1990s junior doctors in Britain routinely worked 100 hours a week, with downward pressures over the past two decades to the current EWTD specified 48-hour working week.

13. See also Chapter 1 (note 6) for other recent critiques of Honoré's position here.

3
(In)equality and (In)justice: The Rights and Wrongs of Sleep

Introduction

Sleep, as the previous two chapters suggest, may well have become increasingly problematised and politicised in recent times. It may also be a vital part of the governance of bodies and the politics of risk, responsibility and blame today. Little, however, has been said so far about the relationship between sleep and broader socio-political issues of inequality, insecurity and injustice, or the way in which sleep, recalling Mills' (1959) now classic formulation of the sociological imagination, constitutes another missing or lost link perhaps between the private realm of personal troubles and broader public issues of social structure.

At one level, of course, sleep remains quite literally the great leveller, rendering us all equally, sooner or later, unconscious bodies as we lay down to rest, thereby easing if not erasing or extinguishing the very distinctions we honour, defend or contest in our waking lives – *'Th' indifferent judge between the high and the low'*, to quote Sir Philip Sidney (1989/1598) or *'the balance and weight that equalises the shepherd and the king, the simpleton and the sage'*, to quote Cervantes (2003/1604–5).[1]

Sleep nonetheless, as we shall see in this chapter, is indeed another important yet all-too-frequently neglected or overlooked aspect of contemporary power relations, inequalities and injustices, which is socially structured and socially patterned in various ways. Key issues in this respect, approached from a variety of different angles and viewpoints in this chapter, include the contested nature of sleep rights and sleep roles across the life course, relations between sleep, autonomy and the 'just' society, the 'dark' side or face of sleep deprivation in the guise of violence and abuse, interrogation or torture, and associated questions to do with sleep, vulnerability and 'bare life'.

To what extent then, returning to a theme largely implicit in the previous two chapters, does sleep figure or feature in contemporary discourses and debates on rights, and if so in what ways? It is to a preliminary or provisional answer to this question that we first turn as a backdrop to the themes and issues that follow.

Defence: sleep and human rights

Although rarely thought of or articulated in these terms, sleep is not simply a universal bodily need, like adequate food, warmth and shelter, but also by virtue of this very fact a basic human right.

Turner's (2006, 2003, 1993a, b) sociological theory of human rights, based on our unavoidable and inescapable bodily or corporeal *vulnerability*, provides a useful starting point here. Sleep, to be sure, may be good for us in all sorts of ways in ensuring or enhancing our capacities and capabilities, but our bodily or corporeal need for sleep nonetheless, from this perspective, also leaves us vulnerable in many ways, including vulnerabilities associated with going to sleep and vulnerabilities associated with staying awake too long or depriving ourselves of sleep – see for example Williams (2007a) for a fuller elaboration of these corporeal matters of sleep and vulnerability and the next chapter (Chapter 4) of this book. It is therefore, we might say, by virtue of this universal bodily need to sleep and the vulnerabilities associated with it, a fact and fate we share with all animal life indeed, that sleep may be thought of and defended or championed as a basic human right.

This in turn, of course, begs further important questions about abuses or violations of various kinds which we shall turn to shortly below. For the moment, however, the key sociological point to note is that that all societies both past and present, by virtue of this basic bodily need and human right to sleep, have to allow for the sleep of their members in one way or another (Aubert and White 1959a, b). Sleep in this respect, sociologically speaking, may be regarded as both a basic human right and a socially institutionalised (i.e. socially sanctioned, socially scheduled) status or role involving a 'periodic remission' (Schwartz 1970) or 'tension-release' (Parsons 1951) from conscious waking social roles, duties and responsibilities, with associated transition roles, rules, rituals or routines to facilitate passage both into and out of the 'sleep role'.

Sociological work, both past and present, has sought to document and detail the basic contours and characteristics of the sleep role – such as exemption from normal role obligations, freedom from noise or disturbance, adherence to normative conventions as to when, where and with whom one may sleep, suitable bedtime attire and so on.[2] The key sociological point for present purposes, however, as Crossley

(2004) rightly stresses, is that these rights and duties or responsibilities may well be assumed or claimed, but are nonetheless increasingly *contested* in social life. They must be *won*, in other words, or at the very least *negotiated* or *renegotiated* in local, contingent, interactional contexts of power and conflict, particularly in the so-called 24/7 era where any such rights may be unravelling fast (Williams 2008; Williams and Crossley 2008; Crossley 2004). It is precisely by virtue of this sociological fact indeed that the politics of sleep is no longer confined, if ever it was, simply to the bedroom, home or neighbourhood, but is now moving out or spilling over into the workplace, the boardroom and even the law courts (Crossley 2004).

Consider, for example, as an instance of legal redress, the *Case of Hatton and Others vs. The United Kingdom* (2001), in which the European Court of Human Rights debated whether or not individuals who lived near Heathrow Airport, London had a right to a sound (i.e. noise-free) night's sleep (European Court of Human Rights 2001). The court, it transpires, ruled by 15 votes to 2 that the finding of a violation of Article 13 constituted in itself sufficient justification for any damages sustained by the applicants, thereby awarding the applicants €50,000 for their costs and expenses (see also Brown 2001). This ruling, to be sure, may have as much if not more to do with night-time noise disturbance than sleep per se. It does nonetheless constitute an important test case, precedent or proof of principle.

Not many grievances of this kind, of course, reach the law courts, particularly the European Court of Human Rights. Some commentators nonetheless envisage or predict a time in the not-too-distant future in which companies will face a growing number of law suits from tired, weary or disgruntled workers, particularly shift-workers, whose well-being if not lives have been seriously endangered through the sleep they have missed courtesy of the long or irregular hours they are required to work (Summers-Bremner 2008: 135). And why not, one may justifiably ask. Why shouldn't sustained sleep loss, debt or deprivation be taken more seriously by employers as well as employees and by society at large, with possible legal redress if need be? If individuals after all, as we saw in Chapter 2, may be prosecuted or sentenced in a court of law for wanton or reckless states of drowsiness behind the wheel, then why shouldn't (chronically) sleep-deprived employees working long or irregular hours, whose lives, as a consequence, are impaired or endangered, turn to the law courts for recompense or redress?

A number of objections, to be sure, may be raised on this count and a number of factors or interests will no doubt continue to conspire or militate against any such future scenario, but that perhaps, to repeat once more, is precisely the point; another prime instance or example of the politics of sleep, that is to say, which serves to discourage or deflect just such a possibility. That such questions or possibilities are now being raised or posed, and that cases of the kind discussed above have already reached the law courts, certainly hints at or points in the direction of a more explicitly fashioned politics of this kind in the (near) future, alongside other forms of political engagement or expression.

It is at this very point, however, that further important sociological questions arise as to how any such sleep rights, claimed or contested, play out across the life course. It is therefore to what we might call the *micro-politics of sleep rights across the life course*, drawing on recent sociological research, that we now turn in the next section of this chapter.

Disadvantage: the micro-politics of sleep rights across the life course

Placing sleep within a life course perspective throws into critical relief important socio-political issues of power, status, inequality and associated issues to do with privacy, autonomy and control, from childhood through to later life (Williams et al. 2010; Arber et al. 2007a).

Despite somewhat rosy, romanticised or idealised constructions of children's bedtimes, particularly those of the world's urban middle classes (Ben-Ari 2008), children's sleep is often a source of considerable anxiety, concern or consternation if not outright conflict for parents and children alike. Whether or not, of course, returning to Chapter 1, this is another prime example or expression of 'paranoid parenting' in contemporary risk culture or society (cf. Furedi 2002), class-related or otherwise, remains a largely open question to date in need of further empirical investigation. There are, to be sure, important historical precedents here that one might point to in the early twentieth century regarding children's sleep, thereby suggesting that the contemporary picture is not entirely new or novel, even if the nature and content of these concerns and anxieties has changed over time – see, for example, Stearns (2003); Stearns et al. (1996); and Chapter 4 of this book.[3]

Today, it seems, children's sleep is increasingly problematised in social, health and/or educational terms (Wiggs 2007). The concern here, in other words, echoing the broader problematisation of sleep as a matter of concern today, is that children are not getting 'enough' sleep, with potentially significant yet all-too-frequently overlooked negative impacts on their attainment, intelligence, behaviour and even obesity levels. This in turn is linked not simply to growing concerns regarding children's over-burdened, over-busy or over-scheduled lives – including early high-school start times in the United States, homework and so on[4] – or the supposed laxity/informalisation of children's bedtimes, but to the ever-increasing technologisation of children's bedrooms as busy if not hyperconnected sites or zones of activity, courtesy of televisions, computers, mobile phones and so on, rather than places for sleep, peace or rest (Venn and Arber 2008; Van den Bulck 2004, 2003). Recent sociological work, in this respect, has documented the complexities of family dynamics and negotiations of sleep within complex and changing household structures and associated issues of autonomy and negotiability as young people make the transition into adulthood (Venn and Arber 2008). This, for example, includes issues of privacy, self-determination and control over the material space of sleep, and various incursions or infringements of these rights (Williams et al. 2007), particularly with respect to siblings, inter-generational power relations, and children's ability to construct their own 'night-worlds' as distinct from those of adults (Moran-Ellis and Venn 2007).

Parents' sleep too, of course, is significantly shaped and influenced by the sleep (or lack of it) of children and young people within the family or household, and associated gender inequalities and ideologies of 'parenting' (Venn and Arber 2008). Recent sociological research, for instance, has drawn attention to the lack of explicit negotiation between parents as to who provides care (both physical and emotional) for children at night-time, which effectively results in a further largely invisible or hidden night shift for women (Venn et al. 2008; Hochschild 1997, 1990).[5] Worries about late-night stop-out teenagers' whereabouts and safety also provide important sources of parental sleep disturbance, together with other potential disruptions such as late-night telephone calls, late-night noise inside or outside the home, doors slamming and so on (Venn and Arber 2008). These problems, moreover, may continue for increasingly prolonged or protracted periods of time in future given cultural trends for young adults to remain in the parental home for longer now due to economic pressures (Venn and Arber 2008; Venn et al. 2008).

If parenthood poses one set of problems in terms of adults' sleep, however, partnerships and the micro-politics of sleeping together pose other potential problems. Sharing a bed as a partner in a relationship, of course, is deeply bound up with notions of intimacy, trust and the culture of 'togetherness' in contemporary Western societies (Hislop 2007).[6] In situations of this kind involving co-presence nonetheless, co-ordination or co-operation is clearly required regarding sleep roles, routines and rituals, which may result in common or complementary patterns in which each party respects the needs or preferences of the other (Crossley 2004). Conflicts, however, may also arise here, or at the very least struggles to accommodate one another's particular needs or preferences, thereby underlining the complex, contingent and ongoing nature of any such co-operation or complementarity (Ibid.). This, for example, may include explicit or implicit negotiation, if not outright struggles or conflict, over aspects of the sleep environment, from the amount of light in the room or when to turn the lights out, to 'appropriate' bedding and bedtimes. The double bed, moreover, may itself become a potential site or source of disturbance, if not a battle zone, courtesy of snoring bed partners, the hogging of bedcovers or the colonisation of too much bed space, nocturnal visits to the toilet, having the television or radio on, and so on (Hislop 2007). These problems in turn are compounded when strategies developed to cope with, say, a snoring bed partner – through prodding, poking or relocating to another room, for example – actually prolong one's own sleep disturbance (Hislop 2007; Venn 2007). While much recent sociological work in this respect has pointed to the *gendered nature of these problems*, particularly women's disadvantaged status in relation to co-sleeping practices and problems (Hislop and Arber 2003a), further work is clearly needed in order to disentangle any such 'gender' effect from the more general effect, or effects in the plural, for they are doubtless multiple, of 'sleeping together' (Crossley 2004).

Paid employment of course, as already noted in Chapter 1, is another prime factor here in the social patterning or structuring of sleep across the life course, not simply in relation to the extensively documented effects of shift work (see, for example, Åckerstedt 2004, 1995), but with respect to all other forms of paid work and their relations to factors such as class and gender. Recent empirical research using the UK Time Use Survey data (ONS 2003), for example, found an inverse relationship between length of working hours and short sleep duration (less than or equal to 6.5 hours), which was stronger for men than women (Chatzitheochari and Arber 2009). Social class was also found to be a significant predictor of short sleep for men in this research, with those at either end of the social spectrum more likely to report short sleep duration. These results, moreover, as Chatzitheochari and Arber (2009) note, suggest a significant gender difference, with working men once again more likely than women to obtain under 6.5 hours of sleep on a typical weekday – see also Sekine et al. (2006).

Other recent sociological work sheds further valuable light on these issues. Paid employment, for example, was identified as one of the main or prime causes of poor sleep, in terms of work constraints and work stresses, in Meadows' (2005) study of men and sleep (see also Meadows et al. 2008a). It also figured strongly in the link these men drew between 'sleep need' and the ability to 'function' in everyday roles (see also Henry et al. 2008). Clearly, however, as Chatzitheochari and Arber (2009) rightly note, it is important to consider here not simply paid work but *other family roles and responsibilities*, and how they impinge on sleep *quality* as well as sleep *quantity* or duration – issues which return us once again to the gendered forms of 'shift work' at home as well as the workplace (Venn et al. 2008) and associated, culturally variable, care-giving roles (see, for example, Bianchera and Arber 2008).[7]

Recourse to a life course approach, however, also throws into critical relief a series of other significant changes, transitions and negotiations regarding sleep throughout adulthood and into later life. This, for example, includes biological or physiological processes associated with ageing, changes in educational and employment status, and changing personal and biographical relationships over time associated with parenthood, partnerships (marriage, divorce, widowhood), friendships and other family relations, all of which may significantly influence or impact on sleep (Williams et al. 2010; Arber et al. 2007a; Hislop and Arber 2003a).

These factors in turn intersect with various 'concerns' or 'worries' across the life course which themselves, as Arber et al.'s (2009) recent study shows, appear to be both more commonly reported by women than men, and significantly gendered by type of concern and worry. 'Financial concerns', for example, were more commonly reported by men in this study, while 'family concerns' and concerns associated with caring for aged parents or relatives more commonly reported by women. Socio-economic status too, once again, appeared to play a significant role here, with strong independent associations found between sleep problems and household income, educational qualifications, living in rented accommodation/housing and not being in paid employment – although income differences in sleep problems were no longer significant when health and other characteristics were adjusted for (Ibid.). While women, moreover, together with the widowed and divorced, reported significantly more sleep problems in this study, these gender differences were halved following adjustment for socio-economic differences, thereby suggesting that socio-economic status inequalities play a major role in accounting for gender differences in sleep problems (Ibid.).

Inequalities in sleep then, as this suggests, constitute another significant yet hitherto largely hidden, private or invisible dimension of social disadvantage across the life course. Related socio-political questions of autonomy and justice also come into view here, which are important to stress. Hale and Hale (2009a), for example, have recently posed the intriguing question of whether or not 'justice is good for your sleep'. Drawing on a variety of empirical research which shows that those with fewer opportunities have poorer sleep habits (see, for example, Hale and Do 2007; Hale 2005),[8] they proceed to argue that those who have more *opportunities* available to them, and hence who have more *control* over their life projects (i.e. people who have a 'distinct track record of self-governance and purpose') are those who have *optimal* sleep durations and better-quality sleep overall. The 'just society' in this respect is a society in which 'the autonomy of its citizens is respected; and a measure of the just society is the degree to which its citizens are sleeping well and are healthy' (Hale and Hale 2009a: 366). Sleep therefore, from this viewpoint, is important not because it gives rise to justice or to a better-functioning democracy or society, but because, like health, it indicates 'the degree to which a functioning democracy provides its citizens with the liberty, opportunity and resources they need to be self-governed'. Justice, in other words, is 'good for your sleep; and it is similarly good for your health' (Ibid.: 367).[9]

Discipline: sleep in institutions

Sleep, as we know, is not simply confined to the privacy or comfort of the home. It also of course takes place in other institutional sites and settings outside the home in which issues of power, privacy, autonomy and control loom large.

Within the normal course or round of adult day-to-day life, for example, as Goffman (1961) reminds us, the individual sleeps, plays and works in different places with different co-participants, according to different rules, relations, rituals and routines. In 'total institutions', in contrast, such as the prison, the asylum, the military barracks or the boarding school, all activities occur in a similar setting, under the same single authority and rational plan, according to clearly defined rules, roles, routines and timetables to which inmates are required to conform.[10] Both sleeping and waking life, therefore, to a far greater degree or extent than normal everyday/night life, remain under the control and surveillance of others.

Total institutions, in this respect, may also be regarded as 'disciplinary institutions' par excellence.[11] Discipline, Foucault (1979) notes, proceeds from the distribution of space and the control of activities through timetables that help establish 'rhythms, impose particular occupations, regulate the cycles of repetition' (Ibid.: 154). The prison, for instance, is an 'exhaustive' or 'omni-disciplinary appa-ratus', involving the *rationalisation, spatialisation* and *tem-poralisation* of bodies, that provides almost total power over every aspect of the prisoner or inmate's life, including sleep.[12]

On the one hand then, one might say, the appeal to sleep in these terms adds very little perhaps to what is already known about the disciplines of institutional life, both past and present. To the extent, however, that this involves the co-ordination and control or disciplining of *both* sleep-ing and waking life within the confines of a *single insti-tutional space*, then it is this perhaps, more than anything else, which sets it apart from the normal course or round of everyday life and qualifies these institutions as 'total' institutions. To the extent nonetheless that sleep consti-tutes a 'release' of sorts for inmates – *The poor man's wealth, the prisoner's release* to recall once more Sir Philip Sidney's (1989/1598) memorable phrase – it introduces further important and indeed intriguing complexities and dimen-sions to the very notion of 'total institutions': issues we shall return to in Chapter 4 when we consider the various ways in which sleep exposes and exceeds the *limits of total rationalisation* and *control*.

The prison, the asylum, the boarding school and the military barracks then, as already noted, are the most obvi-ous cases in point here, no doubt. Less obvious perhaps are those instances of the disciplining of sleep in various other institutional sites and settings, located in the bosom of civil society and wrapped up in the seemingly more benevolent guise of therapy or care, such as the modern-day hospital or nursing home for the elderly. Residents in the latter institutional settings, for example, all too often it seems, have little or no control over the time they go to bed at night or are woken up in the mornings. The 'sporadic' sleep of daytime napping or dozing as a common practice and characteristic feature of nursing homes (cf. Gubrium et al. 1999; Gubrium 1975), in this respect, is joined by the 'regularised' or 'rationalised' sleep schedules associated with going to bed at night and getting up in the mornings. The institutional or institutionalised roles and routines of care home staff and the timings of their shifts, as such, clearly take *priority* or *precedence* here in determining residents' sleep timing, with or without the aid of pharmaceuticals such as sleeping tablets, especially for those who are more physically disabled and in need of more care associated with bedtimes. Residents' surveillance through routine checks, moreover, and associated changes in lighting and noise levels, often disturb residents' sleep (Williams et al. 2010).

A tension, in this regard, is clearly evident between staff concerns with 'risk' and the routine surveillance and control this engenders, and residents' own desire or wish for privacy, autonomy and control at night, including the negotiation of their own timetables of sleeping and waking (see, for example, Martin and Bartlett 2007).[13] To the extent furthermore that the gender mortality/morbidity paradox prevails in the developed world today, whereby women in the main live longer than men but suffer more chronic illness and disability (see Annandale (2009), for example), then women once again may be particularly vulnerable here regarding both sleep disturbance and lack of control over their own sleep in later phases of the life course through institutionalisation of this kind (Williams et al. 2010).

Denial: sleep, torture and interrogation

Here we arrive at a further, altogether 'darker', more disturbing face of sleep disturbance or deprivation in the guise of *deliberate, wilful* or *intentional* attempts to withhold or deny the sleep of others, for the purposes of abuse or control, interrogation or torture.

A number of examples may be pointed to in this regard, both past and present, public and private. Findings from a recent in-depth empirical study exploring the interconnections between patterns of (not) sleeping among women and children living with or recovering from the effects of violence and abuse, for example, suggests that sleep disruption may constitute both a *strategy* and an *effect* of violence and abuse which profoundly affect the lives of women and children (Humphreys et al. 2009; Lowe et al. 2007).[14] Strategies of abuse found in this research, moreover, included some women's sleep being violated through being raped or assaulted while sleeping (Lowe et al. 2007). Children too were sometimes the subject of direct attack through hitting if they failed to go to bed or go to sleep when they were told (Humphreys et al. 2009). More commonly, however, women in this study described the disruption to both their own sleep and their children's sleep as being a result of fear and disturbance associated with the indirect effects of living with domestic violence. All women, in this respect, reported how they adapted, adjusted or modified their sleeping patterns in some way or other in order to minimise risk and maximise their safety in these circumstances of constant fear. This, for example, included trying to stay awake at particularly dangerous or vulnerable times, and trying to play 'catch up' with their sleep at other times when it was safer to do so; snatching sleep, that is to say, whenever and wherever they could. The use of drugs and prescription medications to manage sleep was also commonly reported among these women, though complex and hedged with concerns (Lowe et al. 2007). At stake here then, as this suggests, was an attempt on the part of these women to fit their sleeping patterns around the working life, social habits and sleeping patterns of the abuser in a manner far removed from the normal ways (discussed above) in which couples negotiate their sleeping patterns; a situation, moreover, in which *fear became the guiding principle* and organising factor in any and all such strategies (Humphreys et al. 2009).

Sleep deprivation has also of course, continuing in this vein and elaborating further on the notion of *vulnerability* discussed earlier, been used for military, security or political purposes as an instrument of torture or interrogation which, unlike some other methods, leaves no visible marks or obvious scars on its victims. Sleep deprivation of this kind, indeed, has a long and chequered history as a tried and trusted method of 'softening' people up and getting them to talk, if not confess to just about anything, the irony being that the more prolonged or sustained the sleep deprivation, the more confused or disoriented, if not delusional or deranged, the subject becomes and hence the more unreliable their testimony is likely to be – though that of course may be precisely the point or purpose, rendering its victims all the more pliable or susceptible to manipulation of various sorts. Even moderate sleep deprivation, for example, is known to impair cognitive functioning, including logical reasoning and memory, verbal processing and decision-making, while prolonged sleep deprivation causes short-term memory problems, speech impairments, reduced pain tolerance thresholds and other ailments.

Perhaps the most recent and notable 'outing' of these practices concerns the treatment of US prisoners in Iraq, Guantánamo Bay and Afghanistan (see, for example, Worthington 2007; Rose 2004). 'Sleep adjustment', according to the Pentagon, involves 'altering' the sleep cycles of detainees by reversing day and night, thereby inducing disorientation similar to jetlag. This, for instance, in the well-publicised case of Abu Ghraib, involved the authorisation by the Bush Jr Administration of sleep-adjustment techniques for up to 72 hours. The legality of these techniques has been much contested and debated, with organisations such as Amnesty International arguing that they constitute grave breaches of the Geneva Convention. The European Court of Human Rights and the Supreme Court of Israel, moreover, have both ruled sleep deprivation inhumane and unlawful, thereby further underlining the role of sleep as a basic human right, while the US Obama Administration has pledged a 'new' (post-Bush) era of respecting human rights, including the promotion of safe, lawful and humane treatment of individuals held in US custody and the closure of Guantánamo Bay – the latter albeit a pledge which has yet to materialise a year into Obama's presidency.

What we see here then, to summarise, is yet another important face or facet of the sleep deprivation debate, an altogether darker, deliberate or intentional side which itself, comparatively speaking, casts a long shadow over the other forms of sleep loss, debt or deprivation considered so far in this book and which once again, in the most extreme fashion, raise questions of sleep, vulnerability, human rights and the rule of law.

Dwelling/deracination: sleep and bare life

A final set of issues, for the purposes of this chapter, concerns the rights and wrongs of sleep among those without bed or abode around the world today, whose precarious existence casts further critical light not simply on the embodied vulnerabilities and vicissitudes of sleep but broader political or biopolitical issues of 'bare life'.

Dormancy and domicile or dwelling, of course, are closely related in the normal course of events. Where you sleep, in other words, is in the main where you dwell or reside (cf. Schwartz 1970). For the homeless, however, these links become broken, severed or problematic, particularly for 'rough' sleepers who sleep outside. Sleep indeed, as various studies have suggested, embodies and expresses many important dimensions and dilemmas of homelessness. Duneier's (2000) ethnographic study of life on the sidewalks of Greenwich Village, for example, is revealing on this count in terms of the place of sleep or sleeping in the person's 'overall logic' – people, in this particular case, on the 'margins' of urban American society, who are targeted by politicians, business owners and the police, and who struggle to make a 'decent' living and turn their lives around. Sleeping on the sidewalks in this respect, as Duneier compellingly shows and painstakingly details, may occur for a variety of reasons, such as saving a good vending spot, saving money or drug use (Ibid.: 161–5). For some, moreover, 'sleeping in a bed no longer feels natural' (Ibid.: 168). It is *entrepreneurial* activity more than the person's 'unhoused' status, however, Duneier stresses, that appears critical here to these people's identities, thereby underlining once again the location of sidewalk sleeping within the overall logic of their lives; an 'embeddedness in habitat', in effect, in which sleep must quite literally take its place (Ibid.: 169).

There is then, as this suggests, a certain 'appeal' to life on the streets, entrepreneurial or otherwise, which is also confirmed in Rensen's (2003) ethnographic study of sleeping rough on the streets of Amsterdam. While drugs addiction and mental illness can, in this regard, lead to conduct that perpetuates outside sleeping, the latter also expresses affinities, affiliations or ties to certain settings and the associated 'social scene', including contacts with other homeless individuals and outside sleepers (Ibid.: 105). Sleeping outside indeed, Rensen notes, is almost always 'a compromise'. Rough sleepers moreover, he stresses, remain 'ambivalent' about the meaning of sleep and rest as both important and unimportant in their lives (Ibid.: 101); a 'rare privilege' for the majority of outside sleepers, that is to say, in which bad weather, police control and lack of security regularly conspire against sound sleep or slumber, thereby resulting in a permanent state of tiredness or sleepiness which becomes, in effect, *re-normalised*. What differentiates rough sleepers from the rest of society then, as detailed ethnographic studies of this kind clearly suggest, are the *social conditions* under which they must live, which sleep itself embodies and expresses:

> In society in general people have a stable sleeping place. The non-homeless can fulfil the primary need of rest *without worrying about the rain or cold or other people*: they don't have to find sleeping equipment or a sleeping place. The *certainty of a sleeping room* within a home makes it possible to *separate sleep* to a certain extent from other parts of life such as working and social life... That is the main difference between the homeless and the

non-homeless...Rough sleepers face a specific set of social conditions that makes it *difficult if not impossible to separate rest and sleep from other basic necessities.* (Ibid.: 106, my emphasis)

One may go further here perhaps and suggest that sleep, in such circumstances or situations, is another example or expression of what Agamben (1998) terms 'bare life'. A life, that is to say, of exclusion in which existence is pared to the bone, reduced to bare or naked life, and stripped of all rights by virtue of these very states of exception and exclusion.[15] What Agamben has in mind here, of course, as the very 'paradigm of political space' in which 'politics becomes biopolitics' (Ibid.: 181), is *the camp,* particularly the concentration camps, labour camps and death camps of the Nazi era:[16] a line of argument which includes, no doubt, returning to the previous section of this chapter, the 'bare life' of those contained or detained in places such as Guantánamo Bay. Compared to the spectre of 'the camp' then, sleeping rough may hardly qualify as bare life, particularly if, as both Duneier and Rensen's research seems to suggest, there is a certain 'appeal' or 'logic' to life on the streets, entrepreneurial or otherwise. To the extent nonetheless that participants in these forms of life exist on the margins of society, and to the extent that the lives they live, without bed or abode, involve more or less extreme forms of hardship and deprivation, then sleeping rough too perhaps may be regarded as another example or further expression of bare life. So too no doubt the precarious sleeping as well as waking lives of others around the globe today, such as the slum/street children of Mumbai or Ghana, the forced migrants in refugee camps in unstable militarised border zones where the corporeal boundaries between 'vulnerability' and 'protection' are frequently confused or blurred (Vogler 2008), and the fragile, fickle or fateful sleep of those in other war-torn, poverty-stricken, disease/disaster-ridden parts of the world whose common corporeal fate is indeed 'bare life'.

Conclusion

This chapter, as the reader will no doubt have discerned by now, has shifted focus somewhat from the previous two chapters in order to consider more fully, from a variety of different angles or viewpoints, important socio-political matters of inequality and injustice or the rights and wrongs of sleep around the world today.

From the negotiation and contestation of sleep rights and sleep roles across the life course to the darker face of sleep deprivation in the service of abuse, torture of interrogation, and the bare life of those without either bed or abode in both the developed and the developing world today, the rights and wrongs of sleep, it is clear, constitute another important axis or dimension of the contemporary politics of sleep, albeit a largely hidden, neglected or invisible one.

At once both a basic human right and a sensitive if not profound corporeal expression of power, vulnerability, (in) security, (in)equality and (in)justice, sleep we may safely conclude is something that both *unites* and *divides* us: another vital missing link, recalling Mills (1959) once more, between the private realm of personal troubles and the public realm of social structures.

Notes

1. Others of course cast these levelling powers of sleep in more derogatory terms. Nabokov (2000), for example, refers to sleep in this

egalitarian vein as the 'most moronic fraternity' in which we are all reduced to a state of non-sentience (Nabokov, quoted in Hoffman 2009: 29). See also the fictional character Dr Gregory Duden, in Coe's (1997) novel *The House of Sleep*, discussed in Chapter 5 of this book, who likens sleep to a disease in need of a cure.

2. See, for example, Schwartz (1970) for an early sociological formulation of the sleep role drawing on Parsons (1951) among others, and Aubert and White (1959a, b) for another even earlier sociological interpretation or formulation of sleep. See also Williams and Bendelow (1998), Williams (2008, 2005), Williams and Crossley (2008) and Crossley (2004) for other more recent sociological discussions of these matters.

3. Concerns regarding adult sleep, Stearns suggests, were clearly evident towards the end of the nineteenth century in the context of discourses and debates on stress disorders such as 'neurasthenia' and the general tensions, stresses and strains of modern (urban) life, including the increasing use of electric light and the popularisation of caffeine drinks. It was not until the 1920s, however, that these concerns were significantly picked up in child-rearing manuals and popular parenting magazines, as part and parcel of escalating standards and expert pronouncements on sleep, including strict behaviourist edicts and more permissive advice in the mid-twentieth century by the likes of Dr Benjamin Spock (Stearns 2003; Stearns et al., 1996). See also www.faqs.org/childhood/re-soc/sleep.html (accessed 30 January 2010).

4. Some school districts in the United States indeed, such as Edina, Minnesota, have delayed high-school start times in the morning to allow children more sleep time: a shift, in the case of Edina, from 7.25 to 8.30 AM, which on various measures appeared to boost children's educational performance, motivation and well-being, particularly among the brightest students (see, for example, Martin 2002; Epstein et al. 1998).

5. Venn et al. (2008) in this respect go beyond Hochschild's (1997, 1990) previous sociological notion or formulation of the 'second shift' to delineate in effect a first shift, a second shift, a third shift and a fourth shift: the first shift being daytime work; the second shift undertaken in the evening; the third shift being the emotional activity throughout the first and second shift involved in thinking about the needs of children, partners and/or employment; and the fourth shift being both the emotional activity at night related to children, partners and other family members, and getting up in the night to deal with children's needs or domestic chores (Venn et al. 2008).

6. This adult practice, however, contrasts with the professional discouragement of parent/children co-sleeping in countries such as North America and the UK today. From a global perspective, nonetheless, co-sleeping with children remains a relatively common or culturally accepted/expected practice. Even in the former contexts, moreover, parents may feel strongly that sleeping with their infants or children is 'natural' or the 'right' thing to do, thereby causing resentment in the face of professional advice or intrusions to the contrary. See, for example, Ben-Ari (2008); Tahan (2008); Ball et al. (1999); Lozoff (1995); Caudhill and Plath (1986).

7. The particular intensity of family connections in Italy, for example, and the associated close inter-generational exchanges of informal care, as Bianchera and Arber (2008) show, 'puts into sharp relief how caring delineates the extent and continuity of women's sleep, highlighting how family roles and relationships interact and intersect with sleep' (Ibid.: 131).

8. Measured in terms of sleep duration, with short and long-sleep duration categorised as 'sub-optimal' and mid-range sleep categorised as 'optimal'.

9. This, to be sure, is an intriguing and important argument, but one that rests on a series of debatable assumptions regarding sleep itself, not least the notion that 'one cannot value sleep for its own sake' and that 'one engages in sleep for the purpose of other projects' (Hale and Hale 2009a: 361–4; see also Hale and Hale 2009b). If those, moreover, who have more opportunities available to them and more control over their life projects are those who have better or more optimal sleep, and if sleep in this regard tracks autonomy or self-governance, then how, we might ask, does this square with the previously cited UK evidence by Chatzitheochari and Arber (2009), that those at *both ends* of the social scale or spectrum were more likely to report 'short' sleep, and other more general comparative data on widespread perceptions of time shortages or the absence of genuinely 'discretionary' or 'free time' (cf. Goodin et al. 2008; Hochschild 1997, 1990)? One possibility here perhaps, if this data is correct, might be through *differential forms of stress* linked to social status and associated economies of time. At the very least, however, this suggests a more complex picture or model than Hale and Hale propose at present.

10. Goffman defines the 'total institution' thus:

> a breakdown of the barriers ordinarily separating these three spheres of activity [sleep, play and work]. First, all aspects of life

are conducted in the same place under the same single authority. Second, each phase of the members' activity is carried out in the immediate company of a large batch of others, all of whom are treated alike and required to do the same thing together. Third, all phases of the day's activity are tightly scheduled, with one activity leading at a prearranged time into the next, the whole sequence of activities being *imposed from above by a system of explicit formal rulings and a body of officials.* Finally, the various enforced activities are *brought together into a single rational plan purportedly designed to fulfil the official aims of the institution.* (1961: 17)

11. This therefore suggests further potential points of convergence, not simply (as noted in Chapter 2) between Foucault and Weber, but Goffman too in terms of both the disciplines of the total institution and the rational domination and disenchantment of life for its inmates: an iron cage indeed.

12. See Archer (2002), Fitzgerald and Sim (1979), Cohen and Taylor (1972) and Serge (1970), for example, for other more contemporary accounts of late twentieth and early twenty-first-century prison life.

13. On the darker side of nursing homes, in the guise of bedroom abuse, see for example Lee-Treweek (2001).

14. For other studies either directly or indirectly addressing these issues, see for example: Humphreys and Lee (2006, 2005); Taft et al. (2004); Brokaw et al. (2002); Lemmey et al. (2001); Martin and Mohr (2002); Hathaway et al. (2000); Humphreys et al. (1999).

15. The Foucauldian thesis on biopower and biopolitics indeed, Agamben claims, stands in need of 'correction' or 'completion' on this count in the sense that:

> what characterizes modern politics is not so much the inclusion of *zoē* in the *polis* – which is, in itself, absolutely ancient – nor simply the fact that life as such becomes a principal object of the projections and calculations of State power. Instead the decisive factor is that, together with the process by which the exception everywhere becomes the rule, the realm of bare life – which is originally situated at the margins of the political order – gradually begins to coincide with the political realm, and exclusion and inclusion, outside and inside, *bios* and *zoē*, right and fact, enter into a zone of irreducible indistinction. At once excluding bare life from and capturing it within the political order, the state of exception actually constituted, in its very separateness, the

> hidden foundation on which the entire political system rested. (1998: 9)

See also Rabinow and Rose (2006) for a recent critique of Agamben's conception of biopower.

16. See, for example, Levi's (1987/1958) powerful and poignant personal account of life in the Auschwitz concentration camp.

4
Transgression and Taboo: The 'Sleep of Reason' and the Politics of Release?

Introduction

In this chapter I approach the politics of sleep in a somewhat different corporeal light, one in which corporeal matters of unconsciousness, if not unruliness, transgression and taboo, the dormative and the normative, loom large. Sleep, after all, as the foregoing chapters attest, may very well be disciplined or governed in various ways, but this still leaves largely open and unexplored the degree to which sleep in the final instance, qua corporeal state of unconsciousness, is amenable to discipline and governance in this way, or to put it slightly differently, the degree to which sleep as a loss of waking consciousness ultimately befuddles, confounds, defies, exceeds or in some other way resists any such attempts at discipline or governance. Sleep, that is to say, as a more or less radical albeit reversible form or severance, withdrawal or release, if not refusal or resistance, to the conscious waking rational world and the normative demands and dictates of society both 'outside' and 'within' ourselves.

Discipline and governance, to be sure, operate at multiple levels, both consciously and unconsciously, rationally and affectively. Sleep nonetheless, elaborating on themes largely implicit in previous chapters, constitutes a potentially powerful reminder of our corporeal 'limits', themselves of course contested matters, in relation to the rapidly escalating if not 'excessive' demands and dictates of contemporary social life and living, or to put it the other way around, a potentially potent corporeal reminder of the 'limits' of the conscious waking rational world which sleep, qua corporeal state of unconsciousness if not unruliness, always already exits beyond and hence exposes and 'exceeds'. The 'sleep of reason' indeed, to recall a memorable phrase, albeit one in which the wisdom as much as the will of the body should be remembered if not respected as a site or source of corporeal protest.

The chapter in this respect is best regarded perhaps as a further critical exploration if not a rival or radical reading of sleep that immerses itself more fully in these unconscious if not unruly corporeal matters. Sleep from this viewpoint, I shall argue, both challenges and confirms, underlines and unsettles our conscious waking projects and the dreams, desires and delusions of rational modernity: an 'absent presence' or 'intimate other', in effect, and a powerful corporeal reminder of the complexities and contradictions if not the 'limits' of contemporary forms of governance.

Disappearance: the abyss of oblivion or not-being?

> In my own bed, my sleep was so heavy as completely to relax my consciousness...and when I awoke in the middle of the night...I had only the most rudimentary sense of existence...I was more destitute than a cave dweller, but then the memory...would come like a rope let down

from heaven to draw me out of the *abyss of not-being*, from which I could never have escaped myself. (Proust 2002: 4, my emphasis)

Our starting point here, captured and conveyed so eloquently in the above Proust quote, concerns the absence, blank or void which sleep constitutes in all our lives. Sleep, *phenomenologically* speaking, involves a loss of waking consciousness and a (partial) withdrawal from the world: a 'recessive' mode of embodiment in Leder's (1990) terms, not simply from the world but from ourselves qua conscious waking agents. Your 'night-time journey', as Smith puts it, 'is one in which you *lose yourself for a while*, before meeting up again in the morning. Being human involves an interlude, which we call sleep, between being yourself and being yourself again' (2009: 176, my emphasis). To the extent then that sleep involves a loss of this kind, and to the extent that this by definition involves the absence of even a rudimentary sense of myself qua conscious waking 'self' or 'I', then it is tempting to reformulate Descartes' famous dictum (*cogito ergo sum* or 'I think therefore I am') thus: 'I sleep therefore I am not'. Sleep, however, like other states of unconsciousness, helps furnish by way of contrast our very sense of what precisely it is to have reflective self-consciousness or be a conscious waking agent, just as these self-same states of consciousness help furnish of our sense of what precisely sleep, qua loss of waking consciousness, involves or entails (Williams 2007a).[1]

While sleep nonetheless may appear to constitute an important corporeal 'release', if not *the* most important or radical form of severance or 'periodic remission' there is from the conscious demands and normative dictates of the waking world (cf. Schwartz 1970), including both the social world 'outside us' and the society 'within us' (cf. Cooley 1902), this withdrawal is clearly only ever *partial*. The sleeper, after all, as Merleau-Ponty (1962) rightly reminds us, is still 'in' the world, still attached to it, albeit in a partial state of withdrawal. The sleeper, in other words, is:

> never completely isolated within himself (sic), never totally a sleeper...never totally cut off from the intersubjective world...Sleep and waking, illness and health are not modalities of consciousness or will, but presuppose an 'existential step'. (Merleau-Ponty 1962: 162)

Events moreover, such as the calling of our name or a (loud) noise, may wake us up, qua sleepers, thereby drawing us back into the waking world and underlining sleep's partial, liminal, reversible status.

If we accept that this liminal state is an embodied state, and that *sleep is a bodily transition*, then this in turn serves to illustrate the wider, more general point that our being-in-the-world is irreducibly embodied in a twofold sense: a body, that is to say, that both 'gives us' a world but which also has the *power to call, recall or pull us back from that world*, through a temporary loss of waking consciousness (Williams and Crossley 2008). This *involuntary* aspect of sleep, the fact that sooner or later we all have to sleep, may 'doze' or 'drop off' without realising it, and may *fight* against or *struggle* with various corporeal states of sleepiness, tiredness or insomnia, also therefore highlights the impersonal, organic backdrop to (inter) subjective life (Ibid.). What we see here indeed, as with illness, is that 'normal' waking consciousness emerges out of and hence is dependent upon an organic foundation that is, in effect, *beyond* and *beneath* its own control (Ibid.: 3). Sleep, furthermore, is not something we can, with any degree of precision or predictability, invoke or call up at will. Rather, it is something which *comes of its own accord*, or washes over us, in its own time, albeit in ways we might encourage or help facilitate. As Merleau-Ponty eloquently puts it:

> I lie down in bed, on my left side, with my knees drawn up: I close my eyes and breath slowly, putting my plans out of my mind. But the power of my will or consciousness stops there. As the faithful, in the Dionysian mysteries, invoke the god by miming scenes from his life, I call upon the visitation of sleep by imitating the breathing and posture of the sleeper. The god is actually there when the faithful can longer distinguish themselves from the part they are playing, when their body and their consciousness cease to bring in, as an obstacle, their particular opacity, and when they are totally fused in the myth. There is *a moment when sleep 'comes'*, settling on this imitation of itself which I have been offering to it, and *I succeed in becoming what I was trying to be*. (1962: 163–4, my emphasis)

Sleep then, to summarise, as this provisional phenomenological sketch suggests, provides a powerful corporeal reminder of the involuntary, impersonal if not primordial organic backdrop to (inter) subjective life; a recessive mode of embodiment and a *partial/periodic* form of severance or withdrawal which both affirms and problematises our commitments to the conscious waking world.

Dreams: spiritual and secular struggles

The imagination of the waking consciousness is a civilised republic, kept in order by the voice of the Magistrate; the imagination of the dreaming consciousness is the same republic, delivered up to anarchy (Diderot, the *Encyclopédia* (1965/1751–72), quoted in Solms 2007: 140).

Further important questions arise at this point, concerning both dreams or dreaming and other *in-between* corporeal or dream-like states of consciousness which, once again, seek to problematise if not de-centre or de-throne conscious waking life and bring other states of altered consciousness to the fore.

There are indeed, phenomenologically speaking, a variety of liminal or intermediate corporeal states between (deep) sleep and (alert) waking consciousness that we may point to which, generally without awareness and sometimes *against our explicit will or intentions* (catching us 'unawares' or off-guard, so to speak), we can drift off or lapse into. From this it follows that that our *being-there* in any given situation, by virtue of our embodied subjectivity, is not equivalent to our physical presence or co-presence (Williams and Crossley 2008). We may in such cases say that we are present in body but not in mind or spirit, even though, phenomenologically, our 'not-being-there' is clearly something of a fiction or failure to be there *fully* in body. To 'drift off' in this sense is to *lose one's embodied grasp or grip on* and *involvement in a situation* (Ibid.).

On the one hand then, to repeat, these experiences serve to further sharpen our sense of what it is to be an alert, conscious waking agent (Williams and Crossley 2008). On the other hand, they represent once again another powerful corporeal reminder that our agency is not solely or simply a product of waking consciousness, thereby *complicating our sense of what agency is or is not* and pointing to the possibility of our *inhabitation or involvement in worlds other than the waking world* (Ibid.).

Daydreaming, for example, as a kind of liminal zone between sleep and wakefulness, light and darkness, dawn and dusk, is at once both a rich source of experience and a common if not shared cultural practice which fuels if not foreshadows everyday imaginations, and, perhaps most importantly for our purpose, provides a *potential foil if not point of resistance to systems of routinisation, rationalisation, coercion or control* (Löfgren and Ehn 2007). Daydreams, we might say, permit a form of *'mind wandering* that enables people to travel swiftly from one place to another or from one time to another, without moving a muscle', thereby making it possible once again to live in 'parallel worlds' populated by both 'pleasurable and scary fantasies' and 'imaginary travel' (Ibid.: 18).

Hypnogogic states, as one *descends into* and *emerges out of* sleep, are also instructive on this count: worlds populated by hallucinatory experiences, voices, images, visions and the like which have both inspired and incapacitated the human mind throughout the centuries (Mavromatis 1987). So too lucid dreams, in which, as the name suggests, dreams *are apparent to us as dreams*, we know that we are dreaming, thereby calling into question the conventional view that statements of the kind 'I am asleep' are logically impossible (cf. Malcolm 1959). Plato, Aristotle, Augustine, Nietzsche and Freud, for example, not to mention Shakespeare, Coleridge and Dickens, all in their different ways acknowledged the possibility of the sleeper somehow being 'conscious' of the sleeping state. History, moreover, is littered with acclaimed or professed lucid dreamers, including the Marquis Leon Hervey de Saint-Denys, who in the nineteenth century anonymously wrote *Dreams and How to Guide Them* (1982/1897) – a practice or project which has now gained a more credible or respectable (neuro-) scientific face through figures such as La Berge (1985).[2]

In 'dreams proper', or 'full-blown' dreams, in contrast, if we may call them that, sleep provides the gateway. We need to be asleep, in other words, for dreams like this to occur, which in turn suggests 'sleep dreams' (Mavromatis 1987) as another possible term of reference. The defining hallmark in this case is that dreams of this kind, unlike lucid dreams, are *not apparent* as such, qua dreams, to the dreamer. It was this uncertainty over dreams, for instance, that Descartes was able to exploit to great rhetorical effect in the *Meditations* (1996/1641). How do I know for sure, in other words, that I am not dreaming this right now? Dreams can certainly feel as real as waking experience and often lack any irrefutable sign or signal that they are indeed dreams.[3] Dreams, moreover, as Descartes' dilemma suggests, have provided a rich site and source of conjecture, controversy and consternation if not crisis, throughout the course of human history, including *divine and diabolic, sacred and profane*, not to mention diagnostic or therapeutic reference points in the transition from Classical Greece to the Middle Ages, and from the early modern period through Romanticism to the present day.

One may point in this respect to a transition over time from Ancient notions of dreams as welcome or unwelcome *visitors* or external *intruders* from outside, and associated ideas of dreams 'seen', to notions of dreams as *belonging* to the dreamer and dreams as a *product* of the inner 'psychic life' of the individual; something, that is to say, we *have* or take *possession* of (Pick and Roper 2004: 6–7; Stewart 2004). The psychoanalytic interpretation of dreams as the 'royal road to the unconscious' of course, to invoke Freud's (1900) memorable phrase, is a critical point of reference here in the history of these transitions, albeit one which has subsequently come under fierce attack from a variety of quarters, not least through the neurobiological or neuro-scientific account, if not assault, on dreams – see, for example, Hobson (2002, 1995); Hobson et al. (2000); Flanagan (2000); and Chapter 5 below.

Behind these seemingly linear or straightforward transitions nonetheless, as Pick and Roper rightly remind us, lies a rich and complex history of both *continuity* and *change*, of *oscillations back and forth*, and of 'shifting "viewpoints" within periods and sometimes within the same oeuvre' (2004: 7). At one moment, for example:

> the dream may be contrived as phenomenon intruding from outside, with good and bad thoughts located in clearly defined *dramatis personae;* at other points, even in contemporaneous works and passages of the same text, the dream may be conceived quite differently, the narrator implying that, for all the manifold figures in the dream, it truly *all* belongs to the dreamer, each 'presence' to be integrated with – seen as a product of the *psychic life of the subject.* (Ibid., my emphasis)

Dreams, to be sure, to the present day provide a rich source of *experience, insight* or *inspiration.* History, moreover, as we know, is full of examples or claims regarding the productive link between dreams and creativity, including the role of dreams in: literature, such Robert Louis Stevenson's *Dr Jekyll and Mr Hyde*, Samuel Taylor Coleridge's *Kubla Khan*, Mary Shelley's *Frankenstein*; in science, such as August Kerkulé's discovery of the benzene ring structure and Oto Loewi's Nobel Prize-winning work on the chemical transmission of nerve impulses; and in popular music, such as Paul McCartney's dream inspired song 'Yesterday'.

Yet dreams have also of course, throughout human history, proved a site or source of considerable moral and political controversy, concern or consternation. A whole series of political and cultural assumptions, for example, as Hayward (2004) notes, were implicit in the *secular* interpretation of dreams during the nineteenth century in Victorian Britain, including: (i) the insistence that dreams must be located in the 'interior life' of the individual; (ii) the idea that the unconscious mind could reveal a level of association and connection beyond the conscious mind; (iii) a belief in the 'mythopoetic' ability of the unconscious, particularly the associations it forged with other 'distant memories'; and finally (iv) the inadequacy of oneirocentricism[4] and the need for professional assistance in the 'correct' explication of dreams (Ibid.: 161).

Today perhaps these assumptions may strike us as unremarkable. Their 'mundane' nature and status nevertheless, Hayward argues, 'obscures a whole series of *political struggles* that surrounded the Victorian interpretation of dreams' (2004: 161, my emphasis). Thus while spiritualists, Swedenborgians and superstitious Christians cherished the knowledge dreams imparted, the theory of the subconscious or subliminal mind – pioneered and developed by key members of the Society for Psychical Research (SPR) such as Sidgwick, Gurney and Myers, and facilitated in part through the use of hypnotism as an experimental method to recreate the experience of sleep while maintaining communication with the somnolent body[5] – militated against any such mystical politics associated with the religious or spiritual idea of dreaming (Hayward 2004: 166–8). To the extent indeed, Hayward stresses, that these religious or spiritual ideas of dreaming subverted, sabotaged or at the very least qualified prevailing notions of responsibility and agency, reason and truth, authority and authorisation, self and state, biography and identity, they posed *significant moral and political threats* to a 'consensual society' in which individuals sought to maintain control over their actions and desires (Ibid.: 166).

From this it follows that the very idea of the subconscious or unconscious mind which emerged in the nineteenth century was itself part and parcel of a:

> general strategy for *containing* the power of dreams. It was a *rhetorical mechanism* for *returning* the free floating inspiration of the spiritual vision into the *fleshbound* history of the individual. In its insistence that the discordant fragments of the supernatural must be *surrendered* to a single personal narrative, it matched a transformation that characterised the nineteenth century as whole... [in which] irrational desires, religious events and subaltern actors all disappeared from the historical stage. (2004: 170, my emphasis)

Dreams then, as this suggests, constitute another rich point of reference in the politics or governance of sub/unconscious minds/bodies, both past and present.[6] At stake here indeed, as we have seen, are a history of *struggles*, both secular and spiritual, moral and political, which are not perhaps so much resolved as *rearticulated*, albeit in different guises and in different contexts with different purposes in mind and different projects or visions at stake.

Disturbance: the perils of sleep

Sleep, to be sure, philosophical objections notwithstanding, may be a 'pleasurable' pursuit or pastime.[7] It is also, however, as already noted in Chapter 3, a fragile if not fickle state in which disturbances or disorders of various kinds, and attendant fears or anxieties, if not abject terrors, loom large. A time, that is to say, in which we are not quite 'ourselves', so to speak, or, perhaps more correctly, when we are vulnerable to the potentially capricious whims or dictates of our unconscious if not unruly (nocturnal) bodies with a will seemingly all of their own while our (daytime) selves sleep.

Nightmares, for example, returning to the problem of dreams, are a potent source of fear or terror tied, recalling Goya, to the 'sleep of reason'; a time, in other words, not simply of 'marvels' but of 'monsters'. Fuseli's (1781) *The Nightmare*, for instance, provides a powerful evocation of these themes of demonic visitations, or more specifically of incubi sitting on the chests of sleepers. It is also thought to be one of the classic depictions of sleep paralysis, a terrifying condition accompanied by vivid (hypnagogic) hallucinations and a sense of imminent danger which even to the present day, despite (neuro) scientific explanations, is embodied and expressed through folklore notions such as the 'old hag', 'being pressed', the 'ghost that forces you down' or the 'devil on your back' (see, for example, Weisgerber 2004; Mavromatis 1987).

The resonances here with gothic images of evil and excess, devils and demons, darkness and death, madness and monsters, the spiritual and the supernatural are also, of course, readily apparent (Davenport-Hines 1998). These unwelcome nocturnal 'visitations', however, may not simply terrify us when they happen but leave us terrified at the very thought or prospect of going to bed. Coleridge (1985, 1971), for example, who appears to have been more afflicted than most by the perils of sleep, described sleep as a 'howling wilderness' that 'I dread' given the horrid or tortured visions and creatures that beset him throughout the night.[8]

Other perils or problems of sleep, in contrast, may leave us not so much paralysed with fear or pinned to our beds as propelled into various nocturnal or somnolent states of corporeal action or activity. We may, for example, walk as well as talk in our sleep. Activities such as eating, bathing, urinating, dressing, talking, whistling, dancing, climbing, even driving, engaging in sexual intercourse or committing murder, have also been reported or claimed during episodes of sleepwalking. In July 2005, for instance, a case was reported of a 15-year-old girl in the United Kingdom who was rescued by a fireman after she went sleepwalking and ended up on the arm of a 130-foot crane (Marsh 2005).

The sleepwalker, or somnambulist, was also of course, as Melechi (2003: 164) notes, a familiar or newsworthy figure in Victorian culture. This, for example, recalling themes touched on earlier in this chapter, included various forms of 'artificial somnambulism' into which 'hypnotised' or 'magnetised' subjects may fall, alongside their 'natural' and 'narcotic' counterparts. Somnambulism indeed, as this suggests, was an ill-defined and elastic concept at the time into which 'almost any action undertaken without apparent awareness, and with lack of subsequent recall, might fall' (Ibid.: 166). It also, however, resonated with a broader series of debates, evident at the time, on automatisms, imitation and other mimetic aspects of individual and group behaviours, all of which, in one way or another, pointed to the uncomfortable or troubling truth that *much of what we do we do unthinkingly in a fashion akin to sleepwalking.*[9] With the decline or demise of mesmerism nonetheless, some of the more wild or fanciful, outrageous or outlandish claims associated with these Victorian forms of somnambulism were resolved or rescinded (Ibid.). Somnambulism instead became the province of sleep science and forensic psychiatry and continues, to the present day, to provide a defence against criminal charges such as murder or rape (Ibid. see also Cramer Bornemann 2008).

A tragic case of this kind, for instance, recently hit the news headlines, involving a British man with a history of sleepwalking and other sleep disorders,[10] who strangled his wife of 40 years during his sleep as he dreamt he was tackling intruders (de Bruxelles 2009; Hanlon 2009; Jefferies 2009). Both defence and prosecution had accepted from the start of the trial that Mr Thomas, a retired steel worker from Neath, South Wales and the father of two, was *not* in control of his actions at the time of the killing. The jury therefore had been asked to decide not if Mr Thomas had killed his wife but whether or not he was 'medically insane' at the time he had done so. By the end of the trial, however, the jury were directed to return a not-guilty verdict, thereby allowing Mr Thomas to leave court a free and innocent man.[11] 'In the eyes of the law,' Mr Justice Nigel Davis told Mr Thomas, 'you bear no responsibility for what happened' (de Bruxelles 2009).[12]

Sleeping bodies may be recalcitrant, resistant or unruly in other less dramatic ways too, however. People, for example, may snore in their sleep (of which more below), sometimes quite loudly, the irony being they may be the only one in the house who cannot hear themselves snoring, given that they as the snorer, by definition, are asleep at the time![13] Bodies may also of course, continuing in this 'recalcitrant' or 'unruly' vein, *fall asleep too readily or easily,* as in cases of narcolepsy or *excessive sleepiness,* or *fail to fall asleep,* as in cases of insomnia. In both cases, however, returning to previous phenomenological themes, we *struggle with a body* that is either shutting down before we want it to or not shutting down when we want it to (Williams and Crossley 2008). To the extent, moreover, echoing Chapter 1, that insomnia or sleeplessness is now viewed as a common complaint or symptom of life and living in today's media-saturated, hyperconnected or wired world, then it doubles as both a literal and metaphorical reference point in a relentless if not voracious era that truly *knows no bounds*. Both insomnia and the 24/7 active world, in other words:

> belong to a *regime of desire whose key feature, over-production*, hides their causes... Insomnia produces a *surplus of thought,* and the wired world produces a surplus of information, images and interactive opportunities, and neither our world nor the insomnia it generates seems able to assist us with managing this ongoing surplus. (Summers-Bremner 2008: 133, my emphasis)

The history of insomnia then, from this vantage point, is perhaps best viewed as a history of 'loss' involving an undervaluing of absence or oblivion in contemporary culture on the one hand, and an associated loss of 'nocturnal aptitude' or 'literacy' on the other (Summers-Bremner 2008: 9): an incessant and incandescent age, in short, in which darkness is crowded or drowned out by the glare of artificial light and our busy around-the-clock lives and lifestyles.

Deviance, debauchery and disgust: the dormative and the normative redux

It is precisely at this point that a further series of more explicit questions arises, pertinent to any consideration of

the politics of sleep and the governance of unconsciousness, concerning relations both past and present between
what might be termed 'the dormative and the normative'
(Williams 2007b). Sleep, as we have already seen, may
very well be a basic human right and a socially recognised,
scheduled and sanctioned bodily need, but the legitimacy
of sleep is also of course contextually contingent or variable
in relation to prevailing socio-cultural norms, forms, customs and conventions.

Sleeping at the wrong time or in the wrong place, for
example, as we all know, may incur sanctions of various
kinds given the codes or conventions it flouts or violates
(Williams 2007b). The practice of workplace napping, for
instance, as we saw in Chapter 2, may or may not be greeted
with disapproval, depending on the particular workplace
and associated employment policies and practices in
question. The Japanese custom or practice of *Inemuri*, for
instance, is particularly instructive on this count given the
tolerance or latitude it accords the sleeper or quasi-sleeper in
various public situations or settings (Steger 2003a, b; Steger
and Brunt 2003). It is indeed quite customary and acceptable in Japanese society, it seems, to doze or drop off to sleep
in public (at a lecture, meeting, party or other social event,
for instance), as long as the sleeper or quasi-sleeper is ready
and willing to relinquish 'sleep' at the appropriate moment
when their attention is required.[14] Even here, however, in
keeping with other societies such as China and India that
exhibit a high degree of *tolerance* towards daytime as well as
public sleep or napping, 'there are many occasions', Steger
and Brunt remind us, 'when sleep during social activities is
not allowed' (2003: 19).

It is not simply then, as this suggests, the *when* but the
where and indeed the *with whom* of sleep that matters,

which includes the *distribution* or *spatialisation* of sleep, both past and present, individual and communal, in terms of prevailing norms, forms, bodies and beds. Crook (2008), for example, in an illuminating study of sleep in Victorian Britain, highlights how the evolution of modern sleeping space was informed not simply by ideas of privacy and civility (cf Elias 1978/1939), but also by concerns about the functioning of 'normal' bodies and minds, the governmental agency of space and the moral integrity of the nuclear family. The bed furthermore, he stresses, remained a highly problematic *indeterminate* space, facilitating 'deviant' as much as 'civilised' behaviour and giving rise to all manner of pathologies, perversities, phobias – thereby shedding further valuable light on the reciprocities of 'rule and resistance', 'pleasure and power', which at once 'constitute and imperil' the integrity of the modern body (2008: 15).

We see this, for instance, very clearly in the many social investigations from the 1830s onwards on the 'conditions of the working classes' (e.g. Chadwick 1997/1842; Mayhew 1851), which all in their different ways included a concern with the spatial distribution of dormant bodies, often through 'graphic descriptions of bodies mingling and mixing' (Crook 2008: 20). The concerns and anxieties articulated here, Crook comments, were about moral as much as physical or public health. In such circumstances indeed, 'all manner of bad habits and social ills flourished', such as alcohol, crime, laziness and violence (Ibid.), not to mention the horror or taboo of incest (see, for example, Wohl 1976). These concerns in turn were magnified and multiplied many times over in relation to the common lodging houses, dormitories or 'doss-houses', the very antithesis of respectable domesticity, in which an 'unwholesome mix' of transgressive practices and social pathologies coalesced (Crook 2008), with grotesque echoes and carnivalesque overtones (cf. Bakhtin 1968). Bodies, in other words:

> enjoyed an easiness of presence, possession and perform-ance. No shame was attached to nakedness, nor was there any regard for physical normality. In lodging houses the lame, the blind, the deaf, the deformed were able to mix free of stigma and abuse. To enter a lodging house was to enter a grotesque world of pleasure and perversity, and whatever disgust they elicited was often accompanied by a sense of wonder. (Crook 2008: 31)

'Normal' sleep in this respect, a contested point of refer-ence in any case, to be sure, was very much the excep-tion to the rule in these dens of ill-repute. The Victorian bedroom nonetheless, Crook (2008: 28–9) reminds us, was also a site and source of multiple pleasures, pathologies and phobias, including (middle-class) parental concerns and anxieties over children's sleep, particularly wet-dreaming and masturbation (Hunt 1998) – see also Stearns (2003) and Stearns et al. (1996) on growing concerns and chang-ing standards regarding children's sleep during this time period.

The history of sleeping bodies then, not least the spatiali-sation of sleeping bodies in all their richness, pleasures and perversities, may constitute another important yet hitherto largely neglected or overlooked aspect of the *history of cor-poreal transgression and taboo* (see, for example, Stallybrass and White 1986). Still today, moreover, as Crook (2008: 32) rightly stresses, the bedroom represents a space of consider-able 'struggle' which *defies or resists total rationalisation* given that sleep itself resists total or ultimate rationalisation. While the sleeper qua sleeper, moreover, may convey or display a certain child-like 'innocence', and while one cannot in any fair or just sense be held accountable for one's actions while asleep, the fact that bodies may by daytime or daylight standards behave quite 'badly' if not 'outrageously' while we are 'asleep', may still nonetheless engender certain feelings of awkwardness or embarrassment, guilt or remorse, stigma or shame in waking life, publicly acknowledged or not (see, for example, Meadows et al. 2008b).[15] Sleep, in other words, both confirms and complicates what by daytime standards of civilised conduct we take ourselves, or at least aspire, to be. The dormative and the normative, in short, as this suggests, are intimately related and hence another key part of the politics of sleep and the history of corporeal transgression and taboo.

Darkness: the politics of the night

Here we arrive at a final set of issues to do with darkness, and associated questions concerning not so much unconscious bodies perhaps as unruly bodies and the politics of the night. In many ways, of course, night has always been our deepest, darkest fear. Night, that is to say, as a time in which our visual powers are dimmed or diminished and questions of human vulnerability, frailty and finitude loom large or are perhaps most keenly felt. These fears, moreover, are further compounded or reinforced through long-held or cherished notions of light as 'good', a 'gift' of God and/or a source of self-revelation and enlightenment, for instance, and darkness as 'bad', 'corrupt', 'sinister' or otherwise 'evil': the realm, echoing themes articulated earlier in this chapter, of demons and devils, madness and monsters, not to mention the other, true or ultimate darkness of death itself that 'gets us all in the end, the night that no amount of light will ever illuminate' (Alvarez 1996: 270).[16] The drive to make night bearable or tolerable, in this respect, includes both the human quest through the ages for lighting (cf. O'Dea 1958) and the retreat into the sanctuary or salvation of sleep (Alvarez 1996: 7).

The history of night-time, as this suggests, is a rich and fascinating one, full of ambiguities and anxieties, complexities and contradictions, pleasures and perils within which sleeping and waking life are intimately bound and inextricably entwined. Ekirch (2005), for example, points to a varied and indeed vibrant night-time culture in Western society before the Industrial Revolution, with its own customs, rules, rituals, rites, scents, sights and sounds. At stake here, in other words, was a shadowy, spectral or spiritual realm at 'day's close', filled with real and imagined threats and perils, yet also one full of opportunities and possibilities for people to *escape* the bounds, burdens and banalities of everyday life, to *express* their 'inner impulses' and to realise their 'repressed desires', however 'innocent or sinister in nature' (Ibid.: xxvi). Pre-industrial night-time indeed, as Ekirch clearly shows, was a time of crime and evil spirits, magic and masked balls, ancestral lore and prayers, wool-spinning and storytelling, midnight liaisons and bundling, sleep and dreams, liberation and renewal.

As the physical conquest of 'outer darkness' proceeded through advances in artificial lighting, however, the search moved on into the illumination of 'inner' darkness inside the head (Alvarez 1996: 22), through developments such as psychoanalysis and tools and technologies to monitor and measure electrical signals in the brain (the topic of the next chapter). Night-time, moreover, as Melbin (1989, 1979) notes, has become a 'frontier' of sorts, if not the 'final' frontier, set for colonisation and commercial exploitation in today's 'non-stop' culture characterised by artificial illumination both inside and outside homes and businesses as 'the greatest symbol of modern progress' (Ekirch 2005: 338). Night in the city, for example, now becomes the 'continuation of day by other (electrical) means'; a time of 'leisure and intimacy, family and lovers, hobbies and pastimes ... excitement and celebration' (Alvarez 1996: 259–60). Like the brain, moreover, the city only *seems* to sleep:

> scattered across its darkened cortex are bright points of activity, in police stations, newspaper offices, television studios and whore houses, the night-shift is in place. Firemen and ambulance crews wait for a call, disc jockeys jabber away in their sealed cubicles, bakers pound the dough for the morning bread, the food markets are in full swing, the pubs and cafés around them are packed, and the watchers and listeners whose livelihoods depend on computers and satellites are busy in their terminals: air traffic controllers, the defence establishment, the young tiger and tigresses in the financial district, who monitor figures from the Nikkei and the Hang Seng and talk into two telephones at once. (Alvarez 1996: 261)

It is possible in this respect, as Nottingham (2003: 194) perceptively comments, to discern or detect a certain change or *relaxing* of standards at night-time when one is free or *freer* perhaps to 'loosen' or 'lighten' up and reveal one's 'less serious side'. The politics of the night, in this regard, involves a struggle or contest between those authorities anxious to 'reinforce a code of respectable behaviour' and various ill-defined 'others' who are no less anxious to 'avoid the limitations and boredom of compliance' (2003: 192). The night, in other words:

> not only produces tangible problems for those in author-
> ity and renders their charges less susceptible to political
> appeals, but it can also remind them of a certain moral
> equivocation within themselves. The virtues that lie at
> the heart of citizenship, sobriety, calmness, openness to
> persuasion, an ability to forsake the immediate pleasure
> for longer-term gain, are not at their strongest after dark.
> Night time gatherings are *more disorderly, raucous and*
> *resistant to any but the most basic appeals.* (2003: 195, my
> emphasis)

This, for example, includes various forms of *disorderly or unruly* behaviour on the streets of many cities at night-time, particularly British cities; problems fuelled in no small part by
alcohol and other recreational drugs which keep the police,
ambulance crews and A&E departments busy throughout
the night.[17] Policing the city night, however, as Nottingham
(2003: 210–11) rightly notes, is now accompanied by a proliferation of private security firms and privately employed
doormen or 'bouncers' who regulate entry into all city-centre
pubs and clubs. Of note here too, of course, since the introduction of effective police services in the nineteenth century, is the proliferation of modern-day CCTV cameras (in
which Britain again seems to excel) and which now, in true
neo-Orwellian fashion, appear to be trained on almost every
move we make, both day and night.

Consider, for example, as further evidence of the sorts of
nocturnal 'unruliness' at stake here and the 'remedial' work
required of night-time doorstaff charge with its management,
an extract from Monaghan's field notes on a busy evening

in a large city pub in the run up to Christmas. Incidents recorded during the evening, for instance, included:

> a male customer urinating against a bar; another urinating against a balcony, wetting customers below; a man repeatedly exposing his genitals then complaining when doorstaff insisted he leaves; customers ordering drinks, not paying for them, then physically resisting when being escorted off the premises. A drunken man grabbed my crotch for no apparent reason... Several fights between customers also occurred. A group of young women, who were forcefully ejected by security staff after fighting among themselves, also waited by the front door for some time with the intention of seeking revenge on a doorman (even though he weighed approximately twenty stone). (2002: 4004–5)

If night-time, however, involves a certain dramatic licence or liberty of this kind with respect to everyday normative standards of civilised conduct, it also returns us once again, albeit in a different guise, to questions of 'loss', at once both literal and symbolic, material and metaphoric, regarding night-time and (true) darkness (Summers-Bremner 2008; Alvarez 1996). On the one hand, for example, the gradual colonisation or conquest of night-time and darkness suggests diminished opportunities perhaps for privacy, intimacy and self-reflection, including a 'loss of touch with our dreams as the oldest path or avenue to the human psyche' (Ekirch 2005: 335–9). We are also, however, losing touch with the night sky itself though modern-day forms of light 'pollution' which themselves, in an avowedly political vein, spur various forms of protest or resistance in the guise of organisations or groups such as the International Dark Sky Association (Klinkenborg 2008).[18]

Conclusions

Let me draw this chapter to a close by returning to and spelling out the abiding themes that inform it: corporeal matters, that is to say, of unconsciousness and unruliness, transgression and taboo, the dormative and the normative, if not protest, refusal or resistance.

On the one hand, of course, sleep remains a vital precursor or prerequisite for social and political 'order', without which society and the members comprising it would, quite literally, grind to a halt or cease to function. Without sleep, in short, no 'order'. Yet sleep, as this chapter also suggests, constitutes a corporeal site or source not simply of unconsciousness but unruliness, recalcitrance or resistance, transgression and taboo in relation to the prevailing 'order'. Sleep, that is to say, as a corporeal or somatic state that does not simply exist beyond but exposes or exceeds the bounds or 'limits' of the conscious rational waking world. Or, to put it another way, sleep as a potentially powerful and potent corporeal reminder if not protest regarding the 'limits' of our involvements and investments in the conscious waking rational world and its seemingly endless, if not 'excessive', demands and dictates regarding our time and attention. The 'sleep of reason' then, to be sure, but also perhaps an expression of the 'wisdom' of the body which possesses its own rhythms if not 'reasons', so to speak.

Here once again then, this time albeit through the novel corporeal lens of sleep, we are reminded that the history of human corporeality is not merely one of the *disciplining* or *rationalisation* of bodies, any more than it is one of their *emancipation* or *liberation*. Rather, as Falk (1994: 66) rightly notes, it is a 'paradoxical combination of the two' – see also Stallybrass and White (1986); Bakhtin (1968); Bataille (1987/1962).[19]

One may perhaps go further here, however, and venture two other provocative albeit tentative or speculative conclusions. First, to the extent that society is a consciously held notion or construct, both individually and collectively, and to the extent that sleep involves a more or less radical (albeit reversible) severance or withdrawal from the conscious waking world, then the sleep of any one member of society let alone the sleep of all members of society at once – an improbability if not impossibility admittedly, given that 'some must watch whilst others must sleep' as Shakespeare so aptly puts it – harbours the power and potential to problematise if not liquidate (albeit temporarily) both the social world 'outside' us and the society 'within' us, so to speak (Schwartz 1970; Cooley 1902). Second, if varying corporeal states of sleepiness, drowsiness or partial consciousness, harking back to Chapter 1, are now common if not the 'norm' in the 24/7 era, and if much of what we say and do, even in so-called alert conscious waking life, occurs unthinkingly in a sort of half-conscious or semi-conscious fashion – including auto-feelings or automatisms of various kinds (cf. Wegner 2002) – then sleep (proper) may simply be the most obvious case of a far more intriguing if not disturbing or unsettling truth; namely that societies, as writers such as Thrift (2008) and Castoriadis (2003) intimate, remain only 'half-awake' and therefore that *en-trancement* as much as *enlightenment* is evident if not endemic to societies characterised as much by their 'suggested' qualities (Thrift 2008; Wegner 2002)[20] as the powers of conscious rational minds.[21]

Cast in this light then, to conclude, sleep may justifiably perhaps be regarded as something of an *'absent presence'* or '*intimate other*' within both 'Man' and 'Modernity', self and society; an unconscious if not unruly corporeal matter, that is to say, which simultaneously *underwrites* and *unsettles* if not *undermines* the preferred image of ourselves as conscious rational beings and the prevailing socio-political and moral order, with important implications for the discipline and governance of bodies, both past and present, public and private.

Notes

1. For an intriguing and instructive philosophical debate on these relations, see, for example, Johnstone Jr (1973), for whom sleep provides the necessary and indispensible condition of (self-) consciousness, and Galloway (1977), who argues to the contrary that it is consciousness which makes sleep an intelligible phenomenon, not the other way around. Sleep-related interruptions of consciousness, in other words, from this latter viewpoint, 'are intelligible, if and only if, one is aware of his [*sic*] own consciousness, *prior* to such an interruption' (Ibid.: 110, my emphasis).

2. La Berge, for example, based on a growing body of collaborative scientific work (La Berge and Rheingold 1990; La Berge and Dement 1982; La Berge et al. 1981), has demonstrated that lucid dreaming occurs during unequivocal REM sleep (i.e. the most active period of phasic rather than tonic REM), and that lucid dreaming is a 'learnable skill' through techniques such as MILD (mnemonic induction of lucid dreams). See also Hearne (1990).

3. Descartes of course was not the first, nor the last, to pose this problem: Plato before him and Bertrand Russell after him, for instance, raised similar doubts about the dream–wake distinction. By the time of the sixth Meditation nonetheless, Descartes seems to have regained confidence in his ability to reliably distinguish between these two states, thereby dismissing his own previous doubts as 'laughable', in part because God would not allow him to be so deceived and in part because dreams are 'never joined with all the other actions of life by the memory, as is the case with actions that occur when one is awake' (Descartes 1996/1641, Sixth Meditation: 89).

4. Oneirocentricism pertains to the long tradition of dream interpretations stretching back to the Greeks, including Artemidorus of Daldis'

famous second-century AD text *Oneirocritica* (the fortune tellers' guide to dream interpretation) which remained hugely influential until the early modern period (Artemidorus 1990).

5. While hypnosis, and its predecessor mesmerism, had long since been used (by showmen among others) to illuminate and hence discredit apparently supernatural phenomena, the uses of hypnotism in this context, Hayward notes, served both experimental and rhetorical ends which, at once, sought to challenge both the carnivalesque and mystical theories and interpretations of dreams and associated dream or trance-like states of subconsciousness (2004: 161). See also Melechi (2003) on *Fugitive Minds*.

6. Christopher Nolan's new sci-fi thriller *Inception* is also worthy of mention here, moving forward in time, for the future world of corporate espionage it conjures up and conveys: a world in which thieves invade, manufacture and manipulate people's minds and dreams in order to steal secrets from the unconscious.

7. Sleep, for example, it may be objected, is not strictly speaking something we can never truly 'enjoy' or experience as 'pleasurable' given that we are asleep and hence unconscious at the time. At most, it might be granted, we derive pleasure from the process of *going to* sleep and *waking up* following a 'good' sleep. See, for example, Hale and Hale (2009a, b) on these matters and Chapter 3, note 9 of this book.

8. Coleridge indeed suffered from a number of ailments or illnesses, many opium-related through his use of and withdrawal from the drug. He also coined the term 'psychosomatic' to describe the complex associations between psyche and soma during sleep, yet continued to believe that dreams could be caused by the spirits. See, for example, Ford (2004) on Coleridge and 'The pains of sleep'.

9. Sleepwalking also, of course, figures or features as a theme in many dramatic works, of which Shakespeare's Macbeth – in which Lady Macbeth sleepwalks due to her overwhelming guilt and insanity – is perhaps the most famous example. See Furman et al. (1997), for instance, on Shakespeare and sleep disorders.

10. The defendant apparently had been prone to sleepwalking and other sleep disorders since childhood, including 'night terrors' or *pavor nocturnus* which, it is claimed, triggered this particular tragic incident given that Mr Thomas had come off his regular medication for depression and Parkinson's disease at the time (because it made him impotent).

11. The legal defence here is one of 'automatism' in which the mind is not deemed to be in control of the body. This is a very rare defence,

with fewer than 70 cases worldwide in modern legal history. It is also further sub-divided into 'insane automatism' (which involves psychiatric referral and treatment) and 'non-insane automatism' in which the defendant is judged to be of sound mind and the act is seen as a 'one-off' incident (de Bruxelles 2009; Hanlon 2009).

12. Similar cases of acquittal on grounds of sleep have occurred before, including: (i) a father in the nineteenth century cleared of murder after claiming he dreamt he was throwing his baby to safety; (ii) a man (Mr Jules Lowe) who, in March 2005, was found not guilty of killing his 83-year-old father due to 'insanity' while he was sleepwalking; (iii) a high-profile case in 2002 in which REM guitarist Peter Buck was acquitted of attacking British Airways staff on a transatlantic flight to London due to 'non-insane automatism' brought on by a combination of alcohol and sleeping pills at the start of the flight; and (iv) another recent case in which a man (Mr Leonard Andrew Spencer) was acquitted in Australia of gross indecency and sexual intercourse without consent in relation to a 21-year-old female house guest, after he claimed he was sleepwalking (Ballon 2009; de Bruxelles 2009; Morris 2009).

13. Downloadable 'apps' (such as 'Do I Snore?'), as previously noted in Chapter 2, are now of course available or ready-to-hand courtesy of the iPhone for those wishing to know more about their sleep in the comfort of their own homes. Even then, however, the snorer remains unaware of their snoring while asleep and can only check or audit it upon waking.

14. These very terms of reference, of course, call to mind once again the sociological work of Goffman, particularly his notions of *main* or *side* involvements, and *dominant* and *subordinate* involvements (Goffman 1963), which Steger and Brunt (2003) use to good effect in this context. A case of *inemuri* at a lecture, a meeting or a party, for instance, may profitably be regarded in this Goffmanesque light as a '*subordinate* involvement' to the '*dominant* involvement' which in this particular case, of course, is the social event or gathering in question (Steger and Brunt 2003: 19).

15. On the one hand, Meadows et al.'s research seems to suggest that if the sleeper is considered to be 'unconscious', in a private space and in an intimate relationship, then bodies are free to break the normative boundaries of (waking) acceptable civilised conduct without risking embarrassment. On the other hand, however, they suggest, 'breaking these boundaries does appear to have the potential for biographical or reputational impacts, and audience anger, resentment and conflict'; a potential *mediated* albeit by things such as '*prior normative*

expectations, length and status of relationship, and gender' (Meadows et al. 2008b: 87, original emphasis).

16. The Polish artist Miroslaw Balka's recent installation, 'How shall I move forward?', located in the vast Turbine Hall of the Tate Modern, conjures or conveys many of these complexities, fears and uncertainties as the viewer enters its deep dark cavernous form (a structure resembling a shipping container) and stares into the black void ahead. It is a journey we are left to navigate or sculpt for ourselves, yet one involving both deeply personal and collective or universal meanings, myths and associations (Tate Modern 2009).

17. At the time of writing, the police are pressing the new Tory–Liberal Democrat coalition government to turn the clock back on the 'open all hours' licensing regime introduced by New Labour, given that it does not appear to have had the desired effect of introducing a more 'relaxed' social culture, akin to Southern Europe's approach to alcohol, thereby tempering Britain's 'binge-drinking culture' and cutting alcohol-related crime on the streets (Townsend and Rogers 2010).

18. The 'Vision Statement' of International Dark Sky Association, according to their website (www.darksky.org) is to:

- improve the night-time environment by reducing light pollution through better lighting practices;
- raise awareness about curtailing light pollution, the beneficial effects of doing so, and its solutions;
- educate about the values of environmentally responsible outdoor lighting while collaborating with other like-minded organizations;
- promote responsible legislation, public policy, research, and standards in a professional and scientifically sound manner;
- seek specific solutions that mitigate light pollution.

(www.darksky.org, accessed 6 December 2009)

19. Transgression, Bataille (1987/1962) notes, 'does not deny the taboo but transcends and completes it'.

20. Thrift's (2008) discussions here, of course, indebted as they are to the likes of Wegner (2002) and Castoriadis (2003), are primarily concerned with the politics of affect rather than sleep, particularly affective contagion and related issues of automatisms, imitation and suggestibility. They are nonetheless highly pertinent to the politics of sleep and associated corporeal sleep-like states of (un)consciousness or semi-consciousness.

21. This, of course, is not to deny the powers of the conscious rational waking mind, however limited its 'bandwidth'. It does nonetheless suggest the intriguing possibility that the valorisation of any such powers and potentials, particularly in an era where alertness and cognitive skills are prized, can in part at least be read as a cultural response or reaction to, if not an intolerance or repression of, any such limits. To the extent, moreover, that modernity has always been an 'ambivalent' order (cf. Bauman 1991), founded on both order and chaos, the rational and the irrational, the conscious and unconscious, then this further underlines the complexities of contemporary forms of governance and the powers of persuasion or suggestibility which operate both rationally and affectively.

5

Transformations and Translations: The Laboratory, the Clinic and the Future of Sleep...

Introduction

If sleep is now a 'matter of concern' in contemporary society, if sleepiness has now been transformed into a problematic or 'at-risk' corporeal state, and if we are all now advised, encouraged or cajoled to monitor, manage, modify or optimise our sleep in various ways in line with prevailing mandates or imperatives, then this of course begs important questions about the role of sleep science and sleep medicine within the foregoing storyline regarding the politics of sleep.

This final chapter therefore brings to the fore themes largely implicit in previous chapters concerning the critical roles and relations between biomedicine, bioscience and biotechnology in the contemporary politics or biopolitics of sleep today, from the laboratory to the clinic and into the wider realms or vistas of public and private life. The chapter may also be read as an attempt to revisit and revise or update my previous thinking on these matters, paying particular attention to questions located at the intersection of medical sociology and science and technology studies (STS), concerning the 'biomedicalisation' of sleep and the further light this casts on the biopolitics of sleep today and in the near future.

How then did sleep become an 'object' of scientific or technoscientific interest and inquiry, and to what extent did this pave the way for the subsequent development if not flourishing of more avowedly clinical concerns within sleep medicine in the latter part of the twentieth century? It is to these very questions that we first turn as a critical socio-historical backdrop to the biomedical themes and biopolitical issues that follow.

Brain waves: tracing sleep in the laboratory

A full account of the history of sleep research is of course beyond the scope of the present book, let alone this final chapter.[1] Suffice it to say, for present purposes, that at least four key issues or meta-themes stand out here in the recent history of sleep research.

First, as the loss or negation of experience which for centuries was considered to be a largely *passive* rather than *active* state, sleep it is clear has proved at best problematic and at worst resistant to scientific or biomedical investigation; a mystery whose secrets it seems would not be surrendered easily or given up lightly. Second, while sleep has always of course been a key part of human existence if not experience, and while knowledge of the relationship between sleep and health has been evident for centuries (see Dannenfeldt 1986, for example), the origins of knowledge about sleep until well into the nineteenth century came largely, as Kroker (2007) argues, from evidence grounded in *personal experience* – either one's own or those compiled by physicians and other dream interpreters. Knowing sleep, in other words, was thus for centuries primarily a matter of ' "I" and "thou" and was refracted through the prism of individual experience that depicted sleep as a negative state of consciousness' (Ibid.: 5). Attention to sleep, in the main, occurred in the face of disruptions of various kinds, such as dreams, insomnia and fatigue, all of which related once again to the individual's experiences, sensations, testimonies and self-reports (Ibid.). Third, and perhaps most importantly for our purposes, the practices and techniques that eventually came to constitute the sleep laboratory resulted in the substitution of technical or technological instruments to monitor and measure sleep, thereby effectively bypassing individual or personal testimonies and reshaping sleep as an 'object' of scientific inquiry. Knowing something about sleep in this latter case, as Kroker appositely puts it, implied knowledge originating in the 'sleep of *others*', including both human and animal subjects (2007: 6).[2] A fourth key point flows from these first three points: namely, that what we see here in these transformations are a series of different ways in which sleep is framed, fashioned, figured, formed, traced, tracked, positioned, problematised, understood and unravelled: *different ways*, in effect, *of knowing and visualising sleep*. This, moreover, echoing themes and issues discussed in Chapter 4, includes a dynamic history of oscillating relations or interrelations between sleep and dreaming which themselves are far from simple or straightforward (cf. Pick and Roper 2004).

Our starting point here then concerns the ways in which sleep came to be *known* as an *object* of scientific or technoscientific investigation in its *own right* (rather than a mere *secondary* or *subsidiary* concern), and how, in the process, knowledge about sleep and its very 'nature' *changed, morphed* or *mutated*. This, moreover, includes the *institutionalisation* of this new scientific knowledge of sleep's 'architecture' and 'rhythms' in the very *architecture of the sleep laboratory* and the associated socio-material tools, technologies and relations housed therein to monitor, measure, map, mend or manipulate sleep in this way.

A number of critical or notable developments in the history of sleep research may be pointed to in this regard (Kroker 2007), including: (i) the *encephalitis lethargica* epidemic of the 1920s which brought the concept of a 'sleep centre' in the brain – courtesy of Economo's (1931, 1930, 1928) clinical description and experimental work – to the forefront of neurological research; (ii) the influence of Pavlovian thinking, particularly Pavlov's method of conditioned reflexes, on the study of sleep as a 'generalised inhibition' (Pavlov 1928, 1927, 1923), which in turn fuelled further work on the *physiological* dimensions of sleep; and (iii) the role of the electroencephalograph (EEG) – first developed by the German physician Hans Berger in 1925 (see Berger 1930) – as a research tool which enabled the monitoring and measurement of electrical brain waves (Kroker 2007).

The EEG in particular proved critical here in brokering or bringing about these transformations. Its relevance to the study of sleep nonetheless, as Kroker (2007) rightly notes, was not immediately obvious or apparent. It was not until 1935 that the utility of the EEG as a sleep recording instrument or device was successfully demonstrated, through the work of Alfred Loomis and colleagues in Tuxedo Park New York (Loomis et al. 1935a, b). Tracing sleep through the EEG, in effect, resulted in the identification of what, for the first time in history, came to be categorised as five distinct 'sleep stages' (labelled A–E) through which the sleeping subject's brain cycled throughout the night. This work in turn proved critical to the subsequent uptake of EEG recordings of sleep by other investigators across the United States, notably the work of the physiologist Nathaniel Kleitman whose sleep laboratory at the University of Chicago was not simply the first to be organised around the study of sleep but subsequently 'remained at the heart of the American study of sleep research for decades' (Kroker 2007: 205–6).[3]

These developments in turn occurred in the context of a broader 'revival' of scientific interest in dreams in the 1950s (Kroker 2007), within which the next, and perhaps most significant, development or landmark in the official history of sleep science is located. Although observations had previously been made of rapid eye movement during sleep, the 'discovery' in the early 1950s by Aserinsky and Kleitman (1953) that dreams were associated with rapid eye movements (REM) in sleep, proved critical to the subsequent, though not immediate, changing fortunes of sleep research as a scientifically credible enterprise. As Aserinsky and Kleitman conclude in what has now come to be regarded as a classic or landmark paper in the history of sleep science, published in the same year that Watson and Crick discovered DNA:

> The fact that these eye movements, EEG pattern, and autonomic nervous system activity are significantly related and do not occur randomly suggests that these physiological phenomena, and probably dreaming, are very likely all manifestations of a particular level of cortical activity which is encountered during sleep. An eye movement period first appears about 3 hr after going to sleep, recurs 2 hr later, and then emerges at somewhat closer intervals a third and fourth time shortly prior to awakening. This method furnishes the means of determining the incidence and duration of periods of dreaming. (1953: 274)

Subsequent collaboration between Dement and Kleitman, following Aserinsky's departure form Kleitman's laboratory, carried this work forward through continuous all-night recordings, thereby building up an extensive and systematic body of data on the intricate pattern or architecture of a 'typical' night's sleep, which Dement and Kleitman summarise in the following terms:

> The usual sequence was that after the onset of sleep, the EEG progressed fairly rapidly to Stage 4, which persisted for varying amounts of time, generally about 30 minutes, and then a lightening took place. While the progression from wakefulness to Stage 4 at the beginning of the cycle was almost invariably through a continuum of change, the lightening was usually abrupt and coincident with a body of movement or series of movements. After the termination of Stage 4, there was generally a short period of Stage 2 or 3 which gave way to Stage 1 and Rapid Eye Movements. When the first eye movement period ended, the EEG again progressed through a continuum of change to Stage 3 or 4 which persisted for a time and then lightened, often abruptly, with body movement to Stage 2 which again gave way to Stage 1 and the second Rapid Eye Movement period. (1957: 679)

Sleep then from this moment onwards could no longer be regarded, in scientific terms at least, as a 'passive' state, a time of brain 'idling' or 'inactivity', or even simply EEG 'slowing' (Dement 2000). A basic duality or division was now firmly established between REM and NREM sleep, moreover, with standardised terminology, techniques, technologies and scoring systems established for these 'distinct' sleep stages in human subjects.

It was in this context that the Association for the Psychophysiological Study of Sleep (APSS) formed in the early 1960s. The notion, as Kroker (2007: 13) comments, of a 'marriage' between psychoanalytic concepts and practices and the scientific study of dreams in the 'dream laboratory' was an early aim or ambition for many members of the APSS who conceptualised REM, initially at least, in Freudian terms. The subsequent development of the APSS, however, tells a different story of an increasing move *away* from any such Freudian dreams, desires or ambitions in favour of a more through-going *psychophysiological* emphasis or focus, shorn of psychoanalytic theory, concepts and practices (Kroker 2007). By invoking *sleep rather than dreaming*, in other words:

> the APSS's very name carved out a new space that distinguished laboratory-based research from any Freudian or behaviourist antecedents... Its emphasis was on *defining the parameters of normal sleep* through an *inter*calibration of physiological measures in sleep and wakefulness, and an *intra*calibration of the various sleep stages, whose function remained mysterious. (Ibid.: 332, my emphasis)

That the Association for the Psychophysiological Study of Sleep would later come to be renamed or rebranded as the Associated Professional Sleep Societies is itself revealing in terms of the subsequent shift or transition to more *clinical* concerns, of which more shortly. In both guises or incarnations nonetheless, Kroker (2007) notes, the APSS gave formal organisational or institutional expression not simply to these trends and transformations in sleep research but to the careers of those who, through these new forms of knowledge and associated tools, techniques and technologies, were coming to 'know' sleep in these newly configured ways. No longer construed as the mere 'absence' of wakefulness, to repeat, sleep was now an 'active' process, a dynamic property of the brain, the stages and rhythms (i.e. the architecture) of which could now be discerned, deciphered, detailed and documented through this growing network of expertise, institutionalised through the APSS and the architecture of the sleep lab.

The subsequent decline of interest in dreams or dreaming within this new technoscientific assemblage or configuration of sleep research was far from total, however. Nor, of course, did it dim or diminish interest in dreams and dreaming in personal life or the wider realms of popular culture (cf. Smith 2009 and Chapter 4, this book). Like the return of the repressed with which, in its Freudian guise or psychoanalytic incarnation, it was associated, the battle over dreams has indeed rumbled on, albeit as a somewhat muted or marginal theme inside sleep research and sleep medicine proper.

On the one hand, we may point to the psychophysiological or neuroscientific 'assault', or at least challenge to, psychoanalytic theories and concepts of dreaming, including Jouvet's experiments with cats' brains and other subsequent work on the anatomy, physiology and neurochemistry of dreams and dreaming (Jouvet 1965; Jouvet and Mounier 1960; Jouvet et al. 1959). We see this very clearly, for example, in Hobson and McCarley's (1977) 'activation-synthesis model' – in which REM originates deep within the brain stem courtesy of a small cluster of cells in the *pons* and the work of associated neurochemicals, such as acetylcholine to 'switch it on', and noradrenaline and serotonin to switch it 'off' – a theory, in keeping with the foregoing trends and transformations in sleep science, which effectively turns dreaming into a primarily *neurophysiological/neurochemical* rather than a psychological phenomena. We do not, in other words, contra Freudian renditions of these matters:

> Dream because our unconscious wishes and drives would, if undisguised, wake us up. We dream because our *brains* are activated during sleep, and we do so even if our primitive drives are turned on by that activation. In fact, such drives are not concealed. Rather they are revealed in dreams. It is the specific *neurophysiological details* of that activation process, not psychological defence mechanisms, that determine the distinctive nature of dream consciousness. (Hobson 2002: 158, my emphasis)

Dreams in this respect, alongside fears and phobias, anxiety and depression, anger and rage, become prime expressions of *'brain activation in sleep and waking* that have their own deep and compelling reasons for being' (Hobson 2002: 158; see also Hobson et al. 2000, 1975). These reasons indeed, from this viewpoint, are revealed not through the psychoanalyst's couch and the vagaries of free association, but through the instrumental logic and precision of (deep) brain research in the late twentieth and early twenty-first centuries.[4]

On the other hand, however, we may also point to further attempts to *recover, rescue* or *rehabilitate* psychoanalytic theories and concepts of dreaming in this neuroscientific light, including recent strands of work within the hybrid discipline or enterprise of so-called neuropsychoanalysis. Solms (2009, 2007; Solms and Turnbull 2002), for example (himself a trained psychoanalyst and neuroscientist who has been at the forefront of these developments in recent years), points to the accumulating body of (neuro) scientific evidence which challenges or problematises the division between REM (dreaming) and non-REM (non-dreaming) sleep, in favour of a continuous process of dreaming characterised by variability *within* and *between* sleep stages – see, for instance, Foulkes (1996, 1966). This in turn, Solms suggests, opens a possible doorway or *pathway back to Freud*. Current neuroscientific evidence indeed, from this perspective:

> gives us every reason to take seriously the radical hypothesis – first set out in Freud's book a hundred years ago – that *dreams are motivated phenomena, driven by our wishes.* (2007: 144, my emphasis)

It is also, Solms continues:

> compatible with Freud's concept of when and how the dream process is initiated (i.e. by an arousing stimulus which activates the emotional and motivational systems) and where and how it terminates (i.e. by abstract thinking in the memory systems which is projected backwards in the form of concrete images onto the perceptual systems). (2007: 146)

There has in other words, from this neuropsychoanalytic viewpoint, been an *overestimation* of the part played in dreaming by (REM) mechanisms which do not arise from mental life (Solms 2007: 148).

What we see here then, to summarise, is a series of transformations in the very ways in which sleep and dreams, and their dynamic relations to one another, have been configured and understood during the twentieth century, both *epistemologically* and *ontologically* in terms of shifting forms of knowledge and *institutionally* through the emergence of the sleep laboratory and associated professional organisations such as the APSS which have mobilised around sleep. To speak of the 'architecture' of sleep in this respect is to invoke once again a double point of reference involving both the 'discovery' of distinct sleep stages and their relation to dreams and dreaming, and the architecture of organisations such as the APSS and the modern-day sleep laboratory which may be regarded as prime institutional expressions and loci of this knowledge, including an elaborate array of instruments and (all-night) recording devices designed to measure and monitor sleep. Within this configuration of scientific knowledge and expertise, as we have seen, the 'truth' of sleep could no longer be reliably discerned or validly deciphered from the subjective reports or testimonies of the individuals concerned, or the vagaries of personal experience (cf. Kroker 2007). Rather it came to be known through impersonal instruments such as the EEG to trace the electrical signals or signatures of the brain, and associated standardised criteria and scoring systems within the sleep laboratory, where subjects slept throughout the night while their sleep was continuously recorded courtesy of technicians and sleep scientists.

This in turn, however, suggests a further intriguing facet of sleep research which, as we have seen, first began or set off by tracing the patterns and parameters of 'normal' sleep in an objective way rather than the 'pathological' symptoms generated from individual consciousness (Kroker 2007: 328). How then, we might profitably ask, did this latter-day *clinical concern* with sleep and its attendant pathologies or maladies materialise? It is to this very question that we now turn in the next section of this chapter.

Translating sleep: from the laboratory to the *clinic*

People have doubtless always had sleep 'problems' in one form or another. Associations between sleep, health and hygiene, moreover, date back many centuries, as do proposed 'remedies' or 'treatments' for sleep problems – from praying, dream interpretation and appeasement of the gods, through blood letting, diet, exercise, music and meditation, to medications such as theria, opium and bromide, modern-day pharmaceuticals such as benzodiazepines and the new generation of so-called Z drugs (i.e. zaleplone, zolpidem, zopiclone), and other latter-day forms of intervention such as cognitive behaviour therapy (CBT) (see Dannenfeldt 1986; Thorpy 1991; Kroker 2007, for instance).

The key issue nonetheless, for our purposes, concerns the institutional and epistemological arrangements necessary for sleep disorders to emerge if not flourish in the late twentieth and early twenty-first centuries. How, in other words, could these sleep 'problems' become bona fide medical 'disorders' or 'pathologies', ripe for diagnosis and treatment in the modern-day sleep clinic?

The first potential candidate to qualify on this count was *narcolepsy*. Initially documented and described as an independent disease entity in 1880 by the French physician Gélineau (1880), narcolepsy remained a contested, controversial condition (Kroker 2007), with some considering it a product of a brain lesion located in the 'sleep centre' within the diencephalon (i.e. a neuroanatomical explanation) and others considering it a mental illness (i.e. a psychological explanation or psychogenic emphasis) with somatic manifestations (e.g. Levin 1934; Adié 1926; Camp 1907). This moreover, as Kroker (2007) notes, included psychoanalytic interest in narcolepsy in the immediate post-war period in America, whereby narcolepsy was thought to be a symptom of underlying mental conflicts and the dynamic forces of the unconscious mind.

The sleep laboratory in this respect, as previously noted, helped broker or resolve this conflict through the EEG, which provided a new level of diagnostic precision to the disorder through instrumental means. At stake here, in other words, was a sort of diagnostic 'make over', as Kroker (2007: 344–5) appositely puts it, which happened first in Chicago through the work of Rechtschaffen and colleagues – based on a new diagnostic system of narcoleptic symptoms, EEG recordings of sleep stages and differential diagnosis – the crux of which revolved around the patient's abnormal (i.e. rapid or early arrival) REM periods or profile (see, for example, Dement 2000, 1993; Rechtschaffen et al. 1963). Reconfigured in this fashion, narcolepsy therefore helped establish sleep research and diagnosis through the sleep laboratory as a *'distinct form of medical practice* that was related to, but not reducible to, neurology or psychiatry' (Kroker 2007: 348).

Narcolepsy nonetheless was a relatively rare disorder. *Insomnia*, in contrast, was a far more common complaint. Like narcolepsy, however, insomnia also proved a problematic condition around which sleep medicine could develop or flourish as an independent branch, field or specialty in the late twentieth and early twenty-first centuries (Kroker 2007). On the one hand, to repeat, insomnia clearly trumped narcolepsy as a common or widespread complaint rather than a rare condition. On the other hand, it stubbornly remained an elusive complaint given its ambiguous or dual status as 'part psychological disorder and part somatic complaint' (Ibid.: 395). Insomnia, in other words, was a condition characterised more by controversy than consensus, idiosyncrasy than typicality, regarding its nature and status, including diagnostic difficulties and frequent discrepancies between subjective and objective estimates of sleep loss.

Growing concerns from the 1960s onwards, moreover, regarding the safety and efficacy of prescription hypnotics, particularly the problem of drug 'dependence' (Kroker 2007), changed both the image of the 'insomniac', or person with insomnia, and the fortunes of the sleep laboratory as a place where the safety and efficacy of prescription and over-the-counter remedies for sleep problems could be properly studied and evaluated (see, for example, studies by Kales and Kales 1970; Williams and Agnew 1969; Oswald 1968; Freeman et al. 1965; Oswald and Priest 1965). A 're-tooling' of the sleep laboratory occurred here in effect in this more clinical or evaluative direction (Kroker 2007). The Institute of Medicine (IoM) Report (1979), published a year after Hartman's (1978) influential popular book *The Sleeping Pill* – a book which charged the sleeping pill with contaminating or corrupting the genuine therapeutic encounter between doctor and patient – gave further voice to these concerns, following several decades of critical press coverage of tranquilliser use in medical practice and calls from experts in the field of drug abuse that barbiturates should be banned and prescriptions restricted to alternative sleeping pills (Kroker 2007). Insomnia then, as this suggests, was a nexus or nodal point at this time around which a variety of concerns and agendas converged or coalesced and in which the problems of drug dependence loomed large.

Other important developments in sleep disorders medicine were also occurring at this time, however, including the first systematic attempts to develop *diagnostic classifications* and the spread of sleep clinics across North America (Kroker 2007). Comparison of diagnostic classifications over time are revealing on this count. Within the first *Diagnostic Classification of Sleep and Arousal Disorders* (DCSAD), for instance – published in 1979 by the Association of Professional Sleep Societies (APSS) and the Association of Sleep Disorders Centres (ASDC) – the emphasis, as Kroker (2007: 389) rightly notes, was placed on *symptoms* rather than signs. The DCSAD, in this respect, was organised around two main categories: (i) Disorders Initiating or Maintaining Sleep (DIMS) such as insomnia, or more correctly the insomnia*s* in the plural; and (ii) Disorders of Excessive Somnolence such as narcolepsy.

The 1990 *International Classification of Sleep Disorders* (ICSD), in contrast, which subsequently replaced the DCSAD, effectively dispensed with symptoms in favour of psychophysiological *signs* generated by polysomnography (PSG) and the Multiple Sleep Latency Test (MSLT) (American Sleep Disorders Association 1990).[5] Within this new classificatory system or regime, insomnias and hypersomnias (including narcolepsy) were collapsed into the overall category of *dyssomnias*. These in turn were contrasted to the *parasomnias* (such as sleep paralysis, sleep-walking, sleep bruxism and nightmares), *sleep disorders associated with other disorders* (i.e. mental, neurological and other mental disorders) and finally the tantalising or aspirational category of *proposed sleep disorders* (such as persistent short sleepers, long sleepers, menstrual-associated and pregnancy-associated sleep disorders) for which there is 'insufficient information' at present to confirm their acceptance as definite sleep disorders. Idiosyncrasies regarding the insomniac's symptoms, as such, 'were relegated to the margins of the ICSD' (Kroker 2007: 394).

By 1997, however, some further albeit *minor revisions* were deemed necessary, with the title duly changed to the ICSD-Revised (ICSD-R), and the authorship changed from the 'Diagnostic Classification Steering Committee, Thorpy, MJ, Chairman' to the 'American Academy of Sleep Medicine' (AASM 2001/1997). Since its introduction in 1990, the Chair of the American Association of Sleep Medicine Nosology Committee states in the Foreword to this revised edition, the ICSD has:

> gained wide acceptance as a *tool for clinical practice and research in sleep disorders medicine*. The years between 1990 and 1997 have witnessed *wide-ranging changes in sleep disorders medicine* from many perspectives: the growth of managed health care reform; efforts to better integrate sleep disorders medicine into the community medical specialities; major efforts at improving public awareness of the serious toll of sleep disorder; and – perhaps most importantly – *a rapid growth in our understanding of the pathophysiology and effective treatment of sleep disorders*. (Buysee 2001/1997: v, my emphasis)

Such changes furthermore, it is noted, represent a:

> fundamental challenge to any classification of diseases and disorders... On the one hand, research and clinical developments have clearly changed the way we view sleep disorders, most notably sleep-related breathing disorders. On the other hand, frequent major changes in a classification of disorders can be disruptive for both clinical and research practice... Moreover, *clinical and research progress has varied widely across disorders in the ICSD*. Although we have greatly improved our knowledge about some sleep disorders, the essential features of other disorders (not to mention their epidemiology, pathophysiology, and

treatment) *remain in the realm of expert opinion.* (Buysee 2001/1997: v, my emphasis)

Further significant changes are nonetheless evident by the time of the second ICSD in 2005, a 300-page manual covering more than 80 discrete disorders based on the consensus opinion of more than 100 sleep specialists worldwide (American Academy of Sleep Medicine 2005). These disorders are now organised within the ICSD-2 into eight major categories based on a variety of considerations, including *complaint* (such as insomnia, hypersomnia, parasomnia and sleep-related movement disorder), *presumed aetiology* (such as circadian rhythm sleep disorders) or the *organ system* from which the disorder arises (such as sleep-related breathing disorders), with two appendices for the classification of sleep disorders associated with medical or psychiatric disorder. Classification of sleep disorders within the WHO *International Classification of Diseases* (ICD-9-CM) – now supplanted by the new ICD-10 (WHO 2007) – was also revised at this time in order to establish greater *concordance* between the systems with many, though not all, sleep disorders grouped into a new single series with 'Diseases of the nervous system'. While publication of ICSD-2 and associated changes moreover have made a number of *DSM-IV* sleep codes obsolete, this discrepancy is likely to be addressed when *DSM-V* is published.

Of all these sleep disorders, nonetheless, one in particular, *sleep apnoea*, stands out in the 'making' of modern-day sleep medicine (Kroker 2007). While insomnia, for the reasons discussed above, has indeed proven a problematic condition around which sleep medicine could develop or flourish as an independent specialty, and while the condition as such (despite its high prevalence and the sheer volume of hypnotics prescribed to 'treat' it) became increasingly 'marginal' to the main business of sleep medicine (Kroker 2007: 394),[6] the organic nature and basis of sleep apnoea provided precisely the sort of biomedical platform needed, particularly when construed or constructed as a significant if not major public health problem or issue – see, for example, Phillipson (1993); Pack et al. (2006). This did not occur overnight, however, and was not achieved without a struggle. In order for this problem to emerge indeed as a distinct pathophysiological entity, with considerable biomedical scope or potential for expansion in the clinic and wider public health domain, a variety of negotiations and disputes occurred from the 1980s onwards involving sleep researchers, clinicians, patients and even engineers involved in the design of CPAP technologies, with differing forms of knowledge, experience, expertise; thereby underlining the dynamic creation if not 'invention' of this condition and the technologies devised and deployed to diagnose and treat it (cf. Moreira 2006).

The official backdrop or history to the emergence of sleep apnoea as a recognised clinical condition of course is well rehearsed within the annals of sleep science and sleep medicine. This, for example, includes: (i) a seminal description of so-called Pickwickian syndrome – prompted by Dickens' character Joe, a fat sleepy boy in *Pickwick Papers* (Dickens 1909/1836–7; see also Cosnett 1997) – by Burwell and colleagues in 1956 in the *American Journal of Medicine*; (ii) the subsequent establishment of the obstructive sleep apnoea syndrome (OSAS) diagnostic category during the 1970s (Guilleminault et al. 1973); and (iii) the replacement of tracheotomy by continuous positive airways pressure (CPAP) technology as the treatment of choice in the 1980s (Sullivan et al 1981).

A series of convergences and divergences of opinion, if not disputes, nonetheless, as Moreira (2006) rightly notes, are evident here, particularly between *respiratory medicine* and *sleep medicine* over the precise pathways and mechanisms involved in the condition and the role of the *sleep laboratory* in its detection or diagnosis. This, broadly speaking, can be characterised as a difference between an approach which associated obesity with sleepiness and centred around the presence of clinical symptoms and the composition of blood gases, and an approach which accorded a central role to a sleep disorder (OSAS), detected and diagnosed in the sleep laboratory, as the aetiological agent in the resulting clinical picture (i.e. Pickwickian obesity, somnolence, plethoric (red) face and so on) which pulmonologists observed in their patients (Ibid.). Growing recognition and acceptance of this condition nonetheless, coupled with the progressive use of objective sleep study measures such as the Apnoea/ Hypopnoea Index during the 1980s and 1990s, resulted in a predominance of chest physicians (i.e. pulmonologists/ respiratory physicians) within the American Sleep Medicine Association (ASMA) by the 1990s, who headed up sleep laboratories or clinics. The definition, diagnosis and management of OSAS as a consequence is perhaps best regarded as a sort of hybrid splicing or 'mixture of the two definitions of the condition and the practices of medicine they embody' (Moreira 2006: 58). What emerged from this controversy, in other words, was a:

> *new space of biomedical intervention and representation* that has created a set of objects, entities and practices. These are the outcome of the interaction and the mutual enrichment between two different forms of relating medical knowledge and practice. In the process, collaborative

links between sleep researchers and chest physicians were forged, and novel redistributions of accountability between clinicians, researchers and patients were established. (Ibid., my emphasis)

The development, deployment and uptake of CPAP technologies has also of course, Moreira (2006) stresses, been a critical part of the picture or story here, not simply in terms of the collaborations between physicians and medical engineers it involved and entailed, nor in terms of ensuing controversies over its effectiveness (Wright et al. 1997a, b) and associated struggles to get it approved and funded within healthcare systems such as the NHS, but in terms of the subsequent 'problems' which have come to be framed around so-called patient adherence or compliance and efforts to optimise its usage – see, for example, Cartwright (2008); Engleman and Wild (2003). What we see here, in other words, is a situation in which the apparent scientific/clinical expert consensus as to the benefits of CPAP contrasts with *ongoing problems of use for CPAP patients in everyday or every night life* outside the sleep laboratory or sleep clinic (Moreira 2006).

Patient testimonies of the benefits of CPAP usage nonetheless also constitute a powerful resource which may be deployed to good effect for both professional and public purposes. A recent edition of *Wellcome News* (2009), for example, includes an article on 'life with sleep apnoea'. The article in question features the case of Mr Frank Govan, a retired tax consultant, who for years we are told experienced 'intense tiredness' (or feeling 'zombified', as he describes it) and whose tiredness apparently had become a 'standing joke among his friends'. Mr Govan indeed, readers are informed, once 'fell asleep at the wheel whilst driving his family in the fast lane of the M6. Luckily no one was hurt' (2009: 4). Years of 'fruitless visits' to his GP followed as 'diagnosis remained elusive' until eventually he was referred, thanks to a chance remark by his wife to an ENT consultant at a dinner party, to a sleep specialist and diagnosed with obstructive sleep apnoea. Mr Govan, we are told, now uses a CPAP machine to keep his airways open at night, the effects of which (even 'after just one night of CPAP'), are described as truly 'spectacular'. 'I felt refreshed and my energy had returned,' Mr Govan is quoted as saying. 'I had my life back' (Ibid.).

This personal storyline is in turn embedded in both factual reportage of OSA and CPAP technology, including a 'sleep apnoea at a glance' inset box, and the profiling of Dr Mary Morrell who, readers are told, has 'dedicated her career' to studying the condition. The article also features a picture of Mr Govan wearing his CPAP mask, juxtaposed with a picture of Dr Morrell, and another feature box entitled 'You can't breathalyse for sleepiness', in which it is noted: how OSA is associated with increased *risk* of road traffic *accidents*; how bus and lorry drivers are at a particular risk of sleepiness-related accidents, and; how, according to Dr Charles George, University of Western Ontario, Canada, 'more data are needed for society to establish and accept a "safe" sleep apnoea cut-off for driving akin to that for alcohol' (*Wellcome News* 2009: 5) – see also George (2007).

Obstructive sleep apnoea (OSA) then, to summarise, has indeed relatively speaking proved a relatively effective vehicle or platform for sleep science and sleep medicine to mobilise around as a significant public health issue, not least through its links with obesity and cardiovascular risk and the associated risks and dangers it poses both to self and others in terms of excessive daytime sleepiness. This in turn is rendered all the more significant, as a further

guarantee of the diagnostic significance of the sleep laboratory or clinic, by the fact that many OSA sufferers remain
unaware of the condition, given its occurrence while they
sleep – the only daytime trace or symptom being, as the
above case of Mr Govan suggests, unexplained sleepiness
and associated clinical symptoms detectable or deciphera-
ble by a doctor or specialist. As Dement puts it, in alarming
or arresting terms:

> Apnoea is an *unrecognised killer,* but it is hiding in plain
> sight. Every night more than 50 million Americans stop
> breathing ... It never ceases to amaze me that sleep apnoea
> victims can awaken hundreds of times in a single night
> and remember nothing of that torment. The *severe conse-
> quences* of the disorder and its *very high prevalence make it
> one of the most serious general health problems in America.*
> (1999: 168, my emphasis)

Diagnosed in the sleep clinic, treated through CPAP technology and positioned as a significant public health risk, OSA
then (the 'midnight strangler' as Dement (1999) dubs it), provided sleep medicine with precisely the sort of opportunity
it had been looking for. This, for example, is evident in the
growing number of clinicians certified in sleep medicine,
and the associated growth of sleep clinics in which OSA, the
most commonly diagnosed sleep disorder nowadays, could
be detected, deciphered, diagnosed and treated.

As with the past evolution and emergence of sleep science,
however, these *trends in sleep medicine are more pronounced
in North America* than elsewhere. The *American Academy of
Sleep Medicine* (AASM), for example, now consists of over
7000 physicians, researchers and other healthcare profes-
sionals who specialise in studying, diagnosing and treating

disorders of sleep and daytime alertness such as OSA, narcolepsy and insomnia, with more than 1000 sleep centres and laboratories now formally accredited by the AASM (www.aasmnet.org/). Sleep medicine, as this suggests, is now big business in North America, with significant opportunities for the enterprising physician (see, for example, Norbutt 2004). The typical US sleep laboratory, for instance, according to recent market data, has revenues in the region of US $1.33 million and conducts approximately 1250 sleep studies per year; figures which, when finally tallied and totalled up, amount to a staggering market worth around US $5 billion (Reichen 2009: 485–6).

While OSA continues to be a key condition in much of this clinical work, however, 'circadian rhythm sleep disorders', such as so-called shift work sleep disorder (SWSD), also open up other potential avenues or opportunities for *biomedical expansion*; particularly, returning to themes first aired in the opening chapter of this book, in the so-called 24/7 economy where a significant number of the workforce are engaged in some form of shift work, and where 'excessive sleepiness' becomes an occupational hazard if not the norm.

Excessive daytime sleepiness (EDS), we might say, embodies and expresses precisely the amorphous and ambiguous nature and status of sleep 'problems' today as a 'matter of concern'. Although typically understood in official medical or clinical terms as a *symptom* of other sleep problems or pathologies, or other medical or psychiatric conditions, there are signs moreover that EDS is now being reconfigured within the broader realms of *popular culture* as a problem if not a *pathology* in its own right. Type the keywords 'sleepy', 'sleepiness' or 'drowsiness' into any Internet search engine, for example, as Kroll-Smith (2003: 636) rightly notes, and many if not most hits will portray this as some variant of 'excessive daytime sleepiness'. The impression that this is or may be a distinct disorder moreover, Kroll-Smith argues, is conveyed in a variety of ways, including: (i) omission in discussions of EDS of any obvious or explicit reference to it as a 'symptom'; (ii) the manner in which the very name 'excessive daytime sleepiness' and the acronym EDS imply 'a more significant identity as a bona fide medical disorder'; and (iii) the readily available and multiple websites for online self-diagnostic tests such as the Epworth Sleepiness Scale (ESS) (Johns 1991), which might 'easily assume a somatic reality against which a number becomes a meaningful piece of evidence about the relative presence or absence of a particular disorder' (Kroll-Smith 2003: 637).

Viewed in this light then, EDS stands at the nexus of both *clinical concerns* within the confines of the sleep clinic and broader concerns and imperatives within *popular culture*, which are serving to reconfigure this soporific state and somatic complaint as a novel problem (or *proto-disorder* perhaps) amenable to self-diagnosis on the Internet (Kroll-Smith 2003). This in turn throws into critical relief not simply the apparent *gap* between self-reported sleep troubles and the routine clinical gaze of everyday (front-line) medical practice, but also perhaps, as Kroll-Smith (2003) provocatively suggests, the growing significance of popular culture in the very creation of medical 'problems'.[7]

Medicalisation redux: biomedicine, health and the management of sleep in everyday/night life

Implicit in the foregoing developments and debates are a further series of critical socio-political questions, worth spelling out at this particular juncture, concerning the medicalisation or biomedicalisation of sleep over time. What, in other words, do the foregoing issues tell us about the actual or prospective biomedicalisation of sleep, and what further light does this shed on the governance of alert/sleepy bodies and the biopolitics of sleep and wakefulness in the late modern age? Can particular relays, for instance, be traced or tracked here between sleep science/medicine, self-help and corporate governance in the name of health or virtue, wisdom or well-being, enterprise or enhancement?

Much has been written in recent decades, both inside and outside the academy, on the expansion of medical jurisdiction and control over more and more areas of our lives in the name of health and illness, disease and disorder. Medicalisation, in this respect, denotes the process whereby hitherto 'non-medical' matters become transformed or translated into 'medical problems' such as 'illness', 'disorder' or 'syndromes' of one kind or another (Conrad et al. 2010; Conrad 2007, 2005, 1992). Medicalisation in turn may occur at a number of different *levels* – i.e. *conceptually*, when a medical vocabulary is adopted to describe a problem; *institutionally*, when an organisation adopts a medical approach to a problem; and *interactionally* within the doctor–patient relationship, for instance (Conrad 1992). It may also occur to varying *degrees*, with varying *involvements* on the part of doctors, and is in principle though seldom in practice a *bi-directional* process whereby de-medicalisation may occur over time. While medicalisation moreover describes or denotes a social process, and while some commentators and critics have raised legitimate concerns about the 'over-expansion' of medical control or the 'over-medicalisation' of our lives if not outright cases of 'disease-mongering' (Moynihan and Cassels 2005), medicalisation is ideally a descriptive term that does not necessarily imply a value judgement on these matters. Medicalisation indeed may involve both 'gains' as well as 'losses' and have positive as well as negative faces which are best studied and judged on a case-by-case basis, including the financial 'costs' as well as the personal and social consequences of these processes (see, for example, Conrad et al. 2010).

Recent years have also witnessed a growing number of calls to go 'beyond' medicalisation, at least as conventionally configured and understood within medical sociology, including the aforementioned claim that many forms of medicalisation are now better understood as outright cases of 'disease-mongering' – given the huge profits to be made out of convincing ('healthy') people they are 'sick' and thereby 'selling sickness' for a 'healthy' profit margin (Moynihan and Cassels 2005). Perhaps most significantly of all for our purposes, it is clear that the 'engines' or 'drivers' of medicalisation have shifted over time (Conrad 2007, 2005), not least through the rapid pace of developments in bioscience and biotechnology today, prompting writers such as Clarke et al. (2003) to speak of a shift or transition to a new phase of 'biomedicalisation'. The 'bio-' prefix in this respect is intended to signify a new era of 'technoscientific biomedicine' which is becoming increasingly 'complex', 'multisited' and 'multidirectional', including significant new opportunities to not simply *control* but to *customise* bodies, and which conveys important transformations now taking place in 'both the organisation and practices of contemporary biomedicine, implemented largely through the integration of technoscientific innovations' (Ibid.: 161–2).

A number of points are worth stressing or spelling out in this regard in relation to sleep as both a further elaboration on the foregoing themes and issues considered in this chapter so far, and an update on my previous thinking on the medicalisation of sleep (Williams 2005, 2004, 2002).[8]

First and foremost, sleep very clearly fits more or less readily into the picture here as a rich and fascinating case study of the *changing dynamics of biomedicalisation* over time, and the complexities, controversies, convergence and contradictions contained therein. This, for example, includes not simply the dense, diverse, dynamic relays and relations between the sleep laboratory and the sleep clinic, and the associated tensions, transitions and translations between sleep science and sleep medicine, but a variety of other trends and transformations over time, such as the growing power and influence of the pharmaceutical industry; the blurred or shifting boundaries between therapy and enhancement; the changing role and expectations of patients, consumers and other pressure or advocacy groups; the growing salience and significance of popular culture and new media in construction if not contestation of sleep 'problems' or sleep 'matters' today; and finally the production or potential production, in and through these very processes, of new individual and collective identities and forms of activism.

A number of potential problems and paradoxes also arise here nonetheless, as we have seen, thereby making the biomedicalisation of sleep a far from simple or straightforward process. The historical challenges and problems of transforming sleep into an 'object' of scientific study, in this respect, have been matched by the tensions and difficulties of *translating* sleep into a biomedical problem and matter of public health and safety. Sleep indeed, or at least certain facets and features of it, continues to pose problems for biomedicine, given its peculiarities and paradoxes, while sleep medicine itself is really only now, it seems, *beginning* to emerge from its relatively minor or marginal status as a specialism, within North America at least. Unlike many other forms of diagnosis, moreover, sleep requires the whole patient or proto-patient to surrender consciousness and succumb to sleeping in the artificial, time-consuming, technologically intensive conditions of the sleep laboratory throughout the night in order to record or trace (courtesy of the laboratory technician) and diagnose (courtesy of the sleep doctor or physician) the problem or condition in question (Kroker 2007: 15). If we add to this the aforementioned problem of conditions such as insomnia as a stable base or platform to biomedicalise around; related crises and controversies surrounding the safety and efficacy of sleeping pills; struggles over the precise nature and status of OSA and associated design, development, reimbursement and patient 'compliance' issues regarding CPAP technologies; the fact that specialist or professional 'ownership' over sleep problems or disorders remains patchy and problematic; the often complicated if not chaotic patient trajectories through healthcare; ongoing claims and criticisms regarding the extent of undiagnosed and untreated sleep 'problems' in our midst; and the lack of basic medical education and training in sleep disorders medicine, and one may well be forgiven for concluding that the biomedicalisation of sleep is a non-starter.

For medical writers such as Dement (1999) indeed, picking up on this latter point about the extent of undiagnosed and untreated sleep 'problems' in our midst, 'ignorance' of this kind is the 'worst sleep disorder of all'; a charge which in turn of course serves as a further rallying call or cry regarding the importance of sleep for society in general and the dangers and risks of sleep problems in particular. 'If even the basic facts about sleep,' Dement ventures:

> had been known and understood by the general public and its doctors over the years, there's no way of knowing how many human beings now dead – possibly millions; perhaps even relatives of yours – might be alive today. Never before in human history has a *disparity between the amount of scientific knowledge and the benefits of that knowledge to society* been so tragically vast. (1999: 3, my emphasis)

Perhaps more correctly, therefore, it is safer to say that the biomedicalisation of sleep, for better or worse, remains *partial and incomplete*. An ongoing process, that is to say, subject to ebbs and flows, if not elements, of reversal or resistance. This in turn suggests a need to avoid broad references to the biomedicalisation of sleep in favour of more detailed case or condition-specific forms of analysis. Thus while insomnia, as previously noted, poses ongoing challenges and problems in terms of any simple or straightforward process of biomedicalisation (Williams et al. 2008; Kroker 2007), conditions such as narcolepsy and OSA have indeed proved more fertile soil for the seeds of biomedicalisation to take root and flourish. So too newer conditions such shift work sleep disorder (SWSD), a classic example perhaps of the biomedicalisation of a social problem in which pharmaceutical forms of intervention or governance in the guise of wakefulness-promoting drugs such as Modafinil loom large. There are signs moreover, as we have seen, that excessive daytime sleepiness is now being reconstructed and reconfigured in popular culture at least (i.e. outside the sleep clinic) as a condition or disorder in its own right in ways which invite us to reflect once more upon the extra-institutional, textual or rhetorical dimension of biomedicalisation today in an information society (cf. Kroll-Smith 2003), including the possibilities of *resistance* of various kinds – see, for example, Weisgerber's (2004) study of challenges to biomedicalised understandings of sleep paralysis on the Internet.

A second key issue I wish to flag here returns us to the question of pharmaceuticals as a key biotechnology in the management or governance of sleep(iness) and the role of the pharmaceutical industry in these broader drivers and dynamics of biomedicalisation over time. The (biomedical) management of sleep problems of course includes a variety of therapies other than pharmaceuticals – with non-pharmaceutical interventions such as cognitive behaviour therapy (CBT) now recognised if not preferred as a cost-effective treatment option for insomnia (see, for example, Morgan et al. 2004). Sleeping pills or tablets, nonetheless, are clearly big business, with a global pharmaceutical market for diagnosed sleep disorders estimated to be worth around $4.3 billion in 2005, and some forecasts predicting a 158 per cent increase on these figures to a staggering $11 billion by 2012. 'Underdiagnosed and undertreated', moreover, Reichen (2009: 486) comments with entrepreneurial zeal, 'the sleep disorders market presents a *major opportunity* for pharmaceutical companies'. While many of these sleep medications have been on the market now for over 20 years and are therefore out of patent, and while the pharmaceutical industry in general appears to be suffering something of an innovation crisis – particularly drugs for the central nervous system (CNS) – a number of new sleep medications are also now supposed in the pharmaceutical pipeline, some reportedly now in phase II and phase III clinical trials (Alexander 2009; Reichen 2009), with some commentators and experts predicting a future of 'smarter' drugs that will deliver precise amounts of good-quality slow-wave sleep without the disadvantages of previous generations of hypnotics (Lawton 2006).

The market or potential future market for wakefulness-promoting drugs such as Modafinil (brand name Provigil) is also another key part of the picture here. Initially approved for the treatment of narcolepsy, Modafinil is now officially licensed to treat *excessive sleepiness associated with* obstructive sleep apnoea (OSA) and shift work sleep disorder (SWSD). It is also used off-label for symptoms of sleepiness and fatigue associated with a variety of other conditions. Provigil, according to Cephalon's latest sales figures, has generated more than 12 million prescriptions and over $3 billion in cumulative revenue to date, with Nuvigil (Armodafinil) now approved by the FDA as Cephalon's 'next generation' wakefulness-promoting agent (protected by a US patent which expires in 2023). 'Each day,' Frank Baldino (Cephalon chairman/CEO) states on the Cephalon website:

> millions of people struggle with excessive sleepiness associated with OSA, shift work sleep disorder ... and narcolepsy. These are serious and chronic conditions that impair the body's ability to stay awake, stay alert, and function. Cephalon first recognised the *breadth of this medical need* more than a decade ago. We remain committed to those patients, to the sleep community, and to developing medicines that provide true patient value. (www.Cephalon. com, accessed 15 August 2009, my emphasis)

The Cephalon Nuvigil website, accordingly, includes pictures of office workers, builders and shift workers with arms raised, in triumphant poses with broad grins on their faces, and wraparound banners inviting viewers to 'rediscover wakefulness', with links to further simple (self-administered) online tests such as the Epworth Sleepiness Scale (ESS) (Johns 1991), to find out 'how sleepy' you are (cf. Kroll-Smith 2003), plus prescription advice and opportunities to 'share your story'.

Concerns in this respect are now being voiced in various quarters about the wider lifestyle or recreational market for Modafinil as a, if not *the*, drug of 'choice' in today's 24/7 era, both inside and outside the workplace: the latest pharmaceutical aid or ally, in effect, of the wide or wired-awake world (see, for example, Coveney et al. 2009; Williams et al. 2009; Wolpe 2002). The problem here, in other words, if 'problem' it is, concerns the manner in which Modafinil, like Viagra before it, serves to further blur or redraw the boundaries between the 'medical' and 'non-medical' uses and abuses of these drugs in the name of therapy or enhancement. These issues in turn, however, become all the more complicated in the case of safety-critical occupations, from transport to medicine, where pharmaceutical enhancements of various kinds (in the absence of adequate sleep) may serve legitimate social ends or purposes. Hence Chesire's provocative yet pertinent question: 'Would a pharmaceutically enhanced physician be a better physician?'[9]

These processes of *pharmaceuticalisation* then, if indeed we may call them that,[10] constitute an important strand of the biomedicalisation of sleep and wakefulness today, including a further blurring or reconfiguration of the boundaries between therapy and enhancement or the *customisation* of bodies. They are also, of course, returning to the broader point about the changing dynamics or drivers of biomedicalisation over time, part and parcel of the growing power and influence of the pharmaceutical industry over all our lives today, given industry-sponsored interests in market maximisation. Consider for example, on this latter count, the recent House of Commons Health Committee (HCHC) Report on *The Influence of the Pharmaceutical Industry* (2005), which concluded that:

> What has been described as the 'medicalisation of society' – the belief that every problem requires a medical treatment – may also be attributed to the activities of the pharmaceutical industry. While the pharmaceutical industry cannot be blamed for creating unhealthy reliance on, and over-use of, medicines, it has *certainly exacerbated it*. There has been a *trend towards categorising more and more individuals as 'abnormal' or in need of drug treatment*. (2005: 4, my emphasis)

Here we return to the question of 'disease-mongering' noted earlier: the charge, that is to say, that it is no longer simply a case of the manufacturing of a drug for every disorder, but the manufacturing of a disorder for every drug (Moynihan and Cassels 2005). Clearly not all cases of biomedicalisation or pharmaceuticalisation, however, involve disease-mongering. The gains and losses, risks and benefits associated with these processes of biomedicalisation and pharmaceuticalisation moreover, as I have already emphasised, need assessing on a case-by-case basis – see, for example, Woloshin and Schwartz (2006) for a recent study of restless leg syndrome. The pharmaceuticalisation of sleep and wakefulness nonetheless, in the name of therapy or enhancement, is clearly an important part of the biomedicalisation of sleep and the biopolitics of bodies today, contested or otherwise.

These developments in turn raise a third important series of questions, concerning not simply power but personhood.

To the extent, for example, that these foregoing processes of biomedicalisation and pharmaceuticalisation render sleep a problem or matter of concern today, and to the extent that they influence the very ways in which people come to know, understand, mange or govern themselves qua patients, consumers or citizens, then something potentially powerful if not profound is at work here: new 'biosocial' or 'technosocial' forms of identity and activism, that is to say, both individual and collective in kind (cf. Gibbon and Novas 2008; Clarke et al. 2003). To the extent moreover that sleep is now configured and understood, courtesy of modern-day sleep/neuroscience, as an active state of the brain, and to the extent that sleep medications, in the name of therapy or enhancement, work at the neurochemical level, then sleep constitutes another potential site or source from which, in Rose's (2007) terms, more 'neurochemical' notions of selfhood or personhood and more 'neurochemical' forms of citizenship and activism *may* arise either now or in the (near) future.[11]

A fourth closely related set of issues I wish to flag here concerns the increasingly complex if not contradictory relations between (sleep) medicine, self-help, corporate culture and corporate governance. While discourses regarding the benefits of sleep (and the dangers of sleep deprivation) for health are not of course particularly new or novel, what *is* relatively new, as Brown rightly notes, is 'the connection between corporate policy, management strategy and sleep-related medical and self-help advice' (2004: 174). Here we return to issues first aired in Chapter 2 about the turn, within certain (cognitively rich) sectors of the economy at least, to more 'humancentric', 'worker-friendly' or even 'sleep-friendly' policies and practices (including 'flexi-time' programmes, free gyms or yoga classes, provision or tolerance of workplace napping, and so on), designed to improve work/life balance, reduce stress and ill-health and boost productivity and performance – see Wilson (2004), for example. This moreover, as previously noted, may include the buying or bringing in of outside consultants and therapists to speak to workers about these issues, including organised workshops on sleep-smart or sleep-wise strategies and other tips and recommendations derived from self-help books and 'how-to' manuals. Instructive parallels may be drawn here in this respect between the biomedicalisation of sleepy/alert bodies and enhanced opportunities or possibilities for the 'constant management' of workers both inside and outside the workplace (Brown 2004: 174). Discourses of self-help, biomedicine and corporate management, in other words, in part at least, all depend on appeals to individual 'self-improvement' in which people are 'constantly compelled to monitor and micro-manage every possible aspect of their lives' (Ibid.: 175).

Tensions remain nonetheless, as Brown (2004: 181) rightly notes, between those such as Dement (1999) and Coren (1996), whose prime commitment is the power, promise and potential of sleep on grounds of health, safety and well-being, and those – such as Maas and colleagues (1999); Anthony (1997); Anthony and Anthony (2001); companies such as Alertness Solutions (www.alertness-solutions.com) – for whom sleep promotion or management, courtesy of sleep-'smart' or sleep-'wise' schedules, power naps and the like is primarily about performance and productivity both on and off the job. For Dement indeed, as noted in Chapter 1, modern culture has become an object lesson or living laboratory of (chronic) sleep deprivation, a 'sleep sick society' no less, with profound implications and powerful effects on overall health and vitality, including the immune system response, psychological well-being, quality of life and longevity. It is high time, Dement argues, to start *'taking sleep seriously* as the *foundation of good health'* (1999: 9–10, my emphasis). Prescriptions for our 'sleep sick society' in this respect include basic principles and practices of *sleep hygiene* and *healthy sleep*, learning to manage *sleep crises*, taking 'age into account', and adopting a *sleep-smart lifestyle*. 'Start tonight,' Dement counsels; 'consider it *doctor's orders'* (1999: 433, my emphasis).

A fifth key point, therefore, also comes sharply into view here concerning the increasing focus or emphasis not simply on the problems or pathologies associated with poor sleep, cast in negative terms, but on the power, promise or potential of good sleep, cast in more *positive* terms, as the passport to *health*, *happiness* and *well-being*. A vital matter to repeat, as I have argued throughout the book, which concerns or implicates us all as sleeping as well as waking beings. Sleep in this respect, construed and constructed as an essential ingredient or integral part of health, is thus paradoxically both 'more biomedicalised' through risk factors and (self-) surveillance practices, and seemingly 'less medicalised' as 'the key site of responsibility shifts from the professional ... to include collaboration with or reliance upon the individual' qua patient or user, citizen or consumer (Clarke et al. 2003: 173). This moreover includes a variety of non-biomedical or non-orthodox expertise, such as alternative or complementary therapies, plus a variety of other sleep-related commercial products and over-the-counter remedies designed to assist in the *management* of sleep and the facilitation of a 'good' or 'sound' night's sleep.

Here we return full circle to the notion, first aired in Chapter 2, of the 'well-slept citizen' as moral duty or obligation, something to be worked at or on, and to broader trends and transformations in corporate culture in the neo-liberal era concerning enhanced possibilities or prospects for the *constant management* or *micro-management* of individuals in all spheres of life in the name of self-cultivation, self-transformation or self-improvement (cf. Maasen and Sutter 2007; Rose 2007, 1990; Deleuze 1995; Foucault 1991, 1988). This in turn alerts us to the multiple ways in which sleep, or the promise of sleep to be more precise, is 'sold' in the marketplace. From the sleep clinic to the pharmaceutical and mattress industries, over-the-counter and herbal sleep aids or remedies to how-to books and a host of other sleep-promoting devices, gadgets, methods, mantras, tips, talismans and paraphernalia, the dreams being sold or on offer here appear to converge or coalesce around both *selling better sleep* and *selling sleep better* in order to 'feel better', 'do better', 'perform better', 'live better'; to 'improve' in some way or other, that is to say, aided and abetted by a growing *sleep industry* or 'sleep-industrial complex' (MooAllem 2007; Williams 2005; Williams and Boden 2004). In the United States alone, for example, this 'sleep aids market' (comprising mattresses, pillows, sleep laboratories and annexed services, sleep medications, CPAP sleep apnoea devices, and other retail devices), was worth US \$23.7 billion in 2007 – a growth of 77 per cent since 2000, with a further growth of 36 per cent forecast by 2012 which, if correct, would then amount to a total market of US \$32.3 billion (Alexander 2009: 496).[12]

At stake here then, to summarise, is the further reconfiguration or repositioning of sleep in biomedicalised terms, not simply through discourses of *deprivation* and *disorder*, but through the multiple relays or relations between self-help, biomedicine, corporate culture and corporate governance in the neo-liberal era of the enterprising if not enhanced self. An era, to repeat, where even the seemingly most mundane, personal or private of acts, such as sleep, become something to be cultivated, captured, colonised, worked at or micro-managed in the name of health and happiness, wisdom and well-being, vigilance and virtue, productivity and performance.

Science fact/fiction: sleepless futures?

Here we arrive at a final set of issues regarding the future or possible futures of sleep in the years or decades to come.[13]

At one level, of course, the future of sleep looks pretty much assured. All (animal) life it seems, including us human animals, sleeps and will in all likelihood or probability continue to sleep (see Siegel 2009, for example). Yet sleep, as we have also seen throughout this book, displays a high degree of *plasticity*, albeit within certain limits or parameters, which makes it amenable to management if not modification in a variety of ways in terms of prevailing socio-cultural norms or mandates, particularly those associated with work time, work culture and work ethics. To the extent moreover, as Rose (2007) notes, that the 'vital norms' of life itself are now themselves increasingly amenable to manipulation or modification in the era of biomedical enhancement or optimisation, then this has the potential to radically undermine any fixed notion of biology as 'bedrock' or 'given' – see also Harris (2007); Savulescu and Bostrom (2008); Miller and Wilsdon (2006). We have indeed long since crossed or passed the border, boundary or threshold, itself of course constructed and bound up with the 'purity' myths of modernity (cf. Latour 1993), separating nature from culture or biology from society (Giddens 1991).

A key site here, for example, in which these futures are already actively being explored or exploited, rehearsed or played out, is the military, which itself of course involves important relays and complex relations with biomedicine, bioscience and biotechnology, including the biomedicalisation of the military and the militarisation of biomedicine (Harrison 1999, 1996; Cooter et al. 1998; Montgomery 1991). The translation of sleep into a scientific object or matter of public concern in this respect, and the commodification or customisation of sleep in medical, corporate or popular culture, is paralleled if not surpassed by its transformation into a commodity of war in the military; something to be managed, mobilised, modified, that is to say, in the service of combat and the interests of strategic advantage over one's adversaries or enemies on the battlefield or in the theatre of war.

Sleep deprivation indeed, for obvious reasons, poses a serious strategic challenge for the military, and as such constitutes perhaps the most immediate if not the most important human performance factor in sustained military operations. The military in this respect has long since been interested in new or novel ways to monitor, manage, manipulate or modify sleep in the interests of military efficiency or enhancement and hence the conferral of tactical advantage. Psycho- or neuropharmaceuticals, once again, loom large in this configuration of possibilities, alongside other neurotechnologies associated with the brain and neuroplasticity.

Consider, for example, a recent report entitled *Human Performance* – commissioned by the US Pentagon's *Office of Defense Research and Engineering* (ODR & E) and published by MITRE Corporation in March 2008 – which takes as its starting point rapid developments in the field of neuroscience, psychopharmacology and cognition that provide or promise 'fundamental understanding of linkages among brain activity, electrical and chemical stimulation, and human behaviour' (MITRE 2008: 1). Sleep deprivation, unsurprisingly perhaps, features prominently in the report as both a tactical problem and a target for various neuroenhancement technologies. The most 'immediate human performance factor in military effectiveness', for example, it is noted, is 'degradation under stressful conditions, particularly sleep deprivation. If an opposing force had a significant sleep advantage, this would pose a serious threat' (2008: 23). The 'manipulation and understanding of sleep' therefore, we are told, is 'one part of human performance modification where significant breakthroughs should have national security consequences' (Ibid.).

On the one hand then, as this suggests, sleep deprivation and associated performance 'degradation' is taken as a given on the military battlefield. On the other hand, however, attempts to modify sleep deprivation and/or improve soldiers' performance when sleep deprived is seen less as an option and more as an *obligation* or outright necessity given that lives are at stake and could be saved. The calculus as such, according to this report at least, runs as follows:

The maximum casualty rate depends strongly on the individuals sleep need $\tau 0$. Hence any efforts to improve human performance to minimize $\tau 0$ for given tasks can lead to a significant decrease in the casualty rate of [about] 20 per cent. *Suppose a human could be engineered who slept for the same amount of time as a giraffe [1.9 hours per night].* This would lead to an approximate twofold decrease in the casualty rate. An adversary would need an approximate 40 per cent increase in troop levels to compensate for this advantage. (MITRE 2008: 27, my emphasis)

This report is revealing on other counts too, not least its somewhat awkward or hedged handling of questions concerning the extent of sleep modification already under way in the (US) military to date. The use of 'supplements primarily to ameliorate sleep deprivation and improve physical performance', it is noted, 'is report[ed] to be common amongst US military personnel'. Yet this behaviour, it stresses, while recognised as something of a *'cultural norm* in the US', is *'not endorsed* by the US military' (2008: 33).

Officially endorsed or not, the military are certainly no strangers to the use of simple stimulants such as caffeine, or stronger stimulants such as amphetamines, to combat sleep deprivation and keep soldiers 'wide' if not 'wired' awake. Neuropharmaceuticals such as Modafinil and new generation cognitive enhancement agents currently in development such as ampakines (Lynch and Gall 2006; Lynch 2002), however, add a further important dimension to this pharmaceutical arsenal or arms race, alongside other military-sponsored research to unlock the biological or molecular secret, or secrets in the plural, of how to get by on less sleep.

The *Walter Reed Army Institute of Research* (WRAIR) in Silver Spring, Maryland, for example, has reputedly studied the effects of caffeine, amphetamines and Modafinil on troops kept awake for up to 85 hours (Sample 2004; WRAIR 1997). The French Foreign Legion are also reported to have taken Modafinil as early on as the Gulf War in 1991 (Sample 2004). Researchers at the University of Wisconsin, Madison, meanwhile, are trying to understand how certain animals, such as the migrating white-crowned sparrow, function perfectly well for prolonged periods of time on only a fraction of the sleep they are used to – an intriguing parallel being drawn here between troops on covert or sustained combat missions and migrating birds (Ibid.).

All in all, some 86 proposed 'ergonomic and cognitive aids', according to the aforementioned US MITRE (2008) report, have been evaluated to date, including amphetamines and Modafinil, with ampakines now seen as the smart bet or target of choice. The idea here, as Greg Belenky from the WRAIR tellingly comments, is to *'turn sleep into an item of logistic supply ... to treat it like fuel – how much do people have, how long will it last them, and when do we need to fill them up again'* (Belenky, quoted in Sample 2004). Sleep, in other words, to repeat, becomes a 'commodity of war', much like bombs, bullets and fuel (Sample 2004).

Whether or not of course these developments are another good example or prime expression of the cyborg status (cf. Gray 2000; Haraway 1990) of the modern-day or postmodern soldier is a debatable. To the extent, for example, that sleep in the military is now monitored, measured, managed, manipulated and modified in these ways through a whole array or arsenal of technoscientific paraphernalia – from wristwatches that carefully record and relay how much sleep soldiers get to forms of neuropharmaceutical enhancement and other current or near-future neurotechnologies such as brain stimulation, neural implants and associated technologies for enhanced night vision and the like (see, for example, Ben-Ari 2003) – then the answer may very well be a resounding or unqualified yes. To the extent, however, as Rose rightly reminds us, that many of these developments, in the military as elsewhere, concern *bio-* or *neuro*technological interventions targeted at the vital normativities of life itself and its reshaped, reconfigured or re-engineered possibilities, then they surely render us *'all the more* biological' (2007: 20, original emphasis).

Literature too provides another rich site or source of speculation regarding the future or possible futures of sleep, including both sleep-filled and sleepless futures. H.G. Wells, for example, in *The Sleeper Awakes* (2005/1910), explores and exploits the dormant possibilities embodied and expressed in the case of Graham, who emerges from a 200-year-long sleep during which he has amazingly accumulated enough wealth to make him the owner of the world. At stake here, in other words, as Hancock and colleagues remark, is a novel in which sleep is fast 'becoming transformed into yet another adjunct of both relentless cycles of production and consumption, as well as the reproduction of evermore commercially dependent subjectivities' (2009: 87).

Other literary sources, in contrast, trade or play on various sleepless futures. Jonathan Coe's (1997) popular novel *The House of Sleep*, for instance, features the mad, maverick, half-crazed character Dr Gregory Duden, for whom sleep is considered or likened to a disease in need of a cure. Why despise sleep? Duden is asked, to which he curtly replies:

'I'll tell you why: because the sleeper is helpless; powerless. Sleep puts even the strongest people at the mercy of the weakest and most feeble...[a]...posture of *abject submission*...The brain disabled, the muscles inert and flaccid...the great leveller. Like fucking socialism'. (Coe 1997: 176–7, my emphasis)[14]

Novels within the science-fiction genre also of course conjure up various scenarios or nightmares regarding future 'sleepless' worlds. The critical issue in Ballard's (1992) short story 'Manhole 69', for example, concerns the plight of a group of surgically altered sleepless men, who slowly but surely find the world of permanent consciousness the worst nightmare of all and eventually descend into a catatonic state of psychic zero as the 'walls', a metaphor presumably for consciousness, start to close in on these hapless victims and helpless souls.

Kress' (1996, 1995, 1993) *Beggars* trilogy, in contrast, is set in a near-future United States and the emergence of an ever-growing number of human beings who have been genetically engineered or modified to no longer require sleep – a new class of 'sleepless' and subsequently 'supersleepless', that is to say, who in an intriguing play or parody of values, are beautiful, disease-free, excellent, intelligent and industrious compared to sleeping bodies which are portrayed instead as destructive and 'entropic'. The *Beggars* trilogy in this respect, as Steinberg comments, provides a 'pointed allegory' not only of ' "sleepless" values as embodied, technological and political-economic aspirations, but as emergent from and a basis for a distinctive social order' (2008: 131). As one character tellingly remarks, early on in the first novel:

> Sleep served an important evolutionary function... sleep was an aid to survival. But now it's a *left-over mechanism,* a vestige like an appendix. It switches on every night, but the need is gone. So we turn off the switch and its source, in the genes. (1993: 11, my emphasis)

At stake or on offer here then, glimpsed through these diverse and disparate sources, are a number of futures or possible futures in the making, so to speak. To the extent, moreover, that some of these developments are already with us, both on and off the military battlefield, courtesy of neuropsychopharmaceuticals and other drugs and devices on the horizon in a neuro-age or era, and to the extent that science-fiction *reflects* as well as *anticipates* key trends and transformations in society, then it as much to do with futures present, or partly present perhaps, as futures yet to come. To the extent nonetheless that sleep continues to serve a valuable or vital social as well as biological role as 'time out', a 'tension-release' or a 'periodic remission' from the demands of the waking world (cf. Schwartz 1970; Parsons 1951), and to the extent that a 'good' sleep is a pleasure for many if not most of us, then the notion that sleep may one day become obsolete is unlikely: more a case perhaps of *customisation* or *optimisation* in the era of enhancement than *obsolescence*. On that 'reassuring' note, perhaps we may all rest easy.

Conclusions

At stake here, it is clear, are a series of trends and transformations in sleep science and sleep medicine over the past half a century or so which, in countless ways, constitute another rich and indeed vital part of the politics or biopolitics of sleep today in the late modern age. This, for example, as we have seen, includes the *transformation* of sleep into an 'object' of scientific or technoscientific investigation in the sleep laboratory, the *translation* of sleep through the language or lexicon of 'disorders' into a medical matter diagnosed and treated in the sleep clinic, and more broadly the multiple ways in which sleep, in and through these processes, is part and parcel of the *biomedicalisation* and pharmaceuticalisation of life in the name of therapy or enhancement.

These processes nonetheless, I have argued, remain partial and incomplete to date. At the very least, we may say, they throw into critical relief once again the contested nature and status of sleep today as a matter of concern or problem in the making, both inside and outside the sleep laboratory and the sleep clinic, and the multiple relays between science, medicine and the 'management' of sleep in everyday/night life. This moreover, as we have seen, includes newly forged or reconfigured relations between medico-managerial agendas or mandates, particularly those associated with sleep medicine, self-help and corporate governance and their intersections with prized neo-liberal values of 'enterprise' if not 'enhancement' in all walks of life.

The 'future' of sleep also appears, in a far from trivial or fanciful sense, to be with us already today, both on and off the military battlefield, given the potential now to not simply 'control' but to 'customise' or 'enhance' our bodies in various ways. A scenario in the case of sleep, I have argued, which on the one hand may seek to optimise the *quality* of our sleep, even if its *quantity* declines, and on the other hand may render sleep increasingly 'optional' if not 'obsolete'. Both options of course are ultimately strategies of 'enhancement' or 'optimisation' in effect, albeit with different aims and outcomes in mind.

This in turn highlights a further possible irony or paradox regarding the very role of biomedicalisation in the future of sleep. On the one hand, as we have seen, sleep science and sleep medicine will continue in all likelihood to champion and defend the power and promise of sleep. On the other hand, however, sleep science and sleep medicine also possess the power and potential, through the quest to unlock and unravel the mysteries of sleep and to design new interventions to optimise 'solutions' to sleep problems, to develop or devise ever new ways to downsize or do away with sleep in the (near) future, in part or in whole. Viewed in this latter light then, we might conclude, the 'biomedicalisation' of sleep is itself somewhat Janus-faced, pointing simultaneously in two possible future directions which return us once again to the notion of sleep as a 'final frontier' of sorts. A frontier indeed which looks set to become ever more contested in the (near) future.

Notes

1. See Kroker (2007), for example, for a recent authoritative biography or survey of the transformation of sleep research which I draw on extensively in the early parts of this chapter. Thanks too to Kenton Kroker for helpful conversations/communications on these and related issues over the past few years.

2. The broad, centuries-long, historical sweep of Kroker's (2007) (private to public, subjective to objective) sleep thesis, to be sure, leaves him potentially open to criticism here on various counts – see, for example, Smith's (2009) recent review of Kroker's book in *History of the Human Sciences*. To the extent nonetheless that my main aim or prime concern in this chapter is with trends and transformations in *sleep science and sleep medicine in the twentieth and early twenty-first centuries* it is not necessary to buy wholesale into this broader historical thesis, however productive or provocative it may be. See also previous chapters, particularly Chapter 4, of this book for further historical detail on both the public and private life of sleep and dreams prior to and beyond the modern-day sleep laboratory or sleep clinic.

3. Kleitman's *Sleep and Wakefulness*, moreover, first published in 1939, rapidly established itself as a key reference and authoritative text, covering pretty much everything published on sleep in the field of what subsequently was to become sleep science and sleep medicine.

4. A growing emphasis on the *brain*, as this suggests, is characteristic of these trends and transitions in sleep science over time. Hobson (1995), for example, tellingly captures and conveys this by rephrasing Abraham Lincoln's famous declaration about government. Sleep, Hobson states, is 'of the brain, by the brain and for the brain'. This, he hastens to add, is not to say that other parts of the body do not participate in or benefit from sleep. It is to emphasise nonetheless, he insists, 'that for sleep to occur a highly developed brain is necessary' (Ibid.: 3).

5. Polysomnography involves comprehensive biophysical recordings during sleep, including brain activity (EEG), eye movements (EOG),

muscle activation (EMG) and heart rhythms (ECG). The Multiple Sleep Latency Test (MSLT), in contrast, measures the time taken from the start of daytime naps to the onset of sleep, known as sleep latency, based on the assumption that the sleepier the person is and the heavier their 'sleep load' the shorter the period before sleep onset – with 0–5 minutes rated as 'severe' sleepiness and 15–20 minutes rated as 'excellent alertness' (see, for example, Carskadon and Dement 1977, and Dement 1999).

6. A 'European Insomnia Network' has recently been launched, given these ongoing problems, involving more than 100 researchers and clinicians from 23 countries with the aim to 'accelerate progress in our understanding of the neuroscience of this debilitating condition' and to promote the development of 'better models and pharmacological treatments for insomnia' (Van Somersen et al. 2009: 436). The Royal Society of Medicine, Sleep Medicine Section, also recently organised a day-long meeting in London on 'Insomnia: advances in aetiology and treatment' (17 February 2010), covering a range of topics such as the 'Neurobiology of arousal: relevance to insomnia' (Szabadi); 'Differential diagnosis of insomnia' (Idzikowski); 'Drug treatment of insomnia' (Nutt); 'CBT treatment of insomnia' (Flemming); 'Insomnia in depression' (Wilson); and the 'Influence of gender and socio-economic factors on sleep disturbance' (Arber) (www.rsm.ac.uk/sleep).

7. To the extent nonetheless that biomedicine still remains at the 'definitional centre' or 'core' of these processes (cf. Conrad 2007, 2005) in terms of the official certification or validation of any new bona fide 'disorder', then clearly these claims as to the constitutive or configurational power of popular culture in the making or shaping of a disorder cannot be pushed too far, without important qualifications at least.

8. It is for these very reasons indeed, despite Conrad's (2007) continuing preference for the more limited or specific notion of 'medicalisation', that I use the more extensive technoscientific term 'biomedicalisation' in the remainder of this chapter.

9. Chesire's (2008) own particular response to this question, however, is somewhat equivocal. 'Limited forms of pharmacological enhancement may be beneficial to the practice of medicine,' he notes. When 'pushed to the extreme', however, he continues, 'cognitive enhancement...is likely to be counterproductive. Undue emphasis on the instrumental aspect of medicine would potentially neglect other important aspects of medical professionalism such as striving for humility, compassion, altruism, interpersonal communication, and human wisdom that are always needed at the patient's bedside' (Ibid.: 598).

10. Pharmaceuticalisation in this sense denotes the transformation of human conditions or complaints, capacities or capabilities into opportunities for pharmaceutical intervention. It is, as such, a more specific term than biomedicalisation, which directs attention to the growing power and influence of the pharmaceutical industry in particular in these processes at both the macro (e.g. development, testing, regulation) and micro (e.g. doctor–patient, everyday life) levels of analysis. See, for example, Williams et al. (2011) for a comprehensive analytical framework for the various dimensions and dynamics of pharmaceuticalisation.

11. The emphasis on *may* here is worth explaining further, given that these are far from simple or straightforward matters or possibilities. Rose, for example, is careful to speak of the 'layering' of these more neurochemical or biosocial ways of knowing, understanding and acting on ourselves onto 'other older senses of the self' rather than their displacement or replacement (2007: 222). Yet resistance or rejection is also of course possible, not least when it comes to thinking of ourselves in neurobiological or neurochemical terms. To the extent moreover, as Rose himself notes, that 'different practices and locales embody and enjoin different senses of the self' (2007: 222), then this further underlines the complexities of any such processes of identification or *subjectification* and the need for more fine-grained context-specific empirical studies to tease out these problems and possibilities. See also Lock (2008) for a recent cautionary tale of the limits of 'biosociality' in relation to susceptibility genes for Alzheimer's disease (AD), and other essays on 'biosocialities' in this edited volume by Gibbon and Novas (2008).

12. Some of the most staggering growth here in the US sleep aids market has occurred in the 'sleep laboratories and annexed services' group of products, with revenues of US $2.2 billion in 2000 and a predicted growth of almost 160 per cent to US $5.8 billion until 2012 (Alexander 2009). The product that most tellingly increased sales in this time period, however, was CPAP devices, with a predicted growth until 2012 of 650 per cent from US $600,000 in 2000 to US $4.1 billion (Alexander 2009) – see also Reichen (2009).

13. For a useful recent review of the sociology of the future as a newly emergent sub-field of inquiry, see, for example, Selin (2008). See also Brown and Michael (2003) on the constitutive role of expectations in the mobilisation of various technoscientific futures, including the 'retrospecting of prospects' and the 'prospecting of retrospects'.

14. See also Winterton's (2000) short essay, 'Disappearance, I', in which sleep, in dystopian fashion, becomes illegal.

Afterword: In Search of Sleep ... Or ... The Politics of Sleep Revisited

To speak of sleep, let alone write about the politics of sleep, is a far from simple or straightforward matter, as the foregoing chapters attest. An amorphous, mutating phenomenon within a dynamic field of investments, sleep, as we have seen, is located at the intersection of material-corporeal questions concerning the regulation and governance of bodies and cultural questions concerning meaning and discourse. The site and source of multiple anxieties and aspirations, desires and dilemmas, hopes and fears, facts and fictions, fantasies and projections, which converge, conflict or coalesce in a multitude of forms or fashions. Sleep, as I have argued, doubles as both a *problem* or matter of concern in its own right and a *prism* or *point of articulation* if not *amplification* for a range of other concerns and anxieties, not least our increasingly vexed or troubled relationship to *time* (i.e. time compression, time paucity, time poverty or time scarcity) and the proliferation of doubts, risks and uncertainties associated with life and living in the late modern age.

Tracing or tracking sleep therefore involves its own challenges and complexities as to the very way, or perhaps more correctly the very ways, for they are multiple, sleep comes to be problematised and *politicised*. On the one hand, as we have seen, the politicisation of sleep remains partial, problematic and incomplete if not inchoate and inconsequential. Something that is to say which defies explicit or full-blown politicisation, given that it stubbornly remains a blank or void in all our lives. Consciousness-raising or rallying about an absence or loss of consciousness in this respect, as previously noted, is more than simply a semantic conundrum. Even the biomedicalisation of sleep, on closer inspection, is a far from simple or straightforward process, with many complexities and contradictions. While we all indeed sleep well, poorly or somewhere in-between, the translation or transformation of this seemingly most 'personal' or 'private' of matters into a 'political' matter or matter of 'concern' continues to pose problems for those with any such ambitions in mind.

Yet sleep, as we have also seen, is *always already* indeed a political matter that by all accounts is becoming *ever more politicised* in recent times as a matter of 'concern' or a 'problem in the making' (cf. Wolf-Meyer 2008). From the bedroom to the boardroom, the laboratory to the sidewalk, the clinic to the courtroom, the classroom to the care home, the neighbourhood to the military barracks or battlefield, the prison to the formal corridors of political power, one may point to a variety of ways, places and spaces in which sleep has become or is fast becoming *politicised*.

As to the form or sort of politics at stake here, much of this, on closer inspection, turns out to be biopolitical in character. 'Vital' matters, that is to say, to do with the governance of sleep(iness/lessness), including the very ways in which sleep in all its multiplicity and mutability comes to be known, deciphered, documented, detailed, discussed, debated, disciplined, deployed and distributed in time and space. Like all other aspect of the body indeed, sleep becomes something to monitor, to manage, to work at, to invest in or to improve upon – in the name of productivity, performance, vigilance, virtue, health, happiness, safety, wisdom and well-being or whatever – as active, accountable, responsible citizens and 'enterprising selves' in these neo-liberal or late modern times of ours (cf. Maasen and Sutter 2007; Rose 1996). When sleepiness, for example, becomes transformed into an 'adverse' or 'at-risk' soporific state and a morally culpable or blameworthy corporeal condition (cf. Kroll-Smith and Gunter 2005), when a seemingly 'priva-tised' act like napping becomes transformed into a 'produc-tive' act and a regulated public time-space behaviour as a boost to productivity and performance both inside and out-side the workplace (cf. Baxter and Kroll-Smith 2005), when medico-managerial agendas converge or coalesce around the governance of alert/sleepy or sleeping bodies and the quest for self-improvement (cf. Brown 2004), and when sleep itself becomes a vital 'commodity' or form of 'capi-tal' to be colonised, cultivated, customised or converted into other forms of capital, then we may indeed speak of the biopolitics of sleep. In these and countless other ways, moreover, we glimpse once again the more or less continu-ous nature of contemporary forms of 'control' which quite literally get inside us or under the skin. Sleep, in other words, becomes another prime case or instance not sim-ply of the (self-) governance of bodies but of the more or less subtle and pervasive (extra-institutional) workings of contemporary late capitalist 'control' societies (cf. Deleuze 1995).

As I write this Afterword, for example, a young man, about 18 or 21 years of age perhaps, has just come into the cafe to buy a coffee with his girlfriend wearing a T-shirt (manufac-tured by the 'Obscene 18 Clothing' company according to the tag) which has emblazoned on it for all and sundry to see the following eye-catching statement: 'Damn right I'm good in bed: I can sleep for days'! Now clearly one shouldn't make too much of this. It does nonetheless, in part at least, illustrate perfectly not simply the playful relations between sleep and sex, or even the suggestion that sleep is the 'new' sex if not 'better' than sex, but the transformation of sleep – even when cast or construed if not championed in this case as an unproductive or non-productive act – into yet another opportunity for commercial or corporate capture or exploitation in words and deeds, which people wittingly or unwittingly, willingly or unwillingly, participate or 'buy into' in late capitalist 'control' societies in the name of 'freedom', 'flexibility' or just plain 'fun'.

Yet sleep of course, at one and the same time, is clearly not just another prime instance or example of the governance of bodies per se, but the governance of *(un)consciousness* in all its richness, complexities and contradictions. It is indeed in this very sense that I refer to sleep as an *absent presence* or *intimate other*, something which both *confirms* and *challenges*, *underwrites* and *undermines* our investments in the conscious waking world and the associated modernist dreams or desires of rational containment and control. Here we return then once again to the tensions, productive or problematic, between the *rationalisation*, *colonisation* or *control of sleep* on the one hand, and sleep as something that *befuddles*, *defies*, *exceeds* or *resists total rationalisation*, *colonisation* or *control* on the other hand. A potential site or source of corporeal protest or critique perhaps, or a powerful or potent reminder at least of our corporeal 'limits', themselves of course contested matters, in a rapidly escalating if not excessive, insatiable if not insane world which, to all intents and purposes, never stops.

Viewed in this light then, sleep may very well be regarded as a *final frontier* of sorts, if not *the* final frontier, in the history of humanity or corporeality. To the extent moreover that advances in bioscience, biomedicine and biotechnology, as a 'leading edge' of these developments, promise to further unravel the mysteries of sleep in the decades to come then this, potentially at least, opens up further opportunities not simply to defend or champion sleep through sleep-positive agendas in the 'wired awake' world, but to render it increasingly optional in the age or era of enhancement. A scenario, to be clear, where sleep will never doubtless be done away with altogether (i.e. rendered obsolete, redundant, a relic of the evolutionary past), given the pleasure, sanctuary or salvation it provides for many of us vital and valued 'time out', but where our powers to control and customisation sleep as lifestyle options or choices will in all likelihood grow courtesy of drugs and devices of kinds, some of which are already with us.

Struggles around sleep *rights* then, as this suggests, look set not simply to continue but to escalate or intensify in the near or not-too-distant future. This, moreover, if the foregoing enhancement or optimisation scenarios materialise or take off, will in all likelihood have to include a growing defence or respect for people's *rights not to sleep* on a temporary or even a (quasi-) permanent basis, or at the very least to reduce their sleep need well beyond what is currently deemed either advisable or possible. To the extent furthermore that this was done for good reason – in order, say, to be free of a sleep disorder, to minimise risks in safety-critical occupations, or to maximise time to do other socially or personally valued things in life for which people derived much pleasure or satisfaction – and to the extent that this proved safe for both individuals and society alike, then on what possible grounds, it might be ventured, could we or should we object?

It is not my intention to arbitrate in these debates, or to take a normative stance in these matters, simply to note them as possible trends and tricky questions for the future regarding the sleep-society nexus and the politics or biopolitics of sleep. The proviso nonetheless that any such an 'option' proved safe and was indeed the product of 'free choice' rather than coercion of various kinds, is clearly important to bear in mind and ensure in any and all such future trends or transformations.

It also behoves us to ask, of course, in a more reflexive vein, what role the social sciences and humanities themselves play in these very discourses and debates regarding sleep and society, past, present and future. To the extent indeed that sleep is becoming ever more problematised or politicised in contemporary times, and to the extent that social scientists (myself and this book included), are part and parcel of these developments, discourses and debates, then we may justifiably refer to the co-construction or co-production of the very problems, prospects and possibilities we seek to study. This includes the rehearsal or projection of various possible futures, of the kind sketched in the book, concerning the 'well-slept' or the 'sleepless' society.

Herein then, to conclude, lies a further important dimension and dynamic to the politics of sleep and the role of the social sciences and humanities in these very agendas, positive or negative, critical or reflexive, if not radical. A problem very much 'in the making', to repeat, both inside and outside the academy, the sleep laboratory, the sleep clinic, the school, the workplace, the military camp or barracks, including struggles over futures past, futures present, futures yet to come. In these and countless other ways, to restate the central message of this book one last time, sleep is not simply *political* through and through but increasingly *politicised* in the late modern age or era.

References

Abraham, J.W. (2009) Sociology of pharmaceuticals development and regulation: a realist empirical research programmed, in S.J. Williams, J. Gabe and P.B. Davis (eds) *Pharmaceuticals and Society: Critical Discourses and Debates.* Oxford: Wiley-Blackwell.

Abraham, J. and Davis, C. (2009) Drug evaluation and the permissive principle: continuities and contradictions between standards and practices in antidepressant clinical trial regulation. *Social Studies of Science.* 39: 569–98.

Abraham, J. and Sheppard, J. (1999) *Therapeutic Nightmare: The Battle of the Worlds most Controversial Sleeping Pill.* London: Earth Scan.

Academy of Medical Sciences (AMS) (2008) *Brain Science, Addictions and Drugs.* London: AMS.

Åckerstedt, T. (2004) Sleep – gender, age, stress, work hours, in World Health Organization, Regional Office for Europe. *Technical Meeting on Sleep and Health.* European Centre for Environment and Health, Bonn office, Germany (http://www.euro.who.int/noise/activities).

Åckerstedt, T. (1995) Work hours, sleepiness and the underlying mechanisms. *Journal of Sleep Research.* 4(Suppl. 2): 15–22.

Åckerstedt, T., Arnetz, B.B. and Anderzen. I. (1990) Physicians during and following night call duty-36 hour ambulatory recording of sleep. *EEG Clinical Neurophysiology.* 76: 193–6.

Adié, W.J. (1926) Idiopathic narcolepsy. *Brain.* 49: 257–306.

Agamben, G. (1998) *Homo Sacer: Sovereign Power and Bare Life* [Transl. by D. Heller-Rozen]. Stanford, CA: Stanford University Press.

Agger, B. (2004) *Speeding Up Fast Capitalism: Cultures, Jobs, Families, Schools, Bodies.* Boulder, CO/London: Paradigm Publishers.

Agger, B. (1989) *Fast Capitalism: A Critical Theory of Significance.* Urbana, IL: University of Illinois Press.

Alexander, J. (2009) US sleep market. *Frontiers in Neuroscience.* 3(3), December: 496–7 (www.frontiersin.org).

Alvarez, A. (1996) *Night: An Exploration of Night Life, Night Language, Sleep and Dreams.* London: Vintage.

American Academy of Sleep Medicine (AASM) (2005) *International Classification of Sleep Disorders Diagnostic and Coding Manual, Second Edition (ICSD2).* Chicago, IL: American Academy of Sleep Medicine.

American Academy of Sleep Medicine (AASM) (2001/1997) *International Classification of Sleep Disorders Diagnostic and Coding Manual, Revised (ICSD-R)*. Chicago, IL: American Academy of Sleep Medicine.

American Sleep Disorders Association – Diagnostic Classification Steering Committee, Thorpy, M.J., Chairman (1990) *International Classification of Sleep Disorders: Diagnostic and Coding Manual*. Rochester, MN: ASDA.

Amnesty (2006) Sleep deprivation is torture: Amnesty. *Sydney Morning Herald*, 3 October 2006, Available at www.smh.com.au/news/National/Sleep-deprivation-is-torture-Amnesty/2006/10/03/1159641317450.html (Accessed May 15 2009).

Annandale, E. (2009) *Women's Health and Social Change*. London: Routledge.

Anthony, C. and Anthony W.C. (2001) *The Art of Napping at Work*. London: Souvenir Press.

Anthony, W.A. (1997) *The Art of the Napping*. New York: Larson Publications.

Arber, S., Hislop, J. and Williams, S. (2007a) Editor's introduction: gender, sleep and the life course. *Sociological Research Online*. 12(5) Available at: www.socresonline.org.uk/12/5/19.html (Accessed 5 May 2009).

Arber, S., Hislop, J., Bote, M. and Meadows, R. (2007b) Gender roles and women's sleep in mid and later life: a quantitative approach. *Sociological Research Online* 12(5) Available at: www.socresonline.org.uk/12/5/3.html (Accessed 6 May 2009).

Arber, S., Bote, M. and Meadows, R. (2009) Understanding how socio-economic status, gender and marital status influence self-reported sleep problems in Britain. *Social Science and Medicine*. 68: 281–9.

Archer, J. (2002) *A Prison Diary Vol. I – Belmarsh: Hell*. London: Pan Books.

Aristotle. (2002) Nicomachean ethics, in S. Broadie and C. Rowe [Transl., Introduction and Commentary] *Aristotle: Nicomachean Ethics*. Oxford: Oxford University Press.

Armitage, J. (ed.) (2000) *Paul Virilio: From Modernism to Hypermodernism and Beyond*. London: Sage.

Artemidorus (1990) *The Interpretation of Dreams: Oneirocritica* [Transl. by R.J. White]. Torrance, CA: Original Books.

Aserinsky, E. and Kleitman, N. (1953) Regularly occurring periods of eye motility, and concomitant phenomena, during sleep. *Science*. 118 273–4.

Association of Professional Sleep Societies (APSS) (1979) *Diagnostic Classification of Sleep and Arousal Disorders*. Rochester, MN: Association of Professional Sleep Societies.

Aubert, V. and White, H. (1959a) Sleep: a sociological interpretation I. *Acta Sociologica*. 4: 1–16.

Aubert, V. and White, H. (1959b) Sleep: a sociological interpretation II. *Acta Sociologica.* 4: 46–54.

Bakhtin, M. (1968) *Rabelais and his World.* Cambridge, MA: MIT Press.

Ball, H.L., Hooker, E. and Kelly, P.J. (1999) Where will the baby sleep? Attitudes and practices of new and experienced parents regarding co-sleeping and their newborn infants. *American Anthropologist* 101(1): 143–51.

Ballard, J.G. (1992) *Disaster Area.* London: Flamingo.

Ballon, N. (2009) When the lights go out. *Guardian Weekend,* 5 December 2009, 35–44.

Barkman, P. (2008) Sleepless in SW1. *The Guardian,* 14 October 2008, Available at: www.guardian.co.uk/lifeandstyle/2008/oct/14/healthandwellbeing-labour (Accessed 14 August 2009).

Bataille, G. (1987/1962) *Eroticism* [Transl. by M. Dalwood]. London: Boyars.

Bauman, Z. (2000) *Liquid Modernity.* Cambridge: Cambridge University Press.

Bauman, Z. (1991) *Modernity and Ambivalence.* Cambridge: Polity Press.

Baxter, V. and Kroll-Smith, S. (2005) Napping at work: shifting boundaries between public and private time. *Current Sociology* 53(1): 33–55.

BBC News (2001) Police condemn sleep-deprived drivers. 13 December 2001, Available at: http://news.bbc.co.uk/1/hi/england/1708969.stm (Accessed 6 July 2009).

Beck, U. (1992) *Risk Society.* London: Sage.

Ben-Ari, E. (2008) It's bedtime in the world's urban middle classes, around the world, in L. Brunt and B. Steger (eds) *Worlds of sleep.* Berlin: Frank & Timme, pp. 175–92.

Ben-Ari, E. (2003) Sleep and night-time combat in contemporary armed forces: technology, knowledge and the enhancement of the soldier's body, in B. Steger and L. Brunt (eds) *Night-time and Sleep in Asia and the West: Exploring the Dark Side of Life.* London: Routledge Curzon.

Berger, H. (1930) Ueber das Elekroenkephalogramm des Menschen. *Journal of Psychological Neurology.* 40: 160–79.

Bianchera, E. and Arber, S. (2007) Caring and sleep disruption among women in Italy. *Sociological Research Online* 12(5): Available at: www.socresonline.org.uk/12/5/4.html (Accessed 5 May 2009).

Bianchera, E. and Arber, S. (2008) Women's sleep in Italy: the influence of caregiving roles, in L. Brunt and B. Steger (eds), *Worlds of sleep.* Berlin: Frank & Timme.

Booker, C. and North, R. (2007) *Scared to Death.* London/New York: Continuum.

Bourke, J. (2005) *Fear: A Cultural History.* London: Virago.

British Airline Pilots Association (BALPA) (2009) News: *EU Fatigue Rules Miss ICAO Standards.* Available at www.balpa.org/News-and-campaigns/News/EU-FATIGUE-RULES-MISS-ICAO-STANDARDS.aspx (Accessed 12 November 2009).

British Association of Counselling and Psychotherapy (BACP) (2005) *Insomniac Britain*. Available at www.bacp.co.uk/media/index. php?newsId=300 (Accessed 12 March 2009).

British Medical Association (BMA) (2007) *Boosting Your Brain Power: Ethical Aspects of Cognitive Enhancements*. London: BMA.

Brokaw, J., Fullertone-Gleason, L., Olson, L., Crandall, C., McLaughlin, S. and Sklar, D. (2002) Health status and intimate partner violence: a cross-sectional study. *Annals of Emergency Medicine* 39(1), January: 31–8.

Brown, M. (2004) Taking care of business: self-help and sleep medicine in American corporate culture. *Journal of Medical Humanities* 25(3): 173–87.

Brown, P. (2001) Ruling puts airport night flights in doubt: widespread action likely after European court backs Heathrow resident's right to enjoy a good night's sleep. *The Guardian* 3 October 2001: 10.

Brown, N. and Michael, M. (2003). A sociology of expectations: retrospecting prospects and prospecting retrospects. *Technology Assessment and Strategic Management* 15(1): 3–18.

Brunt, L. and Steger, B. (2008) Introduction, in L. Brunt and B. Steger (eds) *Worlds of Sleep*. Berlin: Frank & Timme.

de Bruxelles, S. (2009) Man with rare sleep illness who killed his wife of 40 years during nightmare is declared innocent. *The Times* 21 November 2009: 10.

Bull, M. (2007) Vectors of the biopolitical. *New Left Review* 45, May–June: 1–12.

Burwell, C.S., Robin, E.D., Whaley, R.D. and Bickelman, A.G. (1956) Extreme obesity associated with alveolar hypoventilation: a Pickwickian syndrome. *American Journal of Medicine* 21(5): 811–18.

Buysee, D.J. (2001/1997) Foreword to the revised edition. *The International Classification of Sleep Disorders, Revised (ICSD-R)*. Chicago, IL: American Academy of Sleep Medicine.

Camp, C.D. (1907) Morbid sleepiness, with a report of a case of narcolepsy and a review of recent theories of sleep. *Journal of Nervous and Mental Disease*. 2: 9–21.

Campbell, D. (2010) The binge working culture is taking its toll. *The Observer*. 16 May 2010, 37.

Cappuccio, F., D'Elia, L., Strazzulo, P. and Miller, M.A. (2010) Sleep duration and all-cause mortality: a systematic review and meta-analysis of prospective studies. *Sleep* 33(5): 585–92.

Carskadon, M.A. and Dement, W.C. (1977) Sleep tendency: an objective measure of sleep loss. *Sleep Research*. 6: 200.

Cartwright, R. (2009) Drowsy society. *Frontiers in Neuroscience* 3(3), December: 466–7 (www.frontiersin.org).

Cartwright, R. (2008) Sleeping together: a pilot study of the effects of shared sleeping on adherence to CPAP treatment in obstructive sleep apnea. *Journal of Clinical Sleep Medicine.* 4: 123–7.

Castells, M. (2000/1996) *The Rise of the Network Society (Second Edition).* Oxford: Blackwell Publishing.

Castoriadis, C. (2003) *The Rising Tide of Insignificancy (The Big Sleep).* Available online at www.notbored.org/RTI.pdf (Accessed 30 August 2009).

Castoriadis, C. (1997) *World in Fragments: Writings on Politics, Society and Psychoanalysis.* Stanford, CA: Stanford University Press.

Caudhill, W. and Plath, D.L. (1986) Who sleeps by whom? Parent-child involvement in urban Japanese families, in T.S. Lebra and W.P. Lebra (eds) *Japanese Culture and Behavior: Selected Readings* (2nd edition). Honolulu, HI: University of Hawaii Press.

de Cervantes, M. (2003/1604–5) *Don Quixote.* London: Penguin Classics.

Chadwick, E. (1997/1842) *Report on the Sanitary Conditions of the Labouring Population of Great Britain* (With a new introduction by D. Gladstone). London: Routledge/Thoemmes Press.

Chatterjee, A. (2006) The promise and predicament of cosmetic neurology. *Journal of Medical Ethics* 32(2): 110–13.

Chatterjee, A. (2004a) Cosmetic neurology: the controversy over enhancing movement, mentation and mood. *Neurology* 63(6): 968–74.

Chatterjee, A. (2004b) Cosmetic neurology: for physicians the future is now. *Virtual Mentor: American Medical Association Journal of Ethics* 6(8): 1–4.

Chatzitheochari, S. and Arber, S. (2009) Lack of sleep, work and the long hours culture: evidence from the UK Time Use Survey. *Work, Employment and Society.* 23: 30–48.

Chesire, W.P. Jr (2008) The pharmaceutically enhanced physician. *Virtual Mentor: American Medical Association Journal of Ethics* 10(9): 594–8.

Clarke, A., Mamo, L., Fishman, J.R., Shim, J.K. and Fosket, J.R. (2003) Biomedicalization: technoscientific transformations of the health, illness and US biomedicine. *American Sociological Review* 68(April): 161–94.

Coe, J. (1997) *The House of Sleep.* London: Penguin Books.

Cohen, S. (2002/1972) *Folk Devils and Moral Panics* (3rd edition). Abingdon: Routledge.

Cohen, S. and Taylor, L. (1972) *Psychological Survival: The Experience of Long-Term Imprisonment.* Harmondsworth: Penguin Books.

Coleridge, S.T. (1985) *The Major Works, Including Biographia Literaria.* Oxford: Oxford University Press.

Coleridge, S.T. (1971) *Collected Letters of Samuel Taylor Coleridge, Vol V 1820–25* (Edited by Earl Lesley Griggs). Oxford: Clarendon Press.

Connolly, W. (2002) *Neuropolitics: Thinking, Culture, Speed.* Minneapolis, MN: University of Minnesota Press.

Conrad, P. (2007) *The Medicalisation of Society: On the Transformation of Human Conditions into Treatable Disorders*. Baltimore, MD: The Johns Hopkins University Press.

Conrad, P. (2005) The shifting engines of medicalization. *Journal of Health and Social Behaviour*. 46: 3–14.

Conrad, P. (1992) Medicalization and social control. *Annual Review of Sociology*. 18: 209–32.

Conrad, P. and Potter, D. (2004) Human growth hormone and the temptations of biomedical enhancement. *Sociology of Health and Illness* 26(2): 184–215.

Conrad, P., Mackie, T. and Mehrotra, A. (2010) Estimating the costs of medicalization. *Social Science and Medicine*. 70: 1943–7.

Cooley, C.H. (1902) *Human Nature and the Social Order* [revised edition 1922]. New York: Charles Scribner's Sons.

Cooter, R., Harrison, M. and Sturdy, S. (eds) (1998) *War, Medicine and Modernity*. Gloucestershire: Sutton Publishing Limited.

Coren, S. (1996) *Sleep Thieves*. New York/London: The Free Press.

Cosnett, J. (1997) Charles Dickens and sleep disorders. *Dickensian* 93(3): 200–04.

Coveney, C., Nerlich, B. and Martin, P. (2009) Modafinil in the media: medicalisation, metaphors and the body. *Social Science and Medicine*. 68: 487–95.

Cox, R.S. (2008) The suburbs of eternity: on visionaries and miraculous sleepers, in L. Brunt and B. Steger (eds) *Worlds of Sleep*. Berlin: Frank & Timme.

Cramer Bornemann, M.A. (2008) The role of the expert witness in sleep-related violence trials. *Virtual Mentor: American Medical Association Journal of Ethics* 10(9): 571–7.

Crawford, R. (1977) 'You are dangerous to your health': the ideology and politics of victim blaming. *International Journal of Health Services* 7 (4): 663–80.

Crook, T. (2008) Norms, forms and beds: spatializing sleep in Victorian Britain. *Body & Society* 14(4), December: 15–36.

Crossley, N. (2004) *Sleep, Reflexive Embodiment and Social Networks*. Paper presented at the first ESRC 'Sleep and Society' seminar, 3 December 2004, University of Warwick, UK.

Cruddass, J. and Gannon, Z. (2009) *A Bitter Pill to Swallow: Drugs for People not Just for Profit*. London: Compass. Available at www.clients.square-eye.com/uploads/compass/documents/compass%20bitter%20pill%20 WEB%20(2).pdf (Accessed 5 January 2010).

Dannenfeldt, K.H. (1986) Sleep: theory and practice in the late Renaissance. *The Journal of the History of Medicine and Allied Sciences*. 41: 415–41.

Davenport-Hines, R. (1998) *Gothic: Four Hundred Years of Excess, Horror and Ruin*. London: Fourth Estate.

Deleuze, G. (1995) Postscript on control societies. *Negotiations*. New York: Columbia University Press.

Dement, W.C. (2000) History of sleep physiology and medicine, in M.H. Kryger, T. Roth and W.C. Dement (eds) *Principles and Practice of Sleep Medicine* (3rd edition). Philadelphia, PA/London: W.B. Saunders Company.

Dement, W.C. (with Vaughan, C.) (1999) *The Promise of Sleep: The Scientific Connection Between Health, Happiness, and a Good Night's Sleep*. London: Macmillan.

Dement, W.C. (1993) The history of narcolepsy and other sleep disorders. *Journal of the History the Neurosciences*. 2: 121–34.

Dement, W.C. and Kleitman, N. (1957) Cyclic variations in EEG during sleep and their relation to eye movements, body motility and dreaming. *EEG Clinical Neurophysiology*. 9: 673–90.

Department of Health (DoH) (2008) *Prescription Cost Analysis, England 2007*. London: Government Statistical Service.

Descartes, R. (1996/1641) *Meditations on First Philosophy with Selections from Objections and Replies* (Ed. by J. Cottingham), Revised edition. Cambridge: Cambridge University Press.

Dickens, C. (1909/1836–7) *The Posthumous Papers of the Pickwick Club*. Volume 2. London: Chapman and Hall.

Dickens, P. (2000) *Social Darwinism*. Buckingham: Open University Press.

Diderot, D. (1965/1751–72) *The Encyclopedia: Selections [by] Diderot and d'Alembert [and] a Society of Men of Letter*. [Transl. with an introduction and notes by N. Hoyt and T. Cassirer]. Indianapolis, IN: Bobbs-Merrill.

Douglas, M. (1992) *Risk and Blame: Essays in Cultural Theory*. London: Routledge.

Douglas, M. (1970) *Natural Symbols: Explorations in Cosmology*. London: The Cresset Press.

Douglas, M. and Wildavsky, A. (1983) *Risk and Culture: An Essay on the Selection of Technological and Environmental Dangers*. Berkeley, CA: University of California Press.

Duneier, M. (2000) *Sidewalk*. New York: Farrar, Straus and Giroux.

Economo, C. von (1931) *Encephalitis Lethargica: It's Sequelae and Treatment*. Oxford: Oxford University Press.

von Economo, C. (1930) Sleep as a problem of localisation. *Journal of Nervous Mental Disease*. 71: 249–59.

von Economo, C. (1928) Theorie du sommeil. *Journal of Neurology, Neurosurgery & Psychiatry*. 28: 437–64.

Ekirch, R. (2005) *A Day's Close; Night in Times Past*. New York: W.W Norton.

Ekirch, R. (2001) The sleep we have lost: pre-industrial slumber in the British Isles. *American Historical Review* 106: 343–86.

Elias, N. (1978/1939) *The Civilizing Process Vol. 1: The History of Manners.* Oxford: Basil Blackwell.

Elliott, J. (1979) Medical news: Physicians prescribing practices criticized: Solutions in question. *Journal of the American Medical Association* 241(22), 1 June 1979: 2353–4, 2359–60.

Engleman, H.M. and Wild, M.R. (2003) Improving CPAP use by patients with the sleep apnoea/hypopnoea syndrome (SAHS). *Sleep* 23 (Suppl. 4): S102–08.

Engels, F. (1999/1845) *The Conditions of the Working Class in England* [Ed. with an introduction and notes by D. McLellan]. Oxford: Oxford University Press.

Epstein, R., Chillag, N. and Lavie, P. (1998) Starting times of school: effects on day-time functioning of fifth-grade children. *Sleep.* 21: 250–6.

European Court of Human Rights (2001) *Case of Hatton and Others vs. the United Kingdom.* 2 October, Strasbourg. [GC] No. 36022/97. Available at: www.echr.coe.int/eng/Press/2001/Oct/Hattonjudepress.htm   (Accessed 21 May 2009).

Falk, P. (1994) *The Consuming Body.* London: Sage.

Fitzgerald, M. and Sim, J. (1979) *British Prisons.* Oxford: Basil Blackwell.

Flanagan, O. (2000) *Dreaming Souls: Sleep, Dreams and the Evolution of the Conscious Mind.* Oxford: Oxford University Press.

Ford, J. (2004) Samuel Taylor Coleridge and 'The pains of sleep', in D. Pick and L. Roper (eds) *Dreams and History: The Interpretation of Dreams from Ancient Greece to Modern Psychoanalysis.* London and New York: Brunner-Routledge.

Foucault, M. (1991) Governmentality, in G. Burchell, C. Gordon and P. Miller (eds) *The Foucault Effect: Studies in Governmentality with Two Lectures by and an Interview with Michel Foucault.* Chicago, IL: University of Chicago Press.

Foucault, M. (1988) Technologies of the self, in L.H. Martin, H. Gutman and P.H. Hutton (eds) *Technologies of the Self: A Seminar with Michel Foucault.* London: Tavistock.

Foucault, M. (1979) *Discipline and Punish: The Birth of the Prison.* London: Tavistock.

Foulkes, W.D. (1996) Dream research 1953–1993. *Sleep.* 19: 609–24.

Foulkes, W.D. (1966) *The Psychology of Sleep.* New York: Scribner's.

Franklin, B. (1855) *Early to Bed and Early to Rise Makes Man Healthy, Wealthy and Wise, or Early Rising: A Natural Social and Religious Duty.* London: Nisbett and Co. Available as pdf document at www.books.google.com (Accessed 5 July 2009).

Freeman, F.R., Agnew, H.W. and Williams, R.L. (1965) An electroencephalographic study of the effects of meprobamate on human sleep. *Clinical Pharmacology and Therapeutics*. 6: 172–6.

Freud (1985/1930) Civilisation and its discontents, in A. Richards (ed.) *Civilisation, Society and Religion: Group Psychology, Civilisation and its Discontents and Other Works, Pelican Freud Library, Vol. 12.* Harmondsworth: Pelican.

Freud, S. (1984/1920) Beyond the pleasure principle, in A. Richards (ed.) *On Metapsychology: The Theory of Psychoanalysis, Pelican Freud Library, Vol. 11.* Harmondsworth: Pelican.

Freud, S. (1976/1900) The interpretation of dreams, in A. Richards (ed.) *The Interpretation of Dreams, Pelican Freud Library, Vol. 4.* Harmondsworth: Pelican.

Frenette, E. (2008) Presenting in the absence of medical need. *Virtual Mentor: American Medical Association Journal of Ethics* 10(9): 544–7.

Fuller, S. (2006) *The New Sociological Imagination*. London: Sage.

Furedi, F. (2005) *Culture of Fear: Risk-Taking and the Morality of Low Expectation* (Revised Edition). London/New York: Continuum.

Furedi, F. (2002) *Paranoid Parenting: Why Ignoring the Experts May Be Best for Your Child*. Chicago, IL: Chicago Review Press, Inc.

Furman, Y., Wolf, S.M. and Rosenfeld, D.S. (1997) Shakespeare and sleep disorders. *Neurology*. 49: 1171–2.

Gabe, J. and Bury, M. (1996) Halcion nights: a sociological account of a medical controversy. *Sociology*. 45(1): 447–69.

Galloway, J.W. (1977) On Johnstone's 'phenomenology of death' and 'philosophy of sleep'. *Philosophy and Phenomenology*. 38(1): 107–13.

Gélineau, J.B.E. (1880) De la narcolepsie. *Lancette Française, Gazette de Hospitaux*. 53: 626–37.

George, C.F.P. (2007) Sleep apnea, alertness and motor vehicle crashes. *American Journal of Respiratory Critical Care Medicine*. 176(10): 954–6.

Gershuny, J. (2005) 'Busyness as the badge of honour for the new superordinate working class', *Social Research*. 72(2): 287–314.

Gibbon, S. and Novas, C. (eds) (2008) *Biosocialities, Genetics and the Social Sciences: Making Biologies and Identities*. London: Routledge.

Giddens, A. (1991) *Modernity and Self-Identity*. Cambridge: Polity Press.

Gleichman, P.R. (1980) Einige soziale Wandlungen de Schlafens. *Zeitschrift fur Soziologie*. 9(3): 236–50.

Gleick, J. (2000) *Faster: The Acceleration of Just About Everything*. London: Abacus.

Goffman, E. (1963) *Behaviour in Public Places*. London: Allen Lane.

Goffman, E. (1961) *Asylums: Essays on the Social Situation of Mental Patients and Other Inmates*. Harmondsworth: Penguin.

Goodin, R.E., Rice, J.M., Parpo, A. and Eriksson, L. (2008) *Discretionary Time: A New Measure of Freedom*. Cambridge: Cambridge University Press.

Goodstein, E. (2005) *Experience without Qualities: Boredom and Modernity*. Stanford, CA: Stanford University Press.

Gray, C.H. (2000) *Cyborg Citizen: Politics in the Posthuman Age*. New York: Routledge.

Greely, H., Sahakian, B., Harris, J., Kessler, R.C., Gazzaniga, M., Campbell, P. and Farah, M.J. (2008) Towards responsible use of cognitive-enhancing drugs by the healthy. *Nature*. 456, 10 December 2008: 702–5.

Green, F. (2001) 'It's been a hard day's night: the concentration and intensification of work in late twentieth-century Britain', *British Journal of Industrial Relations* 39(1): 53–80.

Gubrium, J.F. (1975) *Living and Dying at Murray Manor*. New York and London: St Martin's Press/St James Press.

Gubrium, J.F. and Holstein, J.A. (1999) The nursing home as a discursive anchor for the ageing body. *Ageing and Society*. 19: 519–38.

Guilleminault, C., Eldridge, F.L. and Dement, W.C. (1973) Insomnia and sleep apnea: a new syndrome. *Science*. 181: 856–8.

Hackett, E.J., Amsterdamska, O., Lynch, M. and Wajcman, J. (eds) (2007) *The Handbook of Science and Technology Studies (Third Edition)*. Cambridge, MA: The MIT Press.

Hale, B. and Hale, L. (2009a) Is justice good for your sleep? (And therefore good for your health?). *Social Theory and Health*. 7: 354–70.

Hale, B. and Hale, L. (2009b) Choosing to sleep, in, A. Dawson (ed.) *The Philosophy of Public Health*. Surrey: Ashgate.

Hale, L. (2005) Who has time to sleep? *Journal of Public Health*. 27(2): 205–11.

Hale, L. and Do, D.P. (2007) Racial differences in self-report of sleep duration in a population-based study. *Sleep*. 30 (9): 1092–9.

Hardt, A. and Negri, (2000) *Empire*. Cambridge, MA: Harvard University Press.

Hardy, R. (2009) In my dreams, she forgives me. *Daily Mail*. Monday, 23 November 2009: 22–3.

Hancock, P., Williams, S.J. and Boden, S. (2009) Managing sleep?: The colonization of everyday/night life, in P. Hancock and M. Tyler (eds) *The Management of Everyday Life*. Basingstoke: Palgrave Macmillan.

Hanlon, M. (2009) Nightmares of the unconscious mind. *Daily Mail*. Saturday 21st November: 31.

Haraway, D. (1990) *Simians, Cyborgs and Women*. London: Free Association Books.

Harris, J. (2007) *Enhancing Evolution: The Ethical Case for Making Better People*. Princeton, NJ: Princeton University Press.

Harrison, M. (1999) Medicine and the management of modern warfare, in S. Cooter, M. Harrison and S. Sturdy (eds) *Medicine and Modern Warfare*. Amsterdam: Rodolfi.

Harrison, M. (1996) The medicalisation of war and the militarisation of medicine. *Social History of Medicine*. 9: 267–76.

Hathaway, J.E., Lorelie, A.M., Silverman, J.G., Brooks, D.R., Mathews, R. and Pavlos, C.A. (2000) Health status and health care of Massachusetts women reporting partner abuse. *American Journal of Preventive Medicine*. 19(4): 30207.

Hartman, E. (1979) *The Sleeping Pill*. New Haven, CT/London: Yale University Press.

Harvey, D. (1989) *The Condition of Postmodernity*. Oxford: Blackwell.

Hayward, R. (2004) Policing dreams: history and moral uses of the unconscious, in D. Pick and L. Roper (eds) *Dreams and History: The Interpretation of Dreams from Ancient Greece to Modern Psychoanalysis*. London and New York: Brunner-Routledge.

Hearne, K. (1990) *The Dream Machine*. Wellingborough: Aquarian Press.

Henry, D., McClellen, D., Rosenthal, L., Dedrick, D. and Gosdin, M. (2008) Is sleep really for sissies? Understanding the role of work in insomnia in the US. *Social Science and Medicine*. 66: 715–26.

Hervey de Saint-Denys, L. (1982/1867) *Dreams and How to Guide Them* [Transl. by N. Fry]. London: Duckworth.

Higgs, P. (1998) Risk, governmentality and the reconceptualisation of citizenship, in G. Scambler and P. Higgs (eds) *Modernity Medicine and Health: Medical Sociology Toward 2000*. London: Routledge.

Hinsliff, G. (2004) Stress becomes the No. 1 complain of British workers. *The Observer*. 31 October 2004: 9.

Hislop, J. (2007) A bed of roses or a bed of thorns? Negotiating the couple relationship through sleep. *Sociological Research Online*. 12(5). Available at: www.socresonline.org.uk/12/5/2.html (Accessed 1 June 2010).

Hislop, J. and Arber, S. (2003a) Sleepers wake! The gendered nature of sleep disruption among mid-life women. *Sociology*. 37: 695–711.

Hislop, J. and Arber, S. (2003b) Understanding women's sleep management: beyond medicalization-healthicization? *Sociology of Health and Illness*. 26: 815–37.

Hobson, J.A. (2002) *Dreaming: An Introduction to the Science of Sleep*. Oxford: Oxford University Press.

Hobson, J.A. (1995) *Sleep*. New York: Scientific American Library.

Hobson, J.A. and McCarley, R. (1977) The brain as a dream state generator: an activation-synthesis hypothesis of the dream process. *American Journal of Psychiatry*. 134: 1335–48.

Hobson, J.A., Pace-Shott, E.F. and Stickgold, R. (2000) Dreaming and the brain: towards a cognitive neuroscience of conscious states. *Behavioral and Brain Sciences*. 23: 793–842.

Hobson, J.A., McCarley, R. and Wyzinski, P. (1975) Sleep-cycle oscillation: reciprocal discharge by two brainstem neuronal groups. *Science*. 189: 55–8.

Hochschild, A.R. (1997) *The Time Bind: When Work Becomes Home and Home Becomes Work*. New York: Metropolitan Press.

Hochschild, A.R. (with A. Machung) (1990) *The Second Shift: Working Parents and the Revolution at Home*. London: Piatkus.

Hoffman, E. (2009) *Time*. London: Profile Books.

Holdbrook, A.M. (2004) Treating insomnia: use of drugs is rising despite evidence of harm and little meaningful benefit. *British Medical Journal*. 329, 20 November 2004: 1198–9.

Honoré, C. (2004) *In Praise of Slowness: How a World Wide Movement is Challenging the Cult of Speed*. London: Orion Books.

Horne, J. (2006) *Sleepfaring*. Oxford: Oxford University Press.

House, J. (2009) Calling time on doctors' working hours. *The Lancet*. 373(9680), 13 June 2009: 2011–12.

House of Commons Health Committee (2005) *The Influence of the Pharmaceutical Industry* (Fourth Report for Session 2004–5) London: The Stationary Office Ltd.

Humphreys, C., Lowe, P. and Williams, S.J. (2009) Sleep disruption and domestic violence: exploring the interconnections between mothers and children. *Child and Family Social Work*. 14: 6–14.

Humpheys, J.C. and Lee, K.A. (2006) Sleep of children of abused women in transitional housing. *Pediatric Nursing*. 32(4), July–August: 311–16.

Humphreys, J. and Lee, K. (2005) Sleep disturbance in battered women living in transitional housing. *Issues in Mental Health Nursing*. 26(7): 771–80.

Humphreys, J.C., Lee, K.A. Naylen, T.C. and Marmer, C.R. (1999) Sleep patterns of sheltered battered women. *Journal of Nursing Scholarship*. 31(2): 139–43.

Hunt, A. (1998) The great masturbation panic and discourses of moral regulation in nineteenth and early-twentieth century Britain. *Journal of the History of Sexuality*. 8(4): 575–615.

Institute of Medicine (IoM) (1979) *Sleeping Pills, Insomnia and Medical Practice*. Washington, DC: National Academy of Sciences.

International Dark Sky Association (no data) 'Vision statement'. Available at www.darksky.org (Accessed 6 December 2009).

Jefferies, S. (2009) Night terrors. *Guardian (weekend)*, 5 December 2009: 35–45.

Johns, M.W. (1991) A new method for measuring daytime sleepiness: the Epworth Sleepiness Scale. *Sleep*. 14: 540–5.

Johnstone Jr, H.W. (1973) Toward a philosophy of sleep. *Philosophy and Phenomenological Research*. 34(1): 73–81.

Jouvet, M. (1965) Paradoxical sleep: a study of its nature and its mechanism. *Progress in Brain Research*. 18: 20–57.

Jouvet, M. and Mounier, D. (1960) Effects des lesions de la formation reticular pontique sur le sommeil du chat. *Comptes Rendus des Séances de la Société de Biologie*. 154: 2301–05.

Jouvet, M., Michel, F. and Courjon, J. (1959) Sur un stade d'activité électrique cérébale rapide au cour du sommeil physiologique. *Comptes Rendus des Séances de la Société de Biologie*. 153: 1024–28.

Kales, A. and Kales, J.D. (1970) Sleep laboratory and evaluation of psychoactive drugs. *Pharmacology for Physicians*. 4: 1–6.

Klein, N. (2007) *The Shock Doctrine: The Rise of Disaster Capitalism*. New York: Metropolitan Books.

Kleitman, N. (1939) *Sleep and Wakefulness* (Revised and enlarged edition 1963). Chicago, IL and London: University of Chicago Press.

Klinkenborg, V. (2008) Our vanishing night. *National Geographic*. November: 102–23. Also available at www.ngm.nationalgeographic.com/2008/11/light-pollution/klinkenborg-text (Accessed 29 July 2009).

Klug, G. (2008) Dangerous doze: sleep and vulnerability in medieval German literature, in L. Brunt and B. Steger (eds) *Worlds of Sleep*. Berlin: Frank & Timme, pp. 31–52.

Kodz, J., Davis, S., Lain, D., Strebler, M. and Rick, J. (2003) *Working Long Hours: A Review of the Evidence*. Employment Relations Research Series No.16. London: DTI.

Kodz, J., Kersley, B., Strebler, M.T. and O'Regan, S. (1998) *Breaking the Long Hours Culture*. Institute for Employment Studies Report 352. Brighton: IES.

Klerman, G. (1972) Psychotropic hedonism vs. pharmaceutical Calvinism. *Hastings Centre Report*. 2(4): 1–3.

Kreitzman, L. (1999) *The 24 Hour Society*. London: Profile Books.

Kress, N. (1996) *Beggars Ride*. New York: Tor.

Kress, N. (1995) *Beggars and Choosers*. New York: Tor.

Kress, N. (1993) *Beggars in Spain*. New York: EOS/Harper Collins.

Kroll-Smith, S. (2008) Modern work and the sleepy worker. *Virtual Mentor: American Medical Association Journal of Ethics*. 10(9): 589–93.

Kroll-Smith, S. (2003) Popular media and 'excessive daytime sleepiness': a study of rhetorical authority in medical sociology. *Sociology of Health & Illness*. 25(6): 625–43.

Kroll-Smith, S. (2000) The social production of the drowsy person *Perspectives on Social Problems*. 12: 89–109.

Kroll-Smith, S. and Gunter, V. (2005) Governing sleepiness: Somnolent bodies, discourse and liquid modernity. *Sociological Inquiry.* 75(3): 346–71.

Kroker, K. (2007) *The Sleep of Others.* Toronto: University of Toronto Press.

Kroker, A. and Kroker, M. (1988) *Body Invaders: Sexuality and Postmodern Culture.* Basingstoke: Macmillan.

Kroker, A., Kroker, M. and Cook, D. (1990) Hypermodernism as America's postmodernism. *Social Problems.* 37: 443–59.

Kryger, M.H., Roth, T. and Dement, W.C. (eds) (2010) *Principles and Practice of Sleep Medicine* (5th edition). Philadelphia, PA/London: W.B. Saunders Company.

Kundera, M. and Asher, L. (1996) *Slowness.* London: Faber and Faber.

La Berge, S. (1985) *Lucid Dreaming.* Los Angeles, CA: J.P. Tarcher.

La Berge, S. (1980) Lucid dreaming as a learnable skill: a case study. *Perceptual and Motor Skills.* 51: 1039–42.

La Berge, S. and Dement, W.C. (1982) Voluntary control of respiration during REM sleep. *Sleep Research.* 11: 107.

La Berge, S. and Rheingold, H. (1990) *Exploring the World of Lucid Dreaming.* New York: Ballantine.

La Berge, S., Nagel, L., Dement, W.C. and Zarcone, V. Jr. (1981) Lucid dreaming verified by volitional communication during REM sleep. *Perceptual and Motor Skills.* 52: 727–32.

Latour, B. (2008) *What is the Style of Matters of Concern?* Amsterdam: Van Gorcum.

Latour, B. (2004) Why has critique run out of steam? From matters of fact to matters of concern. *Critical Inquiry.* 30: 225–48.

Latour, B. (1993) *We Have Never Been Modern* [Transl. by C. Porter]. London: Harvester Wheatsheaf.

Latour, B. and Weibel, P. (eds) (2006) *Making Things Public.* Cambridge, MA: MIT Press.

Law, J. (2006) *The Big Pharma.* London: Constable & Robinson.

Lawton, J. (2006) Get up and go. *New Scientist.* 18 February 2006: 34–8.

Leadbeater, C. (2004) *Dream On – Sleep in the 24/7 Society.* London: Demos.

Leder, D. (1990) *The Absent Body.* Chicago, IL: University of Chicago Press.

Lee-Treweek, G. (2001) Bedroom abuse: the hidden work in a nursing home, in M. Allott and M. Robb (eds) *Understanding Health and Social Care: An Introductory Reader.* London: Sage.

Lemmey, D., McFarlane, J., Willson, P. and Maecha, A. (2001) Intimate partner violence. Mother's perspectives of effects on their children. *American Journal of Maternal Child Nursing.* 26(2), March–April: 98–103.

Levi, P. (1987/1958) *If This is a Man and The Truce* [Transl. by S. Wolf with an introduction by P. Bailey and an Afterword by the author). London: Abacus.

Levin, M. (1934) Narcolepsy in the Machine Age: the recent increase in the incidence of narcolepsy. *The Journal of Neurology and Psychopathology*. 15: 60–4.

Li, Y. (2003) Discourse of mid-day napping: a political windsock in contemporary China, in B. Steger and L. Brunt (eds) *Night-time and Sleep in Asia and the West: Exploring the Dark Side of Life*. London: Routledge Curzon.

Lock, M. (2008) Biosociality and susceptibility genes: a cautionary tale, in S. Gibbon and C. Novas (eds) *Biosocialities, Genetics and the Social Sciences: Making Biologies and Identities*. London: Routledge.

Löfgren, O. and Ehn, B. (2007) Daydreaming between dusk and dawn. *Ethnofoor*. XX (2): 9–21.

Loomis, A.L., Harvey, E.N. and Hobart, G.A. (1935a) Electrical potentials of the human brain. *Science*. 81: 1597–8.

Loomis, A.L., Harvey, E.N. and Hobart, G.A. (1935b) Further observations on the potential rhythms of the cerebral cortex during sleep. *Science*. 82: 198–200.

Lowe, P., Humphreys, C. and Williams, S.J. (2007) Night terrors: Women's experiences of (not) sleeping where there is domestic violence. *Violence Against Women*. 13(6): 549–61.

Lozoff, B. (1995) Culture and family: influences on childhood sleep practices and problems, in R. Ferber and M. Kryger (eds) *Principles and Practice of Sleep Medicine in the Child*. Philadelphia, PA and London: W.B. Saunders and Co.

Lupton, D. (1994) Panic computing: the viral metaphor and computer technology. *Cultural Studies*. 8: 556–68.

Lupton, D., McCarthy, S. and Chapman. S. (1995) 'Panic bodies': discourses on risk and HIV antibody testing. *Sociology of Health and Illness*. 17(1): 89–108.

Lynch, G. (2002) Memory enhancement: the search for mechanism based drugs. *Nature Neuroscience*. 5: 1035–8.

Lynch, G. and Gall, C.M. (2006) Ampakines and the threefold path to cognitive enhancement. *Trends in Neurosciences*. 29(10): 554–62

Maas, J.B. (with Wherry, M.L., Axelrod, D.J., Hogan, B.R. and Bloomin, J.) (1999) *Power Sleep: The Revolutionary Program that Prepares Your Mind for Peak Performance*. New York: Harper Collins.

Maasen, S. and Sutter, B. (2007) *On Willing Selves: Neoliberal Politics and the Challenge of Neuroscience*. Basingstoke: Macmillan.

Malcolm, N. (1959) *Dreaming*. London: Routledge and Kegan Paul.

Marcus, S.J. (ed.) (2002) *Neuroethics: Mapping the Field*. New York: The Dana Foundation.

Marcuse, H. (1972/1955) *Eros and Civilization: Philosophical Inquiry into Freud*. London: Abacus.

Marshall, T.H. (1950) *Citizenship and Social Class: and Other Essays.* Cambridge: Cambridge University Press.

Marquez, G.G. (1970/1967) *One Hundred Years of Solitude* [Transl. by G. Rabassa]. London: Jonathan Cape.

Marsh, G. (2005) Girl, 15, rescued after sleep walking up a 30 ft. crane. *Daily Express.* 6 July 2005: 8.

Martin, E. (2000) Flexible bodies: science and a new culture of health in the US, in S. Williams, J. Gabe and M. Calnan (eds) *Health, Medicine and Society: Key Theories, Future Agendas.* London: Routledge.

Martin, E. (1994) *Flexible Bodies: The Role of Immunology in American Culture from the Age of Polio to the Age of AIDS.* Boston, MA: Beacon Press.

Martin, P. (2002) *Counting Sheep: The Science and Pleasures of Sleep and Dreams.* London: HarperCollins.

Martin, P. and Ashcroft, R. (2005) *Neuroscience, Ethics and Society: A Review of the Field.* Background paper prepared for the 2005 Wellcome Trust Summer School on 'Neuroethics.' 26–29 September, St. Anne's College, Oxford, UK. Available at heet://www.wellcome.ac.uk/education-resources/courses-and-conferences/biomedical-ethics-course/html (Accessed 2 December 2010).

Martin, P. and Mohr, P.B. (2002) The incidence and correlates of post-trauma symptoms in children from backgrounds of domestic violence. *Violence and Victims.* 17: 555–67.

Martin, P. and Williams, S.J. (2009) Pharmaceutical cognitive enhancement and society. *Frontiers in Neuroscience.* 3(1), May: 115.

Martin, W. and Bartlett, H. (2007) The social significance of sleep for older people with dementia in the context of care. *Sociological Research Online.* 12(5): Available at: www.socresonline.org.uk/12/5/11.html (Accessed 30 May 2009).

Massumi, B. (2002) Navigating moments. Available as a pdf at www.brian-massumi.com/interviews (Accessed 29 July 2010).

Mavromatis, A. (1987) *Hypnagogia: The Unique State of Consciousness Between Wakefulness and Sleep.* London: Routledge.

Mayhew, H. (1851) *Mayhew's London, Being Selected from 'London Labour and the London Poor'* [First published in 1851]. London: Spring Books.

McCrone, J. (1999) *Going Inside: A Tour Round a Single Moment of Consciousness.* London: Faber and Faber.

McVeigh, T. (2010) 'Sunday blues' ruin weekends for many Britons. *The Observer.* 16 May 2010: 16.

Meadows, R. (2005) The 'negotiated night': An embodied conceptual framework for the sociological study of sleep. *The Sociological Review.* 53: 240–54.

Meadows, R., Arber, S., Venn, S. and Hislop, J. (2008a) Engaging with sleep: male definitions, understandings and attitudes. *Sociology of Health and Illness.* 30: 696–710.

Meadows, R., Arber, S., Venn, S. and Hislop, J. (2008b) Unruly bodies and couples' sleep. *Body & Society*. 14: 75–92.

Melbin, M. (1989) *Night as Frontier: Colonizing the World after Dark*. London: Macmillan.

Melbin, M. (1978) Night as frontier. *American Sociological Review*. 43(1): 3–22.

Melechi, A. (2003) *Fugitive Minds: on Madness, Sleep and other Twilight Affections*. London: William Heinemann.

Mednick, S.C. and Alaynick, W.A. (2009) Enhanced performance: a case for napping at work. *Frontiers in Neuroscience*. 3(3), December: 472–3 (www.frontiersin.org).

Merleau-Ponty, M. (1962) *The Phenomenology of Perception*. London: Routledge.

Miller, C.M. (2008) Lack of training in sleep and sleep disorders. *Virtual Mentor: American Medical Association Journal of Ethics*. 10(9): 560–63.

Miller, D. and Rose, N. (1990) Governing economic life. *Economy and Society*. 19: 1–31.

Miller, P. and Wilsdon, J. (eds) (2006) *Better Humans? The Politics of Human Enhancement and Life Extension*. London: Demos.

Mills, C.W. (1959) *The Sociological Imagination*. Oxford: Oxford University Press.

Mind (2010) *Taking Control of Stress in the Workplace*. Available at http://www.mind.org.uk/blog/3401_taking_control_of_stress_in_the_workplace (Accessed 2 December 2010).

Mitler, M.M., Dement, W.C. and Dinges, D.F. (2000) Sleep medicine, public policy and public health, in M.H. Kruger, T. Roth and W.C. Dement (eds) *Principles and Practices of Sleep Medicine* (3rd edition). Philadelphia, PA/London: W.B. Saunders.

MITRE Corporation (JASON program office)/Office of Defense Research and Engineering (2008) *Human Performance* (JSR-07-625). McLean, VA: MITRE Corporation; Washington, DC: Defense Pentagon.

Monaghan, L. (2002) Regulating 'unruly' bodies: work tasks, conflict and violence in Britain's night-time economy. *British Journal of Sociology*. 53(3), September: 403–29.

Montgomery, S.L. (1991) Code and combat in biomedical discourse. *Science as Culture*. 2: 341–90.

MooAllem, J. (2007) The sleep-industrial complex. *The New York Times*. 18 November 2007. Available at www.nytimes.com/2007/11/18/health/18iht-18sleept.8377935.html (Accessed 5 January 2010)

Moore-Ede. M. (1993) *The 24/7 Society*. London: Piatkus.

Moran-Ellis, J. and Venn, S. (2007) The sleeping lives of children and teenagers: night-worlds and arenas of action. *Sociological Research Online*. 12(5): Available at: www.socresonline.org.uk/12/5/9 (Accessed 1 June 2010).

Moreira, T. (2006) Sleep, health and the dynamics of biomedicine. *Social Science and Medicine*. 63: 54–63.

Morgan, K., Dixon, S., Mathers, N., Thompson, J. and Tomeny, M. (2004) Psychological treatment for insomnia in the regulation of long-term hypnotic drug use. *Health Technology Assessment.* 8(8).

Morris, S. (2009) Cheers from family as husband who killed his wife during nightmare is found not guilty of murder. *The Guardian.* 21 November 2009: 4.

Moynihan R. and Cassels, A. (2005) *Selling Sickness: How the World's Biggest Pharmaceutical Companies are Turning us All into Patients.* New York: Avalon Publishing Group Inc.

Nabokov, V. (2000) *Speak, Memory: An Autobiography Revisited.* London: Penguin.

National Commission on Sleep Disorders Research (NCSDR) (1993) *Wake Up America: A National Sleep Alert.* v. 1, Executive Summary and Executive Report of the NCSDR. Washington, DC.

National Sleep Foundation (NSF) (2009) *Sleep in America Polls: Health and Safety.* Available at: www.sleepfoundation.org (Accessed 21 August 2009).

National Sleep Foundation (NSF) (2008) *Sleep in America Polls: Sleep, Performance and the Workplace.* Available at: www.sleepfoundation.org (Accessed 21 August 2009).

National Sleep Foundation (NSF) (2007) *Sleep in America Polls: Women and Sleep.* Available at: www.sleepfoundation.org (Accessed 21 August 2009).

National Sleep Foundation (NSF) (2006) *Sleep in America Polls: Teens and Sleep.* Available at: www.sleepfoundation.org (Accessed 21 August 2009).

National Sleep Foundation (NSF) (2005) *Sleep in America Polls: Adult Sleep Habits and Styles.* Available at: www.sleepfoundation.org (Accessed 21 August 2009).

National Sleep Foundation (NSF) (2004) *Sleep in America Polls: Children and Sleep.* Available at: www.sleepfoundation.org (Accessed 21 August 2009).

National Sleep Foundation (NSF) (2003) *Sleep in America Polls: Sleep and Ageing.* Available at: www.sleepfoundation.org (Accessed 21 August 2009).

National Sleep Foundation (NSF) (2002) *Sleep in America Polls: Adult Sleep Habits.* Available at: www.sleepfoundation.org (Accessed 21 August 2009).

Nightingale, P. and Martin, P. (2004) The myth of the biotech revolution. *Trends in Biotechnology.* 22(11), November: 564–9.

Norbutt, M. (2004) Waking up to sleep clinics: growing industry offers eye-catching investments. *American Medical Association News.* 5 January 2004 Available at: www.ama-assn.org/amednews/2004/01/05/bisa015.htm (Accessed 5 August 2009).

Nottingham, C. (2003) 'What time do you call this?': change and continuity in the politics of the city night, in B. Steger and L. Brunt (eds) *Night-Time And Sleep in Asian and the West: Exploring the Dark Side of Life.* London/New York: RoutledgeCurzon.

O'Dea, W. (1958) *The Social History of Lighting.* London: Hamish Hamilton.

Office for National Statistics (ONS) (2006) *The Time Use Survey 2005: How We Spend our Time.* Available at: www.statistics.gov.uk/articles/nojournal/time_use_2005.pdf (Accessed 3 January 2010).

Office for National Statistics (ONS) (2003) *The United Kingdom 2000 Time Use Survey Technical Report.* Available at: www.statistics.gov.uk/downloads/theme_social/UKTUS_TechReport.pdf (Accessed 24 August 2009).

Office of Science and Technology (OST)/Department of Trade and Industry (DTI) (2005) *Drugs Futures 2025.* London: DTI.

Organisation for Economic Co-operation and Development (OECD) (2009) *Society at a Glance – OECD Social Indicators.* Available at: www.oecd.org/els/social/indicators/SAG (Accessed 31 January 2010).

Oswald, I. (1968) Drugs and sleep. *Pharmacological Review.* 20: 272–303.

Oswald, I. and Priest, R. (1965) Five weeks to escape the sleeping pill habit. *British Medical Journal.* 2: 1093–5.

Pack, A., Maislin, G., Staley, B., Pack, F., Rogers, W., George, F. and Dinges, D. (2006) Impaired performance in commercial drivers: the role of sleep apnea and short sleep duration. *American Journal of Respiratory Critical Care.* 174: 446–54.

Parsons, T. (1951) *The Social System.* London: Routledge and Kegan Paul.

Pavlov, I.P. (1928) *Lectures on Conditioned Reflexes.* London: Lawrence and Wishart.

Pavlov, I.P. (1927) *Conditioned Reflexes: An Investigation of the Physiological Activity of the Cerebral Cortex.* New York: Oxford University Press.

Pavlov, I.P. (1923) The identity of inhibition with sleep and hypnosis. *Science Monthly.* 17: 603–8.

Petersen, A. (1997) 'Risk, governance and the new public health', in A. Petersen and R. Bunton (eds) *Foucault Health and Medicine.* London: Routledge.

Petryna, A. (2002) *Life Exposed: Biological Citizens After Chernobyl.* Princeton, NJ: Princeton University Press.

Phillipson, E.A. (1993) Sleep apnoea – a major public health problem. *New England Journal of Medicine.* 328: 1271–3.

Pick, D. and L. Roper (2004) Introduction, in D. Pick and L. Roper (eds.) *Dreams and History: The Interpretation of Dreams from Ancient Greece to Modern Psychoanalysis.* London and New York: Brunner-Routledge.

Pilkington, E. (2010) BP rig's alarms were switched off 'to help workers sleep'. *The Guardian* 24 July 2010: 1–2.

Pilkington, E. (2009) The colonel seizes his 15 minutes of fame. 100 minutes later he sat down. *The Guardian* 24 September 2009: 1.

Proust, M. (2002) *In Search of Lost Time/A la recherché du temps perdu* [Transl. by C.K. Scott Moncrieff and T. Kilmartin, Rev. Ed. by D.J. Enright]. London: Vintage.

R v Burgess (1991) 2 ALL ER Rep 769.

Rabinow, P. and Rose, N. (2006) Biopower today. *BioSocieties: An Interdisciplinary Journal for the Social Study of the Life Sciences.* 1(2): 195–218.

Rangel, E.K. (2007) Cosmetic psychopharmacology and the goals of medicine. *Virtual Mentor: American Medical Association Journal of Ethics.* 9(6): 428–32.

Rechtschaffen, A. and Kales, A. (1968) *A Manual of Standardized Terminology, Techniques and Scoring System for Sleep Stages of Human Subjects.* Bethesda, MD: US Dept. of Health, Education and Welfare, Public Health Service.

Rechtschaffen, A. Wolpert, E., Dement, W., Mitchell, S. and Fisher, C. (1963) Nocturnal sleep of narcoleptics. *Electroencephalography and Clinical Neurophysiology.* 15: 599–609.

Reichen, J. (2009) Sleep is money. *Frontiers in Neuroscience.* 3(3), December: 484–5 (www.frontiersin.org).

Rensen, P. (2003) Sleeping without a home: the embedment of sleep in the lives of the rough-sleeping homeless in Amsterdam, in B. Steger and L. Brunt (eds) *Night-time and Sleep in Asia and the West: Exploring the Dark Side of Life.* London: Routledge Curzon.

Richter, A. (2003) Sleeping time in early Chinese literature, in B. Steger and L. Brunt (eds) *Night-time and Sleep in Asia and the West: Exploring the Dark Side of Life.* London: Routledge Curzon.

Rose, D. (2004) *Guantanamo: The War on Human Rights.* New York/London: The New Press.

Rose, N. (2007). *The Politics of Life Itself: Biomedicine, Power and Subjectivity in the Twenty-First Century.* Princeton, NJ: Princeton University Press.

Rose, N. (1996) Governing 'advanced' liberal societies, in A. Barry, T. Osbourne and N. Rose (eds) *Foucault and Political Reason.* London: UCL Press.

Rose, N. (1992) Governing the enterprising self, in P. Heelas and P. Morris (eds) *The Values of the Enterprise Culture: The Moral Debate.* London: Routledge.

Rose, N. (1990) *Governing the Soul: The Shaping of the Private Self.* London/New York: Routledge.

Russell, B. (2004/1933) *In Praise of Idleness* [With a preface by A. Gottlieb with an introduction by H. Woodshouse]. London: Routledge.

Salkeld, L. (2009) Freed, the 'decent man' who killed his wife as they slept. *Daily Mail*. 21 November 2009: 31.

Sample, I. (2004) Wired awake. *Guardian*. 29 July 2004: 6.

Sample, I. and Evans, R. (2004) MoD bought thousands of stay awake pills in advance of the war on Iraq. *The Guardian*. 29 July 2004: 1.

Savulescu, J. and Bostrom, N. (ed.) (2008) *Human Enhancement*. Oxford: Oxford University Press.

Schwartz, B. (1970) Notes on the sociology of sleep. *Sociological Quarterly*. 11: 485–99.

Seale, C., Boden, S., Williams, S.J., Lowe, P. and Steinberg, D.L. (2007) Media constructions of sleep and sleep disorders: a study of UK national newspapers. *Social Science and Medicine*. 65: 418–30.

Sekine, M., Chandola, T., Martikainen, P., Marmot, M. and Kagamimori, S. (2006) Work and family characteristics as determinants of socio-economic and gender inequalities in sleep: the Japanese Civil Servants Study. *Sleep*. 29: 206–16.

Selin, C. (2008) The sociology of the future: tracing stories of technology and time. *Sociology Compass*. 2/6: 1878–95.

Serge, V. (1970) *Men in Prison*. London: Gollancz.

Shilling, C. (2003) *The Body and Social Theory* (2nd edition). London: Sage.

Siegel, J.M. (2009) Sleep in the animal Kingdom. *Frontiers in Neuroscience*. 3(3): 394–95.

Sidney, Sir P. (1989/1598) *Sir Philip Sidney: The Major Works including 'Astrophil and Stella'* (ed. By K. Duncan-Jones). Oxford: Oxford University Press.

Singh, I. and Rose, N. (2006) Neuro-forum: an introduction. *BioSocieties*. 1: 97–102.

Smith, R. (2009) Kenton Kroker's 'The Sleep of Others' (Book review). *History of the Human Sciences*. 22: 108–12.

Smith, R. (2007) *Being Human: Historical Knowledge and the Creation of Human Nature*. Manchester: Manchester University Press.

Smith, R.J. (1979) Study finds sleeping pills overprescribed. *Science*. 204: 287–8.

Smith, R.R. (2009) *Breakfast with Socrates: The Philosophy of Everyday Life*. London: Profile Books Ltd.

Solms, M. (2009) Freudian dreams today. *Frontiers in Neuroscience*. 3(3), December: 453 (www.frontiersin.org).

Solms, M. (2007) The interpretation of dreams and the neurosciences, in Deutsches Hygiene-Museum/Wellcome Collection (ed.) *Sleeping and Dreaming*. London: Black Dog Publishing.

Solms, M. and Turnbull, O. (2002) *The Brain and the Inner World: An Introduction to the Neuroscience of Subjective Experience*. London: Karnac.

Stallybrass, P. and White, A. (1986) *The Politics and Poetics of Transgression*. London: Macmillan.

Stearns, P. (2003) *Anxious Parents: A History of Modern Childrearing in America*. New York: New York University Press.

Stearns, P.N., Perrin, R. and Glarnella, L. (1996) Children's sleep: sketching historical change. *Journal of Social History*. 30: 345–66.

Steger, B. (2008) 'Early to rise' making the Japanese healthy, wealthy, wise, virtuous and beautiful, in L. Brunt and B. Steger (eds) *Worlds of Sleep*. Berlin: Frank & Timme.

Steger, B. (2003a) Negotiating sleep patterns in Japan, in B. Steger and L. Brunt (eds) *Night-time in Asia and the West: Exploring the Dark Side of Life*. London: Routledge Curzon.

Steger, B. (2003b) Getting *away* with sleep – social and cultural aspects of dozing in parliament. *Social Science Japan Journal*. 6: 181–97.

Steger, B. and Brunt, L. (2003) Introduction: into the night and the world of sleep, in B. Steger and L. Brunt (eds) *Night-time and Sleep in Asia and the West: Exploring the Dark Side of Life*. London: Routledge Curzon, pp. 1–23.

Steinberg, D.L. (2008) Reading sleep through science fiction: the parable of Beggars and Choosers. *Body & Society*. 14(4), December: 115–35.

Stewart, C. (2004) Dreams and desires in ancient and early Christian thought, in D. Pick and L. Roper (eds) *Dreams and History*. London/New York: Routledge.

Stickgold, R. (2009) Sleep: the easy road to cognitive enhancement. *Frontiers in Neuroscience*. 1(3), May: 104–05.

Stores, G. and Crawford, C. (1998) Medical student education in sleep and its disorders. *Journal of the Royal College of Physicians of London*. 32(2): 149–53.

Stradling, J.R. and Davies, R.J.O. (1997) Obstructive sleep apnoea: evidence for efficacy of continuous positive airways pressure is compelling. *British Medical Journal*. 315: 368.

Strohl, K.P. (2008) Keeping sleepy people off the road: the responsibility of drivers, doctors and the DMV. *Virtual Mentor: American Medical Association Journal of Ethics*. 10(9): 578–84.

Strong, P.M. (1990) Epidemic psychology – a model. *Sociology of Health and Illness*. 12: 249–59.

Summers-Bremner, E. (2008) *Insomnia: A Cultural History*. London: Reaktion Books.

Sullivan, C.E., Issa, F.G., Berthon-Jones, M. and Eves, L. (1981) Reversal of obstructive sleep apnea by continuous positive airway pressure applied through nares. *Lancet*. 1: 862–5.

Taft, A., Broom, D.H. and Legge, D. (2004) General practitioner management of intimate partner abuse and the whole family: qualitative study.

British Medical Journal. DOI: 10.1136/bmj.38014.626535.OB (published 6 February 2004): 1–4.

Tahan, D.A. (2008) Depth and space in sleep: intimacy, touch and the body in Japanese co-sleeping rituals. *Body & Society.* 14(4), December: 37–56.

Tate Modern (2009) *The UniLever Series: Miroslaw Balka How It Is.* London: Tate Modern.

Taylor, B. (1993) Unconsciousness and society: the sociology of sleep. *International Journal of Politics and Culture.* 6: 463–71.

Thompson, E.P. (1967) Time, work discipline and industrial capitalism. *Past and Present* 38(December): 56–97.

Thorpy, M. (1991) History of sleep and man, in M. Thorpy and J. Yager (eds) *The Encyclopaedia of Sleep and Sleep Disorders.* New York: Facts on File.

Thrift, N. (2008) *Non-Representational Theory: Space/Politics/Affect.* London: Routledge.

Thrift, N. (2005) *Knowing Capitalism.* London: Sage.

Thrift, N. (2000) Still life in nearly present time: the object of nature. *Body & Society.* 6(3–4): 34–57.

Thrift, N. (1997) The still point: resistance, expressive embodiment and dance, in S. Pile and M. Keith (eds) *Geographies of Resistance.* London: Routledge.

Thrift, N. (1996) *Spatial Formations.* London: Sage.

Thrift, N. (1995) A hyperactive world, in R.J. Johnston, P.J. Taylor and M. Watts (eds) *Geographies of Global Transformation.* Oxford: Blackwell.

Tomlinson, J. (2007) *The Culture of Speed: The Coming of Immediacy.* London: Sage.

Townsend, M. and Rogers, R. (2010) Bottoms up: continental café culture was never meant to be like this... *The Observer.* 20 June 2010: 5.

Turner, B.S. (1997) From governmentality to risk: some reflections on Foucault's contribution to medical sociology, in A. Petersen and R. Bunton (eds) *Foucault, Health and Medicine.* London: Routledge.

Turner, B.S. (1993a) *Max Weber: From History to Modernity.* London: Routledge.

Turner, B.S. (1993b) Postmodern culture/modern citizens, in B. van Steenbergen (ed.) *The Condition of Citizenship.* London: Sage.

Turner, B.S. (1992) *Regulating Bodies: Essays in Medical Sociology.* London: Routledge.

Turner, D., Robbins, T.W., Clark, L., Aron, A.R., Dawson, J. and Sahakian, B.J. (2003) Cognitive enhancing effects of modafinil in healthy volunteers. *Psychopharmacology.* 165(3): 260–9.

University of Warwick (2009) *The University of Warwick Around the Clock Twenty Four Seven.* Coventry: University of Warwick.

Van den Bulck, J. (2004) Television viewing, computer game playing, and Internet use and self-reported time to bed and time out of bed in secondary-school children. *Sleep.* 27(pt. 1), February: 101–04.

Van den Bulck, J. (2003) Text messaging as a cause of sleep interruption in adolescents, evidence from a cross-sectional study. *Journal of Sleep Research.* 12(3), September: 263.

Van Eeden, F. (1913) A study of dreams. *Proceedings of the Society for Psychical Research.* 26: 431–45.

Van Somersen, E.J.W., Pollmächer, T., Leger, D., Espie, C., Bassetti, C. and Riemann, D. (2009) The European Insomnia Network. *Frontiers in Neuroscience.* 3(3), December: 436 (www.frontiersin.org).

Venn, S. (2007) It's okay for a man to snore: the influence of gender on sleep disruption in couples. *Sociological Research Online.* 12(5). Available at: www.socresonline.org.uk/12/5/1.html (Accessed 28 July 2008).

Venn, S. and Arber, S. (2008) Conflicting sleep demands: parents and young people in UK households, in B. Steger and L. Brunt (eds) *Worlds of Sleep.* Berlin: Frank & Timme, pp. 105–29.

Venn, S., Arber, S., Meadows, R. and Hislop, J. (2008) The fourth shift: exploring the gendered nature of sleep disruption in couples with children. *British Journal of Sociology.* 59: 79–97.

Virilio, P. (2000) *The Information Bomb* [Transl. by C. Turner]. London: Verso.

Virilio, P. (1991) *The Lost Dimension: Zero Gravity* [Transl. by D. Moshenberg]. New York: Semiotext(e).

Virilio, P. (1986/1977) *Speed and Politics: An Essay on Dromology.* New York: Semiotext(e).

Vogler, P. (2008) Sleeping as refugee? Embodied vulnerability and corporeal security during refugees' sleep at the Thai-Burma border, in L. Brunt and B. Steger (eds) *Worlds of Sleep.* Berlin: Frank & Timme.

Wainwright, D. and Calnan, M. (2002) *Work Stress: The Making of a Modern Epidemic.* Buckingham: Open University Press.

Wainwright, M. (2002) Dozing driver who caused 10 deaths gets five years. *The Guardian.* 12 January 2002: 1.

Wajcman, J. (2008) Life in the fast lane? Towards a sociology of technology and time. *British Journal of Sociology.* 59(1): 59–77.

Walsh, J. and Englehardt, C. (1999) The direct economic costs of insomnia in the US. *Sleep.* 22 (Suppl. 2): S386–93.

Walter Reid Air Institute for Research Staff (WRAIR) (1997) *Sleep, Sleep Deprivation and Human Performance.* Bethesda, MD: WRAIR, Dept. of Behavioral Biology. Available at: wrair.www.army.mil/depts/behavbio (Accessed 23 July 2008).

Warren, T. (2002) Gendered and classed working time in Britain: dual employee couples in higher/lower level occupations, in G. Crow and S.

Heath (eds) *Social Conceptions of Time: Structure and Process in Work and Everyday Life.* Basingstoke: Palgrave Macmillan.

Weber, M. (1974/1930) *The Protestant Ethic and the Spirit of Capitalism* [Transl. by T. Parsons, foreword by R. Tawney]. London: Unwin University Books.

Wegner, D.M. (2002) *The Illusion of Conscious Will.* Cambridge, MA: MIT Press.

Weisgerber, C. (2004) Turning to the internet for help on sensitive medical problems: a qualitative study of the construction of a sleep disorder through online interaction. *Information, Communication & Society.* 7(4): 554–74.

Wellcome News (2009) Take my breath away. 61(December): 4–5.

Wells, H.G. (2005/1910) *The Sleeper Wakes.* Harmondsworth: Penguin.

Widerberg, K. (2006) Embodying modern times: investigating tiredness. *Time and Society.* 15(1): 105–20.

Wiggs, L. (2007) Are children getting enough sleep? Implications for parents. *Sociological Research Online.* 12(5): from www.socresonline.org.uk/12/5/13.html (Accessed 1 June 2010).

Williams, R.L. and Agnew, H.W. (1969) The effects of drugs on the EEG sleep patterns of normal humans. *Experimental Medicine and Surgery.* 27: 53–64.

Williams, S.J. (2008) The sociological aspects of sleep; progress, problems, prospects. *Sociology Compass.* 2(2): 639–53.

Williams, S.J. (2007a) Vulnerable/dangerous bodies? The trials and tribulations of sleep, in C. Shilling (ed.) *Embodying Sociology: Retrospect, Progress, Prospects.* Oxford: Blackwell.

Williams, S.J. (2007b) The social etiquette of sleep: some sociological observations. *Sociology.* 41(2): 313–28.

Williams, S.J. (2005) *Sleep and society: sociological ventures into the (un)known.* Abingdon: Routledge.

Williams, S.J. (2004) Beyond medicalization-healthicization? A rejoinder to Hislop and Arber. *Sociology of Health and Illness.* 26(4): 453–59.

Williams, S.J. (2002) Sleep and health: reflections on the dormant society. *Health.* 6(2): 173–200.

Williams, S.J. and Bendelow, G. (1998) *The Lived Body.* London: Routledge.

Williams, S.J. and Boden, S. (2004) Consumed with sleep? Dormant bodies in consumer culture. *Sociological Research Online.* 9(2). Available at: www.socresonline.org.uk/9/2/willliams.html (Accessed 5 June 2010).

Williams, S.J. and Crossley, N. (2008) Introduction: sleeping bodies. *Body & Society.* 14(4), December: 1–15.

Williams, S.J. and Martin, P.A. (2008) Risks and benefits may turn out to be finely balanced. *Nature.* 457, 29 January 2008: 532.

Williams, S.J., Meadows, R. and Arber, S. (2010) The sociology of sleep, in F. Cappuccio, M. Miller and S. Lockley (eds) *Sleep, Health and Society: From Aetiology to Public Health*. Oxford: Oxford University Press.

Williams, S.J., Seale, C., Boden, S., Lowe, P. and Steinberg, D.L. (2009) Waking up to sleepiness: modafinil, the media and the pharmaceuticalisation of everyday/night life, in S.J. Williams, J. Gabe and P.B. Davis (eds) *Pharmaceuticals and Society: Critical Discourses and Debates*. Oxford: Wiley-Blackwell.

Williams, S.J., Seale, C., Boden, S., Lowe, P. and Steinberg, D.L. (2008) Medicalisation and beyond: the social construction of insomnia and snoring in the news. *Health*. 12(2): 251–68.

Williams, S., Lowe, P. and Griffiths, F. (2007) Embodying and embedding children's sleep: some sociological comments and observations. *Sociological Research Online*. 12(5): Available at www.socresonline.org.uk/12/5/6.html (Accessed 5 May 2009).

Williams, S.J., Martin, P. and Gabe, J. (2011) The pharmaceuticalisation of society? An analytical framework for future study. *Sociology of Health & Illness*.

Willis, T. (1692) *The London Practice of Physick*. London: Thomas Basset.

Wilson, H. (2004) Sleep your way to the top. *The Guardian*. 16 February 2004 (Office Hours): 5.

Winterman, D. (2004) Sleeping on the job. *BBC News Online Magazine*. 7 September 2004. Available at: news.bbc.co.uk/1/hi/magazine/3631040.stm (Accessed 2 April 2010).

Winterton, J. (2000) Disappearance, I. *The World and Other Places*. London: Vintage.

Wohl, A.S. (1976) Sex and the single room: incest among the Victorian working-classes, in A.S. Wohl (ed.) *The Victorian Family: Structure and Stresses*. London: Croom Helm.

Wolf-Meyer, M. (2008) Sleep, signification and the abstract body of allopathic medicine. *Body & Society*. 14(4), December: 93–114.

Wolpe, P. (2002) Treatment, enhancement and the ethics of neurotherapies. *Brain and Cognition*. 50: 387–95.

World Health Organization (WHO) (2007) *International Classification of Diseases and Related Health Problems* [10th Revision]. Geneva: World Health Organisation. Available at: apps.who.int/classifications/apps/icd/icd10online (Accessed 5 January 2010).

World Health Organization (WHO) Regional Office for Europe (2004) *Technical Meeting on Sleep and Health*. Bonn: European Centre for Environment and Health. Available at: www.euro.who.int/noise/activities (Accessed 30 June 2009).

Worthington, A. (2007) *The Guantanamo Files; Stories of the 774 Detainees in America's Illegal Prison*. London: Pluto Press.

Wright, J., Johns, R., Watt, I., Melvitla, A. and Sheldon, T. (1997a) Health effects of obstructive sleep apnoea and the effectiveness of continuous positive airways pressure: systematic review of the research evidence. *British Medical Journal*. 314: 851–60 (plus Editorial 'Deep and shallow').

Woloshin, S. and Schwartz, L.M. (2006). Giving legs to restless eggs: a case study of how the media make the people sick. *Public Library of Science – Medicine*. 13(4): e170 Epub 11 April 2006 (Accessed 3 December 2010).

Wright, J., Johns, R., Watt, I., Melvitla, A. and Sheldon, T. (1997b) Obstructive sleep apnoea: Author's reply. *British Medical Journal*. 315: 551.

Index

193

'May I present  **Heston?' Adan** **pleasantly.**

Miranda swayed. The ~~could not be~~ happening. Events had moved with the speed of some dreadful nightmare from which she must awaken. Then Heston slipped a hand beneath her elbow. 'Until tomorrow, dearest,' he said tenderly. 'Your uncle and I have much to discuss. . .settlements. . .the announcements in the morning papers. . .'

Miranda gazed at him in horror, but his expression was impassive. She had put herself in Heston's power, and she could think of no way to escape.

After living in southern Spain for many years, **Meg Alexander** now lives in Kent, although, having been born in Lancashire, she feels that her roots are in the north of England. Meg's career has encompassed a wide variety of roles, from professional cook to assistant director of a conference centre. She has always been a voracious reader, and loves to write. Other loves include history, cats, gardening, cooking and travel. She has a son and two grandchildren.

Recent titles by the same author:

HIS LORDSHIP'S DILEMMA
FAREWELL THE HEART
THE SWEET CHEAT

MIRANDA'S MASQUERADE

Meg Alexander

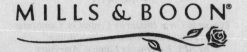

MILLS & BOON®

DID YOU PURCHASE THIS BOOK WITHOUT A COVER?

If you did, you should be aware it is **stolen property** as it was reported *unsold and destroyed* by a retailer. Neither the Author nor the publisher has received any payment for this book.

All the characters in this book have no existence outside the imagination of the author, and have no relation whatsoever to anyone bearing the same name or names. They are not even distantly inspired by any individual known or unknown to the author, and all the incidents are pure invention.

All Rights Reserved including the right of reproduction in whole or in part in any form. This edition is published by arrangement with Harlequin Enterprises II B.V. The text of this publication or any part thereof may not be reproduced or transmitted in any form or by any means, electronic or mechanical, including photocopying, recording, storage in an information retrieval system, or otherwise, without the written permission of the publisher.

This book is sold subject to the condition that it shall not, by way of trade or otherwise, be lent, resold, hired out or otherwise circulated without the prior consent of the publisher in any form of binding or cover other than that in which it is published and without a similar condition including this condition being imposed on the subsequent purchaser.

MILLS & BOON and MILLS & BOON with the Rose Device are registered trademarks of the publisher.

First published in Great Britain 1997
Harlequin Mills & Boon Limited,
Eton House, 18–24 Paradise Road, Richmond, Surrey TW9 ISR

© Meg Alexander 1997

ISBN 0 263 80125 X

Set in 10 on 12 pt Linotron Times
04-9705-80954

Typeset in Great Britain by CentraCet, Cambridge
Printed and bound in Great Britain
by BPC Paperbacks Limited, Aylesbury

Chapter One

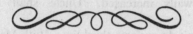

'I'll make him sorry he ever offered for me!' With a cry of anguish, Frances Gaysford threw herself upon her bed and burst into a storm of tears.

'That shouldn't be too difficult, Fanny,' her twin observed dispassionately. 'Just let Lord Heston see you now and he'll cry off at once. The end of your nose is as red as your eyes...'

'Oh! Oh! Unfeeling! I might have known you'd make a joke of it...my own *sister*! You don't care in the least, Miranda.'

'I might if I believed in this Cheltenham tragedy. Come to your senses, love. Harry Lakenham will never marry you. Even if he were of age, he won't wed to disoblige his family.'

'We are promised to each other...' Fanny raised her head, the drowned blue eyes looking enormous in the delicate oval of her face. 'His heart will not change, and nor will mine...'

'But yours has changed three times in the last three months! I have lost count of the men to whom you've sworn undying devotion.'

'This time it's different. In the past...well...it was

but an illusion. Now I know the meaning of true love.'

'Perhaps so. In the meantime, you had best get up and bathe your face. Heston will be here at noon. You have less than an hour to change your dress, which, I may say, is sadly crumpled...'

'I won't see him. I can't. I am not well enough.' Fanny's wails increased. 'Uncle shall make my excuses...'

'He won't do so for a third time. Both Mr Mordaunt and Sir Patrick Caswell were insulted when you claimed the headache, and then they saw you later at the Opera.'

'Could I help it if I felt a little better later in the day? I should not have taken either, in any case...a widower on the one hand, and a middle-aged country squire? I can't think what Uncle was about to allow them to address me.'

'He hopes to see us comfortably settled, Fanny. Was that not his object in giving us this season? Mama could not afford it—'

'I know! Pray do not go on about it. He has been kind, but doubtless he has his reasons...'

'What can you mean?' There was a note of anger in Miranda's voice, and Fanny looked uncomfortable.

'Don't get upon your high ropes!' she said defiantly. 'With Father gone, Uncle will not care to have our family foisted upon him. He would marry us to anyone.'

'That is both ungenerous and untrue! You might at least see Heston. Uncle does not insist that you accept him...only that you listen to his offer.'

'How can I? My heart is broken...' With a gesture worthy of a tragedy queen, Fanny raised herself upon one elbow and covered her eyes with a drooping hand.

Miranda recognised the scene at once. It was part of the repertoire of the latest actress to take the town by storm.

'What do I care for money or position?' her sister mourned. 'I should be happy in a cottage with my darling.'

'Stuff and nonsense!' Miranda said decisively. 'Sometimes you put me out of all patience with you. You in a cottage? I can just see you feeding chickens and cleaning out the pigs. Remember how you hated life in Yorkshire. . .the plain food, no new clothes, an outside privy, and the cold? Have you forgot the cold?'

'No, of course not, but it will not come to that. Harry has expectations. All we need is a little time. . . He will see his grandfather—'

'Do be sensible, Fanny! It will not serve, you know.'

'You have always been against him. How can you be so cruel? Why must I be sacrificed to that ugly dotard? Heston is a freak. . .a mountain. . .a positive Alp! He has neither manners nor wit to recommend him. Oh, why could he not take you?'

This suggestion was too much for Miranda. Her sense of humour bubbled to the surface. 'Fanny, you will be the end of me! Do you believe that this. . .this monster, as you call him, would make me an ideal husband?'

'Of course not!' Fanny sniffed. 'And you need not laugh. I doubt if any man would suit you. You treat them all as if their compliments are meaningless.'

'Most of them are, and I won't be taken in by flattery.'

'It isn't all false. We are not ill-looking, you and I. When a gentleman expresses admiration it is not kind in you to put him out of countenance by speaking out so plain. You frighten them away, you know.'

'I'll try to mend my ways,' Miranda promised. 'Now, dearest, do get dressed. Much as I should like to help you, Lord Heston has not offered for me. He has asked to see Miss Gaysford, and you are the elder. . .'

'Only by twenty minutes. It isn't fair!' Fanny gazed at her twin, a look of speculation in her eyes. 'He would not know the difference,' she said thoughtfully. 'We might play a trick on him, if you were to take my place.'

Miranda stared at her. 'I wonder that you could suggest it,' she said in dismay.

'But we have exchanged places all our lives. It cannot signify for a mere half-hour. It could do no harm.'

'I doubt if Lord Heston would see it so. It would be insulting, Fanny. Think of the scandal if we were to be found out? This is no childish game. The scandal would be unbearable—' She stopped. Fanny had given way to a series of hiccuping sobs. They were a certain prelude to an attack of hysteria. She looked up helplessly as her aunt came into the room.

'Why, what is this, my dears?' Mrs Shere gathered Fanny to her ample bosom. 'There, my love, pray don't distress yourself. When your sister marries, she will not be lost to you, and you will be wed yourself before the year is out.' She stroked her niece's copper curls with a gentle hand.

'I. . . I'm sorry, Aunt.' Fanny lifted a drooping head. 'I do not mean to be a watering-pot.' The glance she threw at Miranda was one of triumph. Mrs Shere had mistaken one twin for the other, as she had often done before.

Miranda was about to correct her when Fanny caught at her hand. 'You will come back at once and tell us what Lord Heston has to say?' she pleaded.

'Of course she will.' Mrs Shere beamed upon the twins. 'His lordship has arrived, and we must not keep him waiting.' She took Miranda's arm and led her from the room.

'Aunt, please wait! I have something to say to you.'

'Not now, my love. It must wait until later. This is not the time. . .' She hurried ahead, along the corridor and down the staircase, pausing only when they reached the door to the salon.

'You were right to wear the white sprigged muslin.' She considered Miranda with a critical eye. 'It is most becoming. I could wish that these short hairstyles were not so much the vogue, but there, we must be in the fashion. Be kind to Lord Heston,' she whispered finally. 'Gentlemen, too, can be nervous on these occasions.'

She opened the door and led her niece towards the man who stood by the window.

He turned as they entered and came towards her, bowing first to her aunt and then to herself.

Miranda felt a slight twinge of amusement. Anyone less nervous she had yet to see. A sharp glance from beneath his black brows had assured her of that.

She held her breath as she waited for his first words. Would he see through her deception? Then it became apparent that he too had mistaken her for Fanny. As he exchanged civilities with Mrs Shere, Miranda kept her eyes upon the carpet.

At last she nerved herself to look at him more closely. Immensely tall and built in proportion the perfect tailoring of his coat and breeches could not disguise his heavily muscled shoulders and thighs. He moved with the easy grace of an athlete.

Even the most partial would not have termed him handsome. Crowned by a mass of thick black hair, cut

in the fashionable 'Brutus' style, his face had a vitality
of its own. The heavy jaw and a slightly crooked nose
merely added character to his expression.

At this moment, that expression was unfathomable
as his eyes met hers. She was startled. Hard and bleak
as the grey of a winter sea, they roved over her with
indifference.

It must be her imagination. She had seen him before,
of course. His height alone made him conspicuous in
any gathering. His lordship did not dance, and seemed
to find no pleasure in feminine company.

'Who is that man?' she had asked her friend,
Charlotte Fairfax. She had been half-piqued and half-
amused when he had thrown her a single glance and,
clearly unimpressed, had turned away.

'Heston? He is one of the richest men in London.
Don't cast your handkerchief in his direction, my dear.
You would be wasting your time.'

'Why is that? Has he a reputation?'

'Not that I can discover, but he is a mis—a mis—
well, one of those men who has not time for women.
He thinks only of gaming, horses, and curricle racing.'

'How very dull of him!' Miranda had watched as his
lordship had strolled idly through the chattering throng
and had made his way to the card tables in the adjoining
room.

'Miranda, never let anyone hear you say so! Heston
is a Corinthian and quite at the top of the tree. He is
the idol of the younger set and a member of the Four-
Horse Club.'

'Remarkable! Are we supposed to admire him
because he wears a Belcher handkerchief, a nosegay in
his driving coat, and a spotted cravat? How ridiculous!
It seems more like fancy-dress to me.'

'Please, I beg of you...' Charlotte had drawn her friend into the shelter of an alcove, and had cast an anxious look about her. 'Do guard your tongue, Miranda. You must not speak your mind so openly. Someone will overhear you. Gentlemen have their odd notions, and we must accept them.'

'I suppose so...' Miranda had given her hand to the gallant who had come to claim her for the quadrille and had promptly forgotten Lord Heston's existence.

It was strange to see him again under these circumstances. She had been as puzzled as Fanny by his sudden decision to call upon their uncle. Fanny had met him once, when he was introduced to her by Harry Lakenham, and had taken him in instant dislike. Why, then, did he wish to offer for her hand? She was deep in thought when her aunt recalled her to the matter in hand.

Mrs Shere rose to her feet. Ignoring Miranda's imploring look, she murmured something about leaving the two young people to get to know each other and left the room.

A silence fell, which his lordship made no attempt to break.

'Won't you sit down, my lord?' Miranda asked in desperation. Standing over her as he did, Lord Heston seemed to fill the room.

'Certainly, madam.' Heston took a seat on the other side of the fireplace. 'I imagine you can guess why I am here?'

Miranda coloured. 'My uncle said that you had asked to speak to me in private. I confess I was surprised...'

She heard an ugly laugh. 'Were you? You do not suppose that Lakenham's friends would allow him to contract a *mésalliance* without making some attempt to save him?'

Miranda gazed at him in stupefaction.

'Come, now! Don't play the innocent with me. Will you deny that the boy has been fool enough to promise marriage?'

Miranda found her voice at last. 'What has that to do with you?' she demanded. 'You are not his guardian.'

'True, but I am connected with the family. The details need not concern you. It is enough for you to know that I am here on behalf of Harry's grandfather, Lord Rudyard.'

The cool effrontery of this statement made Miranda burn with rage. Heston was insolence personified.

'The decision must rest with Lord Lakenham,' she snapped.

'On the contrary, it rests with you. Harry has refused to give you up. Nothing his grandfather could say will alter his resolution. . .'

'Then, sir, you are wasting your time!'

'I think not. It is up to you to make the break. You must cry off at once. It is contemptible to take advantage of a young man's inexperience. I must appeal to your better nature. . .'

Miranda gave him a limpid look. 'What makes you think I have one? On the contrary, I have a fancy for a title and a fortune.' Anger had betrayed her into indiscretion, but she did not care. Who did this pompous creature think he was, issuing demands and insulting her with every word?

'I see!' His voice was soft, but there was an underlying note of menace. 'Well. . .let us get down to cases. . . how much?'

Fury threatened to choke Miranda, but she kept her eyes upon the carpet. 'La, sir, I don't see an objection to the match,' she simpered. 'My family is perfectly respectable—'

'I know your background,' Heston snapped. 'You are penniless and your uncle is in trade.'

'The money cannot matter. Harry will have a handsome fortune when he comes of age.' The great blue eyes peeped up at him through long dark lashes. 'As to the trade. . .well. . .no one need find out. When Harry and I are wed, I shall not spread it abroad.'

'Strumpet! Make no mistake, ma'am, you shall not marry him.'

'Who is to stop me, sir? When Harry knows of your visit here, he may insist on an elopement.'

'Such a marriage would be annulled.'

'But think of the scandal, my lord! And then, you know, I might present his family with an heir.'

Heston did not mince his words. 'The child would be a bastard. Will you saddle yourself with a burden such as that for life? I ask you again. . .how much?'

'I could not think of such a sordid bargain,' Miranda said demurely. 'With every tender hope dashed, I might go into a decline. . . No amount of money would be of use to me if that should happen.'

'It might soothe your final moments, madam. They are like to be upon you more quickly than you realise if you do not stop this trifling.'

'Threats, sir? I might have known it!' Miranda raised a hand to her brow in one of Fanny's more theatrical gestures. 'Your reputation is not unknown to me, my lord. You are said to be the hardest of men, even in your dealing with the fair sex.'

'You may believe it. I have had dealings with your

sort before. Every harpy in the country converges upon London in the Season, hoping to entrap some innocent boy. This time you won't succeed.'

'No!' She favoured him with her sweetest smile. 'You are mistaken, sir. Harry's letters have made his sentiments clear. . .'

She heard a muttered curse. 'Letters, too? I wonder that the lad escaped his leading-strings. You have kept them all, I take it?'

'Naturally. How could I find it in my heart to part with them? Harry is so poetical. My eyes, so he says, are like the brightest stars in the heavens, and he compares my skin with that of the softest peach.'

She heard a snort of disgust.

'Hardly original, madam!'

'But most sincere!' Miranda peeped up at him again, and then wished that she had not done so. His face was dark with anger, and there was a strange glitter in his eyes. For a moment she wondered if she had gone too far, but his lordship's insults had made her reckless.

'We are wasting time,' he announced. 'Tell me what price you set upon your charms. Shall we say five thousand pounds?'

She managed a coquettish laugh. 'Does Lord Rudyard set so little store upon his family honour?'

She was unprepared for what happened next. Heston was out of his chair in a single lithe movement. Her chin was gripped in an iron hand and the harsh dark face came close to hers.

'Amazing!' he said softly. 'The face of an angel, and a heart as hard as that of any common doxy. Aye, you're a beauty, you little vixen. I suppose you must peddle your wares.'

Miranda struck out sharply and caught him full

across the face. The imprint of her fingers showed up
clearly on his cheek, but he merely laughed. She lifted
her hand again, but this time he caught her wrist with
such force that she gave a cry of pain.

'Temper!' he reproved. 'Let us not turn this interview
into a common brawl. You would have the worst of it,
I promise you. Now, madam, pray consider. Lakenham
is not the only catch in London. With money you might
buy a house in which you and your sister might.. .er. . .
entertain without the trouble of a husband.'

As the implications of this speech came home to her,
Miranda flushed to the roots of her hair. She reached
out blindly and caught up a heavy vase, but he was too
quick for her. The pressure of his fingers forced her to
put it down.

'Insulted, my dear? I had not supposed it possible.
Pray do not feel obliged to throw this delightful object.
Your uncle would find your behaviour somewhat
eccentric.'

'You are despicable,' Miranda cried. 'You came here
under false pretences. My uncle would never have
received you or allowed you to be alone with me had
he not believed that you intended to make me an offer.'

'Have I not just done so?' His face was bland as he
resumed his seat.

'You worm! You Corinthian! How dare you suggest
that way of life to my sister and myself? Words cannot
express what I should like to say to you.'

'True! The title of Corinthian is, you know, regarded
as a compliment. Perhaps your vocabulary is a little
lacking in force?' He was very much at his ease as he
lounged back in his chair.

Miranda longed to wipe the sneer from his lips. 'I
wonder that you did not make your offer to my uncle,'

she said in icy tones. 'You may regard him as a counter-
jumper, but he would soon have disabused you of the
idea that I am a—'

'A lightskirt?' he supplied helpfully. 'I had considered such a course, Miss Gaysford, but I had not
met you then. I decided to give you the benefit of the
doubt, not knowing if your uncle was aware of
Lakenham's entanglement. For all I knew, you might
have been some simple country miss who fancied
herself in love with him.'

'You do not think so now?' There was a dangerous
sparkle in her eyes.

'Not for a moment.' Again she heard the ugly laugh.
'It is more likely that you are all in this together. . .your
aunt. . .your uncle. . .and your sister.'

Miranda felt that she must explode with rage. How
she longed to crush him. . .to grind her heel into that
mocking face. She wanted to strike at him, to wound
him as he had wounded her. He would pay for these
insults, no matter what the cost.

'Silent, my dear? Am I to suppose you robbed of
speech? A temporary condition only, I feel sure. I am
prepared to give you a little time to consider my
proposition.'

He rose then and strolled over to the window,
apparently convinced that the outcome of this meeting
would be as he wished.

Miranda's mind was racing. She should have ordered
him out of the house, but she longed to pay him back
in his own coin. Yet how was she to do it? Oh, if she
could but see this proud and arrogant creature grovelling at her feet.

Suddenly, the solution flashed into her mind. It
would be dangerous, but it was worth it just to see him

squirm. For once this haughty member of the nobility would find himself at a loss. A little smile lifted the corners of her mouth, but when she looked at him her face was composed.

'You are mistaken, sir,' she told him. 'My aunt and uncle know nothing of this matter. They do not accompany us into Polite Society.'

'I had supposed as much.' Heston's sneer grew more apparent. 'I wondered how you got the entrée, but I supposed there are enough impoverished gentlefolk about to introduce you at a price.'

'Quite so! Alas, when one is of indifferent breeding, it is necessary to make shift as best one can.' Something in her voice made him eye her with suspicion, but her expression told him nothing. 'Only my sister knows of Harry's attachment to me.'

'Hmm! Well, that is of little consequence. You may change your mind, I suppose.'

'My sister will wonder at it. You were right in thinking that we are penniless, she and I, and it is true that our mama hopes that we shall marry well enough to restore the family fortunes.'

'That, at least, is honest,' he said grudgingly. 'Your ambitions are no worse than those of many another in the marriage market.'

'Oh, you do understand. I felt sure you would when I explained.' Any member of Miranda's family could have warned Lord Heston of the danger in that charming smile, but his lordship fell into the trap.

'I may have been a little hard on you,' he admitted. 'My remarks were not those of a gentleman, and for that I crave your pardon.'

'They are forgotten.' Miranda beamed at him. 'I could not take the money, sir, even had I wished to do

so. How might I have come into possession of such a
large sum?'

'I see that it might have been a problem.' He smiled
at her, and Miranda was satisfied. He would not smile
for long.

Heston resumed his seat. 'Give up Lakenham,' he
pleaded. 'With your beauty, half the men in London
will offer for your hand.'

Miranda dimpled. 'Are you referring to my starry
eyes and my peach-like skin, my lord?'

'Now you are making sport of me. Harry was a fool
to put his sentiments in writing. If these young sprigs
would learn to avoid the pen, much trouble might be
avoided.'

'How right you are! Perhaps the letters should be
burned. . .?'

'That would be generous, indeed! Now, I do not
mean to be offensive, but if you will oblige Lord
Rudyard in this matter you may consider me your
servant, ma'am. I will do my best to further your. . .
er. . .'

'My career?' she said innocently.

'I was about to say your ambitions. I am not without
influence—'

'Pray say no more!' Miranda waved his words aside
with an airy gesture. 'You have persuaded me. I shall
give up Harry Lakenham.'

He came to her then and raised her fingers to his
lips. His relief was apparent.

'I had hoped that you would see the good sense of
such a course,' he told her warmly. 'Harry will mourn
his loss for a time, but the young are resilient. I shall
invite him to my place in Warwickshire—'

'Before our wedding, my lord? There will not be much time.'

Heston frowned. 'Have you not this moment assured me that you will give him up?'

'I have, and I meant it. I was not speaking of Harry, my lord. I have decided to make you the happiest man alive... I accept your offer of marriage.' Modestly she kept her eyes upon her folded hands.

He was silent for so long that she thought he had misunderstood her. Then he spoke.

'I made you no such offer,' he said quietly.

'That is not my understanding, nor my uncle's. You said all that was proper to him, I believe, when you asked his permission to address me. I must suppose that you gave him some indication of your circumstances and went into the matter of a proper settlement?'

'I see that I have underestimated you, Miss Gaysford. In answer to your question, I did not explain my circumstances to your worthy relative. There seemed to be no need—'

'Of course not! How very stupid of me! Your wealth is common knowledge, is it not? How foolish I should be to pin my hopes upon a young man not yet in possession of his fortune when I might have the use of yours. I daresay you could buy and sell Lord Rudyard. Is that not correct?'

Heston bowed. 'There is one small point which you may have overlooked. How are you to coerce me into making you my bride, or is that an indelicate question? Will you tear your gown and accuse me of rape, or have you some other plan in mind?'

'There will be no need for such dramatics, sir. We

have made an excellent start. This household is at present agog to know the results of our tête-à-tête.'

'I see! I might have had second thoughts, upon reflection. Had you considered that?'

'You, my lord? I think not! You are known to be a man of firm resolution. Alas, so is my uncle. He is an Alderman, as you must know. I fear he would advise me to sue for breach of promise.'

Miranda felt a little breathless even as she spoke those hasty words. Heston had goaded her beyond endurance, and now she had gone much further than she had intended. She had hoped only to shatter his composure, to crack that icy mask of hauteur, and to pay him out for his offensive remarks. She felt a twinge of panic. To threaten such a man was the height of folly and she knew it. She waited for the explosion which must follow.

'Breach of promise? That would never do!' Somehow his calm words frightened her more than if he had shouted at her.

She looked up to find that he was smiling. It was more terrifying than anything she could have imagined. Though his lips were curved in a wolfish grin, there was no amusement in his eyes. They were as hard as stone. He reached out and pulled the bell-rope. Then he issued a swift order to the servant who came in answer to his summons.

'Ask Miss Gaysford's family to join us,' he said briefly. Then he strode over to Miranda and pulled her to her feet.

'So you would try a fall with me, would you? Don't say you haven't been warned. I'll teach you a lesson you won't forget. . .'

His arms slid about her and he kissed her with such

force that the breath was driven from her body. Miranda struggled wildly, but she was powerless against his strength. She clenched her teeth as he tried to force her lips apart, arching away from him until she thought her spine must crack.

He released her only as the door opened to admit her aunt, her uncle, and a startled Fanny.

Clamping her to his side with an arm that felt like a band of iron, he turned to face them.

'You may wish us happy,' he said pleasantly. 'May I present the future Lady Heston?'

Chapter Two

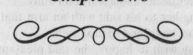

Amid the babel of congratulations, Miranda was conscious only of Fanny's stricken face. An imperceptible shake of her head brought her sister to her side. On the pretext of kissing her, Fanny drew her to the window-seat.

'Miranda, how could you?' she murmured brokenly. 'You know I cannot marry him.'

'Nor shall you! It is a fate I would not wish upon my worst enemy. Don't look so startled. I'll explain later.'

Her mouth was bruised and swollen, but she managed a crooked smile as Heston came towards them with two glasses of champagne. He accepted a third from a nearby servant and turned to Alderman Shere.

That gentleman advanced towards Miranda, his rubicund face glowing with pleasure. He took her hand and drew her to her feet. Then he raised his glass.

'To the betrothed couple! My dear young people, we wish you all the happiness in the world!'

Miranda swayed. This could not be happening. Events had moved with the speed of some dreadful nightmare from which she must awaken.

Then Heston slipped a hand beneath her elbow,

holding her upright by main force. 'Until tomorrow, dearest,' he said tenderly. 'Your uncle and I have much to discuss. . .settlements. . .the announcements in the morning papers. . .'

Miranda gazed at him in horror. He could not mean to continue with this farce. Her eyes pleaded with him to release her. . .to make some excuse. . .but his expression was impassive.

What had she done? She must have been mad to think that she could worst him. She felt that she had opened Pandora's box, only to let out all the evils in the world. She had put herself in Heston's power, and she could think of no way to escape.

'Dearest, you look a little pale,' he murmured with exaggerated concern. 'It is the excitement, I expect. I shall leave you in the care of your aunt. . .' He pressed a chaste kiss upon her cheek.

His lips seemed to burn her skin, but she did not flinch, although she longed to jerk her head away. Heston's smile was jovial as he took her uncle by the arm and left the room.

'My dear love, what a match for you!' Mrs Shere embraced her niece.

It was all too much. Miranda burst into tears.

'There. . .his lordship was quite right. How thoughtful he is! You are overwrought and it is not to be wondered at. The future Lady Heston? Your mama will be beside herself with joy. It is more than even she had hoped for you.'

Miranda could not speak, and her aunt began to look a little anxious. 'Will you not lie upon your bed for an hour or two? Perhaps a tisane. . .and a hot brick for your feet?'

'Thank you... I am being foolish, I expect, but I do feel a little strangely.' Miranda dabbed at her eyes.

Fanny, too, appeared to be suffering from shock. She put her arm about her sister's waist and hugged her.

'Let us go upstairs and then you may rest,' she said.

'What a pair you are!' Mrs Shere regarded her nieces with a benevolent eye. 'This is an occasion for rejoicing, not for tears. Ah, well, I know how close you are. You will not care to be separated, even by marriage. Off you go! I will send up your luncheon on a tray, and you shall not stir from your room until this evening.'

'Miranda, what has happened?' Fanny swung round upon her twin as soon as they were alone. 'I was never so shocked in all my life when I heard that you had accepted Heston. How could you betray me so?'

'I didn't,' Miranda told her dully. She ached all over and was convinced that when she slipped out of her gown her arms and shoulders would be black and blue. 'That brutal creature! He should be whipped at the cart's tail!'

'But...but...you are betrothed to him.'

'No, I am not,' Miranda snapped. 'He tricked me... at least I think he did. Oh, Fanny, I am so confused... I don't know what happened. I was hoping to frighten him, you see.'

Fanny gasped. 'You must be mad! What did you say to him? What have you done? You lost your temper, didn't you? When you fly into alt, you never guard your tongue!'

'Nor does he. If you must know, he did not come to make you an offer at all.'

'Then why did he ask to see me alone?'

'He came to buy you off. Harry has been to see his

grandfather, who will have nothing to say to the connection. Heston is Lord Rudyard's envoy, come to save his grandson from a fortune-hunting harpy who is tainted by the smell of trade.'

Fanny's face grew scarlet. 'Cruel!' she whispered in a failing voice. 'Has he persuaded my darling to give me up?'

'No, he has not.' The sight of her sister's distress fuelled Miranda's sense of outrage. 'You had best hear the whole of it, Fanny. You won't like it, but I feel you should know what Heston was about.'

Her recital was interrupted at frequent intervals by Fanny's moans and sobs. It was not until the letters were mentioned that she raised her head.

'There are no letters,' she wailed. 'Harry has never written to me. When he picks up a pen, he cannot think of anything to say.'

'It is of no importance. I offered to burn the letters in any case when I offered to give him up.'

'You did that? Then my life is over. . .' Fanny buried her head in the pillow and gave way to despair.

'At nineteen? Really, Fanny, where is your spirit? You cannot think I meant it?'

'Heston must have been delighted!'

'He was, but his delight lasted for no more than thirty seconds.'

'I don't understand you. How could that be?'

'His rapture was short-lived when I said that I would marry him instead—'

Fanny screamed. She was on the verge of a strong attack of hysterics, but Miranda held her hands.

'No, listen to me. I meant it only as a joke. Well, not perhaps a joke, but I could not bear his insults. I wanted to pay him back, to shock him out of his smug complacency.'

'Oh, do not say so! I cannot bear it. What folly to defy a man like that! He had not even offered for you. . .for me, I mean.'

'I pretended I thought he had. I even—'

'Even what? There cannot be more!'

'I'm afraid there is. I mentioned. . .er. . .an action for breach of promise.'

Fanny lay still. Her face was white to the lips. 'Then we are ruined. Have you no sense at all? Heston is the most ruthless creature alive. Have you not heard what is said of him? A threat is merely a challenge.'

'I know it now. It was a stupid thing to do, but I had no idea that he would take me at my word and move so fast. You were all in the room before I had time to think.'

'What did you expect?' Fanny's voice was bitter. 'Did you imagine that he would flee the house with his tail between his legs? You do not know him. He will be revenged on all of us. And when the announcement appears in the *Gazette*, Harry is sure to call him out.'

Miranda was dismayed. 'I hadn't considered that. Can you get a message to him?'

'What can I say? He will think me faithless. . .and all we needed was a little time.'

'Ask him to call this evening. If we can contrive to leave you alone, you could explain—'

'Explain what? That I am to marry a dotard?'

'Heston isn't exactly a dotard, Fanny. He can't be more than thirty, but that is beside the point. You are not going to marry him. Can Harry keep a secret? You might tell him what has happened.'

'Tell him the whole, you mean?' Fanny grew

thoughtful. Then her eyes began to sparkle. 'He would think it a famous jest, and it would throw Lord Heston off the scent. If only he may not discover that he is betrothed to the wrong person. When Harry comes of age in December he may do as he pleases. . .it would give us the time we need.'

'You must warn him to be careful. He must appear to be broken-hearted. Still, loving you as he does, he must wish only for your happiness.'

The twins exchanged a glance of pure mischief. Then Fanny's face clouded.

'What of you?' she asked. 'Can you support Lord Heston's company for a time?'

'I intend to do so. For the moment he believes that he holds the upper hand, but I shall find some way to crush his. . .his pretensions.'

Miranda had recovered her composure and now she began to dwell with pleasure upon the delightful prospect of seeing Lord Heston grovelling at her feet, begging for mercy.

Quite how this desirable state of affairs was to be achieved she had no idea, but she would think of something.

'Do be careful, dearest,' Fanny pleaded. 'You are so reckless when you fly into the boughs, and Heston is a dangerous man. There is a sort of black glitter about him. . .about his eyes, I mean.'

'His eyes are grey,' Miranda said shortly. 'He thinks himself a god, you know. A Corinthian, forsooth! What has that to say to anything? He may be a famous whip, and the idol of a pack of silly boys because he boxes at Gentleman Jackson's saloon, and can afford to buy his clothes from Schweitzer and Davidson. I have seen no evidence of honour or of a pleasing character in him.'

'That is what I mean. He is unscrupulous. Oh, love, I fear he means to harm you.'

'He won't do so,' Miranda told her stoutly. 'Now you must write to Harry without delay. Ellen will take it for you. There is not much time if you wish to avoid a duel.'

This terrifying thought was enough to send Fanny to her desk at once. When Ellen came up with a tray she was told to slip out with the message during the afternoon.

'I do feel hungry.' Miranda lifted the lid from a tureen of asparagus soup and began to serve her sister.

'I don't know how you can eat.' Fanny pushed her plate away. 'This is all such a tangle. Heston cannot mean to marry you.'

'Of course not! He intends to frighten me. Would he wed the niece of a mere Alderman. . .a nobody? His pride would not allow it. Well, he will learn. This nobody will prick the bubble of his conceit. These chicken patties are delicious. . .won't you try one?'

Fanny was persuaded to nibble at a little of the food and to take a glass of wine. Then, worn out by the events of the last few hours, she fell asleep.

Miranda took up her book, but she could not read. Heston's lightning reaction to her attempt to worst him had shaken her to the core of her being.

She drew a hand across her swollen mouth, as if by doing so she could wipe out the memory of that brutal kiss.

She had never been handled so roughly in her life. The man was a monster. He must have known that she was merely teasing him, but he had not spared her.

She slipped out of bed and walked over to the mirror. Dark bruises showed up clearly on her milky skin. He would be made to pay for each one of those marks, and pay in full.

She wondered if he would go ahead with his plan to announce the betrothal in the morning papers. If so, the world would take him for a fool if he mistook the name of his bride-to-be. Then she frowned. That solution would not serve at all. She and Fanny shared the same initials.

Fanny had been christened Melissa Frances, whilst she had been named Miranda Ferne. Not for the first time she wondered what had possessed their mother to indulge in such flights of fancy.

It could not be helped. Miss M. F. Gaysford might be either of them when the name appeared in the *Morning Post* and the *Gazette*.

In any case, it was important that Heston should continue to believe that he was betrothed to Fanny. She would play out this charade for the present. Meantime, Fanny might grow out of her infatuation with Harry Lakenham. That would be the ideal solution. Then she herself could cry off from her supposed engagement, and let the world believe that she had jilted Heston.

Even so, she felt dispirited. Nothing had worked out as she had hoped.

She and Fanny had been in transports when their uncle had offered them a Season. It was true that they had enjoyed the balls, the drums, the routs, visits to the Tower to see the King's Beasts, the Grand Firework Displays and the Balloon Ascents, yet not all the efforts of Lady Medlicott, the faded gentlewoman who was their chaperon, had served to produce the type of offer upon which their mama had set her heart.

If only Mrs Gaysford had not been so taken with the

story of those Gunning girls. The famous Irish beauties had taken London by storm more than fifty years earlier. Elizabeth Gunning had married the Duke of Hamilton, and Maria Gunning had become the bride of the Earl of Coventry. Mrs Gaysford could think of no reason why her own girls should not enjoy similar success.

Instead, Fanny had fallen in and out of love with a succession of young officers, dazzled by their splendid appearance in their regimentals, and not one of them a suitable match for her.

Her own heart had remained untouched. Such offers as had come their way had been from middle-aged worthies, warm enough in the pocket to overlook a lack of dowry, but scarcely calculated to arouse the interest of two lively nineteen-year-olds.

She laid aside her book as her aunt entered the room.

'That's better.' Mrs Shere looked with approval at Fanny's sleeping figure. 'Your sister will be more herself when she awakens. The excitement was too much for her, and it is not to be wondered at. Who could have supposed that Lord Heston would offer for her?'

Miranda managed a faint smile. 'It was surprising,' she agreed. 'Ma'am, may I ask you something?'

'What is it, my dear?'

'Would you object if Lord Lakenham were to speak to Fanny alone. . .that is, if he calls upon us?'

Mrs Shere looked mystified.

'The thing is that he has conceived a tender for Fanny. It is but calf-love, yet it would be kind if you could allow her to tell him herself of her betrothal.'

Miranda felt ashamed of herself. It was not at all the

thing to be deceiving this gentle woman who had been so kind to them.

'I don't know, Miranda. I cannot think that Lord Heston would agree to such an interview...' Mrs Shere was clearly troubled.

'Ma'am, he need not know. If Lakenham were to call, you would not turn him away?'

Mrs Shere smiled. 'You know your uncle better than that, my dear. No military man is ever refused admittance to this house. Shere is only too well aware of what we owe to Wellington's armies.'

Miranda kissed her aunt's cheek. 'How good you are,' she said warmly.

Her kiss was returned, and Mrs Shere patted her cheek. 'It will be your turn next,' she announced. 'Then how happy your mama will be. Your uncle has sent off to her already with the news, but Fanny must write too.'

'So soon?' Miranda was startled. Events were moving so fast that they were overtaking her.

'Of course, my love. She must not read it first in the *Gazette*. That would be most improper. We shall not make the announcement until she has given Fanny her blessing. You had best wake her. Were you not to go to the play tonight?'

'I think we should cry off,' Miranda told her. 'I doubt if Fanny will be up to it.'

'You are right. A quiet evening at home would be best. I will send a message to Lady Medlicott, and your uncle will be pleased. He wishes to speak to Fanny about arrangements for her marriage.'

Her parting words did nothing to reassure Miranda. She was becoming entangled in a web from which it was growing more and more difficult to free herself. At least she had ensured that Fanny would be at home if Harry came in answer to her summons.

Later that evening she and Fanny walked into the dining-room, dressed alike in pale blue muslin. Alderman Shere greeted them with a beaming smile.

'You are both in looks tonight,' he announced. 'Alike as two peas in a pod! I'm blessed if I know how Lord Heston could tell you one from the other.'

Miranda stiffened. It was merely one of their uncle's endearing jokes, but it was uncomfortably close to the truth.

'Well, well,' he continued. 'Come and sit you down. We have much to celebrate. Fanny, you are a lucky girl. I confess you might have knocked me down with a feather when his lordship called on me. The finest catch in London, and he has offered for you.'

Fanny's enchanting smile peeped out. She dimpled as he chucked her under the chin.

'That's a good girl,' he said approvingly. 'Those sparkling eyes tell me all I need to know. Swept off his feet, was he? My dear, I hope he will make you happy. I was a little worried at first, if the truth be known. I had heard him spoken of as high in the instep and a cold fish, but you have not found him so, I imagine.'

His eyes twinkled as a blush rose to Fanny's cheeks.

'Nay, I won't tease you further. Now you shall take a glass of wine.' He signalled to the footman and sat down.

Though not as wealthy as many of his friends, the Alderman kept a good table, and prided himself upon the excellence of his cook.

He made short work of a dish of mushroom fritters, followed by a slice or two of tongue braised in Madeira wine. This was followed by a serpent of mutton with green peas. A succulent pigeon pie was waved aside in favour of a curd pudding.

To Miranda, the meal seemed endless. She looked across at Fanny and frowned a warning. Her twin was trying without success to hide a feeling of suppressed excitement. Miranda hoped that her aunt and uncle would put it down to the supposed betrothal.

She took a little of the delicately flavoured Floating Island pudding. It was one of her favourites, but tonight she found it tasteless. She sighed with relief when Mrs Shere withdrew, leaving the Alderman to his port.

'Aunt, the drawing-room feels so warm. May I open the windows?'

'Certainly, my dear. On a night like this we shall not take a chill.'

Miranda threw open the long French doors and walked on to the terrace with Fanny by her side.

'Will Harry come tonight?' she murmured in an undertone.

Fanny nodded. 'He told Ellen that he would. Oh, this is famous!'

'Is it? I don't like to deceive our aunt and uncle.'

Fanny pouted. 'You haven't changed your mind already? You will go ahead with our plan?'

'I won't fail you,' Miranda said with some asperity. 'There is the door-knocker. It must be Harry.'

As Fanny disappeared into the drawing-room, Miranda pressed her fingers to her burning cheeks. What on earth was she to do?

For a moment she was tempted to make a clean breast of the whole, in spite of her promise to her sister. Yet it could serve no useful purpose. Reproaches would be heaped upon the twins from their mama, to say nothing of the humiliation which must fall upon her relatives. She was forced to admit it. . .she was caught in a trap of her own making.

When the door opened to admit Harry Lakenham and his friend, John Helmsley, both girls made their curtsies. Then Miranda walked over to the spinet. 'Aunt, shall I play for you?' she asked.

'Would you dearest? That would be pleasant, and if Mr Helmsley would be kind enough to turn the music for you. . .? Lord Lakenham, I fear I am sitting in a draught. Might I ask you to close the window a little? Fanny will explain the catch.'

Miranda threw her aunt a look of gratitude as Fanny and her lover moved out to the terrace. They were gone for so long that Mrs Shere grew agitated.

Miranda looked up at John Helmsley. 'Will you forgive me, sir?' she said. 'I am a little tired tonight.'

She closed the instrument and walked towards the window. As she peered into the night she caught a glimpse of Fanny's gown, pale against the darkness of the shrubbery. Harry Lakenham and her sister were locked in each other's arms.

Miranda walked towards them. 'Are you quite mad?' she hissed. 'You will ruin everything.'

Harry seized her hand and kissed it. 'Thank you!' he said in fervent tones. 'You have saved us!'

'I shall not be able to do so if you continue to behave so foolishly. For heaven's sake, take care, my lord. Don't forget that you have your part to play in this.'

Miranda grasped Fanny's arm and led her sister back indoors. They were followed by Harry who was striving to give the appearance of a rejected lover.

'Dear boy!' Mrs Shere said fondly. 'You will not

desert us, even though Fanny is to wed? You are always welcome here, you know.'

Harry sighed, but his eyes were dancing, and Miranda took him to task at once.

'Do you take your leave,' she urged in an aside. 'You look like the cat with its paw in a pot of cream.'

Obediently he signalled to John Helmsley and they moved towards the door. There he blew her a kiss behind her aunt's back, laughing as she frowned at him.

'Have I missed our guests?' The Alderman walked through from the dining-room. 'You should have called me, wife.'

'They could not stay, my love.'

The Alderman beckoned Fanny to his side. 'Lord Heston agrees that we must wait to hear from your mama before the announcement appears, but the world will learn of your good fortune before the week is out. Don't trouble your head about settlements and so forth. I have undertaken to discuss those with him. You will not find him ungenerous, I believe.'

Fanny nodded as he beamed at her. Then he settled himself more comfortably in his chair, legs planted firmly apart, with his plump little hands resting on his knees.

'There is one other thing,' he continued. 'You are not to trouble your head about the cost of bride-clothes and the other female fripperies which you'll need. Those shall be my gift to you. We shall send you off in style.'

Fanny looked uncomfortable, but she murmured her thanks and kissed him, colouring as she did so.

'No need to be embarrassed about it,' he told her kindly. 'I could wish I might do more, but sadly, dowries are beyond my means—'

'Sir, you have been more than generous,' Miranda broke in swiftly. 'You have your own boys to consider. Is not George to transfer from a line regiment?'

Her uncle nodded. 'I must set up Frederick, too, when he is done with Oxford. . .'

'You must be very proud of them.'

'Aye! I want to give them a better start than I had myself.' He looked across at her aunt. 'Still, we haven't done so badly, Emma, have we?' A look of affection passed between them, and Miranda sprang up to kiss them both.

How unjust it was of Heston to sneer at these good people. They were more honourable than he would ever be. Her determination to humiliate him grew even stronger as she looked at their two lined faces.

She said as much to Fanny when they were alone.

'I hope you know what you are about,' her twin said doubtfully. 'Harry was delighted. He says that Heston needs a set-down, but I cannot help but fear for you. I wish that you may not get yourself into a scrape.'

Miranda stared at her in disbelief. 'I am already in a scrape,' she cried. 'I should never have agreed to take your place.'

'Thank heavens you did so. Had Heston insulted me as he did you, I should have fainted on the spot. I did not tell Harry the whole of it, but he was already planning an elopement.'

'Fanny, you would not! Think of the scandal. . .the disgrace! It would break Mama's heart, and my uncle would blame himself for not taking better care of you.'

'Well, it need not come to that if you will but keep Heston occupied.' Fanny drew her bedgown over her head and began to tie the ribbons of her nightcap. 'He must not know the truth until we are safely wed, so do take care not to betray yourself.'

'Heston cannot wish for my company,' Miranda said with decision. 'I doubt if he would consider it amusing to take me about.' In that she was mistaken.

Both girls were sitting by the window on the following morning when a high-perch phaeton drew up at their door. Heston threw the reins to his tiger, and ran lightly up the steps.

Miranda felt sick with apprehension, but apart from her heightened colour there was little to betray that emotion when Heston was shown into the room.

She took her sister's hand as they rose to greet him. She and her twin were dressed alike in white sprigged muslin with blue ribands in their hair. This was the test. Would he be able to tell them apart?

To her astonishment, he did not hesitate. He strode straight towards her and took her hand.

'My love!' he uttered in throbbing accents. 'An hour apart from you seems like a lifetime. . .' He drew her to him, kissed her fingers, and pressed a chaste salute upon her cheek.

She longed to free herself, but with Mrs Shere's indulgent eyes upon her she was forced to submit to his caresses.

'Make haste, my love,' her aunt urged gently. 'If Lord Heston hopes to take you for a drive, he will not wish to keep his horses standing.'

'Quite right, ma'am!' Heston bowed to indicate his pleasure at her understanding. 'Sadly, the phaeton is unsuitable for more than one passenger, but you have no objection to my taking your niece to the Park?'

'Of course not! We have promised ourselves a shopping trip to Bond Street.' She glanced at Fanny. 'You will enjoy that, will you not, my dear?'

Fanny's smile of agreement was unconvincing. She had nothing to say either to her aunt or to Lord Heston.

'Miss Gaysford, have you seen the Elgin Marbles? They are very fine, I assure you. Perhaps on another occasion you may care to accompany us to the British Museum?'

Fanny murmured an inarticulate reply, which caused her aunt to stare, but she was saved from further embarrassment when Miranda reappeared.

'Charming! Quite charming!' His lordship put up his quizzing-glass to inspect the neat little figure who stood before him. 'How well that shade of bronze becomes you! The bonnet, too! It is quite a triumph! I shall be the envy of every man in town.'

'You are too kind, my lord.' Miranda gritted out the words through clenched teeth, feeling rather as if she were a slave on sale in an Arab market.

'Not at all! My words come from the heart!' With a bow to the two ladies, Heston gripped her elbow and ushered her from the room.

He handed Miranda up into the phaeton, and dismissed his tiger. 'I shall not need you, Jem.'

Miranda was at a loss to account for the astonishment on the lad's face, but Heston did not appear to notice it. He took the reins and turned the splendid pair of chestnuts south in the direction of Piccadilly.

That thoroughfare was crowded, but, as Miranda soon realised, his lordship was capable of driving to an inch. With careless ease he avoided the press of hackney carriages, a stately landaulet, and a smart barouche.

He stopped for a crossing-sweeper, moved on and then was forced to swerve as a curricle, clearly in

inexperienced hands, shot out from the southern end
of Bond Street.

Heston did not hesitate. He was past the plunging
horses in an instant as Miranda gasped.

'My apologies, ma'am. I trust I did not frighten you.
The town is overfull with the arrival of the Allies for
the Gala Celebrations.'

'You did not,' Miranda told him with more dignity
than truth. Her knuckles were white as she gripped the
side of the vehicle.

'Liar!' he said smoothly.

'Did you seek my company merely to insult me?'
Miranda's face was pale. The day was warm and the
stench in the streets was overpowering. She began to
wish that she had provided herself with a nosegay to
counteract the vile odours, but she had not done so.
The near-collision had disturbed her, and suddenly she
felt sick.

'You will feel better when we reach the Park,'
Heston predicted. 'London can be trying on a hot day.
Bear up, my dear. When we are settled in
Warwickshire, I shall not insist that you come to town
again.'

'Warwickshire?' Miranda was perplexed.

'My country seat. Had you forgot? With your children about you, you will not yearn for the pleasures of
the capital.'

'My children?'

'Naturally. Why do you look surprised? I am hoping
for a full quiver, as the saying goes. At least four boys
and perhaps a girl or two. I won't promise to keep you
company in the Season, but you will not mind that.'

Miranda eyed him with acute dislike.

Chapter Three

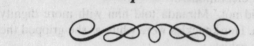

'My love, must you give me dagger-looks?' Heston continued smoothly. 'Have I said something to offend you?'

Miranda did not answer him.

'Lost your tongue? You surprise me! Yesterday you had so much to say. Must I crave your pardon for being so indelicate as to mention the main purpose of our marriage? I had not thought your sensibilities quite so nice. You are not, I must hope, of a frigid disposition?'

'No, I am not! How dare you speak of such things to me?' Miranda cried hotly.

'There must be no misunderstanding between husband and wife.' Heston's tone was sententious. 'The physical side is, after all, an important part of marriage.' He looked down at her then, assessing her from head to toe, and Miranda flushed to the roots of her hair, feeling naked beneath his gaze.

'There! I have put you to the blush. How unforgivable of me!' With a cynical grin his lordship drove his phaeton into Hyde Park. 'Do you think you could manage a smile or two, my dear? My friends must not be led to believe that we have quarrelled at this early stage in our relationship.'

Miranda tried to compose herself. Anger threatened to overwhelm her, but her voice was calm as she replied, 'I shall play my part, my lord.'

'Of course you will, and very prettily, too.' Heston bowed and smiled as he slowed the horses to a walking pace, and threaded his way past other carriages.

Thankful to find his attention diverted from herself, Miranda looked about her. She was not too green to realise that the passers-by included the cream of Polite Society. She saw a look of surprise on several faces, and wondered why everyone was staring so. She was not long kept in ignorance.

A cavalier reined in beside them and swept off his hat.

'Adam, you sly dog! I might have known. . .'

'Might have known what?' his lordship answered mildly.

'That you are not the misogynist we suspected. Here you are, with the loveliest girl in London—'

'Ah, yes. May I present my cousin to you, my dear? This is Thomas Frant.'

Miranda was disarmed by the cheerful smile with which the young man greeted her. He was short and stocky, but he had a pleasant open face. A dusting of freckles across his snub nose emphasised a pair of bright blue eyes.

Miranda gave him her hand.

'I won't say I'm surprised,' Thomas told her gaily. 'Who could resist you, ma'am?'

'Who, indeed? My love, you have made yet another conquest.' Heston gathered up the reins and prepared to move on, apparently oblivious of the effect of his tender words upon his cousin.

Thomas caught him by the arm. 'Adam, you ain't thrown the handkerchief at last?' he said in awed tones.

'You may believe it!' Heston replied. 'As you said yourself, my dear Thomas, who could resist such beauty?' He gazed down fondly at Miranda as he spoke.

'Good God, Adam!' Thomas was brought to his senses by the cool expression in his cousin's eyes. 'Beg pardon, ma'am. I meant no offence. . .but Adam ain't in the petticoat line, not as a rule, I mean.'

'You have said quite enough. In confidence, Thomas, Miss Gayford and I are recently betrothed. You will keep it to yourself for the moment. . .?'

'Of course! Of course!' Thomas was so astonished that he grabbed sharply at his reins, causing his mount to jib. 'Not a word! You may rely on me.' He moved away.

'I hope we may,' Miranda said in scathing tones. 'Did we not agree, my lord, that no one was to know of our betrothal, until my mother had been informed?'

'You feel she may object? Oh dear, I hope not. You see, Thomas, charming though he is, is possibly the worst gabster in London. He is incapable of keeping a secret.'

'You knew that, and yet you told him?'

'A lamentable oversight on my part. . .due, perhaps, to my longing to acquaint the world of our happiness. Will you forgive me, dearest?'

Miranda's anger threatened to overcome her. Heston was taunting her, utterly sure of himself. He would soon learn that he had met his match.

'Of course!' She smiled up at him. 'I am so happy to know that you care nothing for the opinion of the *ton*.'

Heston raised an eyebrow. 'Would you care to explain yourself?'

'I was thinking only of the possible consequences to you, of such a connection, sir. I'm sure you understand me. The betrothal of such a notable Corinthian as yourself to a mere nobody, moreover one who is related to a cit? I fear it may have a sad effect on your position in society.'

Heston laughed aloud. 'If you believe that, you will believe anything. My credit will survive the worst *mésalliance*. I am known to be eccentric, and I do as I please, as I hope to prove to you.'

Miranda turned her head away. Yet again this unpleasant creature had managed to have the last word. She was still fuming when they were hailed by a well-known voice.

'Lakenham, by all that's holy!' Heston drew his carriage to a halt. 'How are you, my dear boy? What a surprise to find you here! I had not thought that you rose till noon.'

'I could not sleep.' Viscount Lakenham was much in danger of overacting, Miranda thought to herself. She wished him elsewhere with fervour as he looked at her with a mournful expression.

The boy was a fool, and Heston must be sure to see through his pretence of abject despair. She stole a fleeting glance at her companion, to find him all concern.

'Liverish this morning, are you?' Heston said cheerfully. 'Take my advice, my lad, and change your wine merchant.'

Lakenham threw him an angry look and was about to address Miranda.

'No, you shall not delay us,' Heston protested. 'Miss Gaysford finds the heat oppressive. I have promised to take her home. My regards to your mother.' He whipped up his horses and left the Park by the West Gate.

'Harry looks somewhat subdued,' he remarked idly as they rejoined the traffic in Piccadilly.

'Are you surprised, my lord?'

'I had not thought to see him so dejected merely because you are in my company. You have not found his jealousy excessive?'

'Sir, he knows the truth. My aunt allowed me to tell him of our. . .of our betrothal.'

'You assured me yesterday that she was unaware of Harry's infatuation.'

'She was. . .but my sister explained to her that it was but calf-love, scarce worth a mention. We. . . I thought it best that he should learn the news from me.'

'Hoping to save his skin, my dear? You may be easy in your mind. I shall not allow him to call me out. In any case, I doubt if he would be so foolish.'

'You are a marksman too, Lord Heston? How very splendid! You put all my acquaintance in the shade. . .'

'Ah, yes, but then your acquaintance is not large, and, dare I say it, a little questionable?'

Miranda did not rise to the bait, though it took a supreme effort not to do so. She gave him an innocent look, thinking as she did so that if she were a man she would have called him out herself for that remark.

'Quite so!' she murmured. 'But now that I am to rise in the world, your friends will be mine, I trust. It can

only be an improvement.' Her tone left him in no doubt
that she did not think so for a moment.

To her fury he laughed again.

'Well done!' he said. 'A palpable hit, my dear. I must
learn not to lead with my chin when sparring with you.'

Miranda did not trouble to reply. Instead, she gazed
at the passing scene which never failed to fascinate her.
Piemen shouting their wares, flower-sellers and a group
of quarrelling jarveys striking out at the beggars who
barred their way, all contrasted sharply with the
fashionable exquisites who lounged along the pave-
ments. Women dressed in the height of fashion lounged
in their barouches, accompanied in many cases by their
beaux, riding alongside.

Heston was hailed again and again, and Miranda
found herself subjected to many a hard stare, both
from the occupants of the carriages and their
companions.

'You seem to be creating something of a stir today,
my lord,' she murmured wickedly.

'I cannot claim the credit for that. Much of it is due
to you. Did I not say that every man in London must
envy me? Think what a furore you will arouse at the
play tonight.'

'I do not intend to visit the play this evening,' she
told him stiffly.

'No? What a disappointment for your sister and your
aunt! They were looking forward to it.'

'You asked my aunt?' Miranda was astonished. She
had not supposed that Lord Heston would care to be
seen with someone so far beneath him in status.

'Naturally. . .and your uncle, too. You must not think
me lacking in courtesy, my dearest. Sadly the Alderman

has another engagement, but your aunt felt free to accept my invitation.'

Miranda's mouth set in a mutinous line.

'I do not care to go.'

'But you will, my dear, you will. That is, unless you decide to plead the headache. That would be unworthy of you. I had not supposed you capable of cowardice.'

Miranda's eyes flashed and her chin went up, but they had arrived at their destination, and she had no opportunity to utter the angry words which sprang to her lips.

Heston handed his reins to the groom who came down the steps towards them and handed Miranda down from the phaeton with great solicitude.

'Until tonight, then?' Oblivious of the passers-by he saluted her with a tender kiss upon her cheek and sprang back into the carriage.

Miranda stalked indoors without a backward glance, to find that Fanny and Mrs Shere had returned from their shopping expedition. The hall was littered with bandboxes and parcels.

'Did you enjoy your drive, my dear?' Mrs Shere did not wait for an answer. 'We have been so busy you would scarce believe it! Pray come upstairs and see what we have bought for you. How fortunate that you and your sister are the same size and colouring. What becomes one of you must suit the other. . .'

Still chattering, she led the girls upstairs.

'See now, is this not delightful?' She held up a gown of sea-green gauze over an underslip of satin.

'It looks expensive,' Miranda said doubtfully.

'It was, but your uncle will not care for that. He is not a penny-pincher, and we must consider what is due to Lord Heston.' She began to rifle through the other boxes, drawing out filmy undergarments, long kid gloves, silk stockings and handkerchiefs trimmed with Valenciennes lace.

Fanny was in raptures when she found herself the proud possessor of a matching gown. She flung her arms about her aunt and kissed her.

'There, it is little enough, my dear girl. It will cheer you up, I hope, and your uncle likes to see you dressed alike. You both look so charmingly together. . .'

Miranda tried to smile, but such generosity served only to depress her spirits further. She longed to end the deception, but she could not find the courage to do so.

Fanny was quick to sense her mood.

'Was it very bad?' she asked when Mrs Shere had left them. 'Surely Heston did not continue to insult you?'

'What makes you suppose that he will give up now? His lordship is enjoying himself, knowing that I cannot escape.'

'Harry said that he had seen you. We met him in Bond Street.'

'Fanny, you must speak to him. He should not have sought us out. You are fond of telling me that Heston is a dotard, but he is far from being feeble-minded, I assure you. Harry's manner was such as to make him question me later, and should he ever suspect that we have changed places. . .'

'Harry thought he gave a very good performance as a rejected lover,' Fanny said defensively.

'Perhaps he should be on the stage! It would be better if he returned to his grandfather for a time. He is sure to give us away.'

'No, I won't be parted from him!'

'Very well, but you must both be more discreet. You can't be seen together. Lord Heston intends that Harry shall sever all connection with our family. It won't serve if he thinks that you are now the object of his attentions.'

'I suppose I may meet him in company?' Fanny sulked.

'If you do so, pray take care! Last evening, for example, if anyone but myself had found you in the garden, all would have been lost. I won't go on with this charade if you don't play your part.'

'I thought you wanted to punish Heston.'

'I do, but you must help me. The insults were addressed to you, you know.'

'Oh, very well!' Fanny dismissed the matter from her mind, and began to peacock round the room with a shawl of Norwich silk thrown about her shoulders.

'There is another thing,' Miranda added quietly. 'I cannot like all this expense. Uncle cannot well afford it.'

'Of course he can! Did he not insist? And Aunt Emma enjoyed herself so much this morning. She tells me that she has always longed for a daughter. I don't see how you can stop her.'

'We might mention that Mama would wish to be consulted.'

Fanny stared. 'Have you written to her?'

'I have not,' Miranda said with a heavy heart. 'I don't know what to say.'

'Well, Uncle will think it strange of you. You might mention that Heston has offered, and that you hope for her blessing. You may be sure it will be given. Nothing could be more certain.'

'And what then?'

'Why ask me? You were so set on getting back at Heston. Surely you have some plan?'

'I have not, and well you know it. As far as I can tell I am simply getting deeper into the mire.'

'You'll think of something,' Fanny told her comfortably. 'After all, you always do. We have been in scrapes before and you have got us out of them.'

Miranda was not attending. 'Fanny, don't you find it strange that Heston never mistakes us one for the other?' she said thoughtfully. 'He came to me at once this morning.'

'Nor does Harry,' her sister replied. 'Have we not always found it so in men who care for us? Oh, I see what you mean. . .' Fanny looked startled.

'Exactly so! Heston must be the exception. Do you suppose that he can have noticed the mole behind my ear? It is the only difference.'

'He must have done. He seems to see everything. I must confess he frightens me. His eyes are so penetrating. . .they seem to look into my mind.'

'I hope you are wrong. I would not have him know what is in my mind.'

'Let us forget him,' Fanny cried impatiently. 'Shall we wear our new gowns tonight?'

'That is Aunt's intention, I believe.'

'She was pleased to be included in the invitation. She refused at first, you know, but Lord Heston can be most persuasive. He insisted. . .'

'And why not, pray? The world may consider that Aunt Emma married beneath her, but her birth, like our own, is unexceptionable.'

Fanny began to giggle. 'I love you when you get upon your high ropes, dearest. Have you told Lord Heston of our worthy connections?'

'No, I have not!' Miranda snapped. 'I intend to make him squirm. Let us see if he can carry off this affront to his consequence.'

She looked at her sister and dimpled. 'If I thought that Aunt Emma would permit it, I should try to look as vulgar as possible, with plumes, and feathers, and gauds. I should even paint my face. . .'

'Miranda, you wouldn't?' Fanny was shocked. 'Aunt would send you to wash it off.'

'I know.' It was with regret that Miranda abandoned the idea. 'But Heston need not think that he will find me biddable, hanging upon his every word as if it were. . .were the laws of the Medes and Persians. . .'

'I expect he has never heard of the Medes and Persians and nor have I. What have they to do with anything?'

'Nothing, love. Let us go down. We shall be late for luncheon.'

She was thoughtful as she toyed with a dish of buttered eggs, and took so little of a proffered platter of cold meats and salad that her aunt was moved to protest.

'My dear, this will not do! If you go on in this way you will be naught but skin and bone, and that will not please his lordship.'

Obediently, Miranda allowed herself to be helped to another slice of beef from the sirloin, and forced herself to take a little of the Celerata cream which followed.

At last Mrs Shere rose from the table, announcing that she planned to rest for an hour or two, and indicating that the twins should follow her example.

'But, Aunt, we intended to go to Richardson's, to change our library books,' said Fanny. 'That is, if you have no objection.'

'Very well, but you shall take the carriage, and Ellen must go with you. Now do not dawdle about, my dears. I believe that you should lie upon your beds for at least an hour before you dress this evening.'

Both girls kissed her and went upstairs to put on their bonnets.

'I could wish that Aunt did not treat us as a couple of dowagers,' Fanny grumbled. 'Where is the harm in walking on such a pleasant day?'

'I expect she was thinking only of our comfort. In any case, it will give you more time to find another of those dreadful Gothic romances.' Miranda's eyes twinkled. Fanny's passion for romantic fiction had made her the butt of their elder brother's jokes for years.

She was too preoccupied with her own search for something to read to pay much attention to Fanny when they reached the library. She had taken out much of the stock already, including *Evelina* by Fanny Burney, and the works of Samuel Richardson. Her eye fell upon a copy of *Tom Jones*, but then she decided against it. Aunt might not approve. The book was considered too explicit to be thought suitable reading for an unmarried girl, even though the author, Mr Fielding, was a magistrate.

Poetry? No, she was no admirer of Lord Byron, though his works were all the rage. *Ivanhoe* looked promising, and there could be no objection to any of the works of Sir Walter Scott. She would lose herself in the story, and it would help her to forget her present troubles.

'I will take this,' she said decisively. 'Have you found anything, Fanny?'

There was no reply. Fanny had disappeared. Miranda was untroubled, thinking that her sister had wandered into another part of the shop. Then she saw Ellen. Their abigail was standing by a deep recess and her furtive expression warned Miranda that something was amiss.

As she approached she heard the murmur of voices. Anger threatened to consume her as she recognised that of Harry Lakenham.

'You may wait in the carriage, Ellen,' she said sharply. As their maid scurried away, Miranda walked towards the lovers.

They were standing in the shadows, oblivious of all about them. Harry's arm was about her sister's waist and her head was resting on his shoulder.

'I see now why you were so anxious to change your library book, Fanny. When did you make this assignation?' Miranda's tone was so cold that Fanny fired up at once.

'It is not an assignation,' she cried hotly.

'What else would you call a clandestine meeting? Did I not beg you most particularly to take care?'

'It is all my fault,' Harry intervened. 'I persuaded Fanny when we met this morning. Do not be cross with her. It is I who deserve your censure.'

Miranda ignored him. 'You had best return to the carriage, Fanny, but before you go I have something to say to both of you. If Lord Lakenham appears at the play tonight, I shall not help you further.'

'You would go back upon your word?' Fanny stared at her in consternation.

'You have not kept yours. I mean it, Fanny. I will put an end to this ridiculous charade.'

Pausing only at the counter to record the loan of her book, she marched out of the shop.

Aware of the coachman on the box, Miranda did not trust herself to say more until they reached the privacy of their bedchamber. Then she swung round upon her twin.

'How could you deceive me so?' she demanded. 'Have you no sense at all? Suppose Lord Heston had seen you?'

'There was no danger of that.' Fanny's face was sullen. 'Harry said that he was gone to Tattersall's to look at bloodstock. You do not suppose that he spends his time in libraries, do you?'

'I have no idea how he spends his time, nor do I care, but he is not blind. You know how gossip travels among the *ton*. Any of his friends might have seen the pair of you together.'

'It was unlikely,' Fanny protested. 'Harry is no reader, nor are his friends. . .'

'Then how strange that he should enter a library. . .it must give rise to comment.'

'Suppose it did? I am supposed to be you. Heston could not take exception. . .'

Miranda eyed her twin in disbelief. 'You think not? Heston would no more countenance a match with you than with me.'

'He can't forbid a mere friendship. Harry might have sought me out to comfort him for his loss. . .'

'And we all know what that can lead to. You put me out of all patience with you. I meant what I said. If Harry appears tonight, you may say goodbye to all your hopes.'

'He won't,' Fanny sulked. 'You made it clear that he must not, though I do not see how you can stop him.'

'You don't? I could cry off from this supposed engagement, Fanny, having mistaken my own heart. It happens every day, and it must come to that in the end.'

'Not yet, I beg of you!' Fanny began to whimper. 'I will be good, you'll see.'

'Very well, but don't be such a watering-pot.' Miranda looked at the clock. 'I shall take Aunt's advice and rest for an hour. You had best do the same. I suppose you had no time to choose another book?'

In silence Fanny held out *The Mysteries of Udolpho* for her sister's inspection.

Miranda smiled. 'That will do very well,' she said. 'Better to frighten yourself with that than with thoughts of Heston's anger if he should discover how we have deceived him.' She picked up her own book and was soon deep in the story.

Before she knew it, it was time to dress and not all her worries could quite destroy her pleasure in her new gown. It was a perfect fit, and over the slender column of the under-dress the pale green gauze whispered softly to the ground, caught at the bosom with matching ribbons.

She gazed at the mirror-image of herself as Fanny twisted and turned before the glass.

'Have you ever seen anything so beautiful?' Fanny whispered reverently. 'We have never worn anything so expensive!'

Miranda grimaced. 'We did not pay for the gowns, I must remind you.'

'I know it, but may we not enjoy our finery just for tonight? Oh, if Harry could but see me now. . .'

'You must pray that he does not,' her sister told her

sternly. She frowned at Fanny and was about to repeat her warning when Mrs Shere came to find them.

'Why, Aunt, how fine you are this evening!' Fanny caught the older woman by the shoulders and turned her round. 'You will put us in the shade. . .'

Mrs Shere shook her head in a disclaimer, though she was pleased. Her dark grey silk was trimmed at the neck with rows of French lace, and she carried a shawl of the same material. The garment was beautifully cut, and it did much to disguise the outlines of her ample figure.

'Nonsense, my dear, you are too kind. I admit that, before we married, your mama and I were used to have a fondness for the latest modes, but I have grown stout, I fear.'

'No, ma'am, Fa—my sister does not exaggerate.' Miranda caught herself before she made a fatal slip. 'You look charmingly. . .that gown is so becoming. . .'

She felt that she was babbling in fright. She had come so close to giving herself away. Would Aunt Emma notice?

'Well, we owe it to Lord Heston to appear at our best,' Mrs Shere told her. 'Most certainly he cannot find fault with either of you, my dears. I have not seen you look so well before. The gowns were a good choice, were they not?'

'They were.' Miranda kissed her warmly. 'I hope that our uncle will be pleased with the results of his generosity.'

'He is gone out to dine,' her aunt announced. 'Lord Heston invited him, you know, but he felt that he owed it to his lordship's consequence to refuse. I was a little undecided on my own account, but Heston insisted.'

'And why should he not?' Miranda cried. 'We may

not be of noble birth, not persons of consequence, but
we have some pretensions to gentility, and our family
is respectable.'

'Of course, my love! You must not think me insen-
sible of our connections, though my family has cast me
off...'

'More fool them!' Miranda cried inelegantly. 'There
are no better people alive than you and my uncle...
To spurn you just because you married for love...? It
is past all bearing.'

'It is an old story, and we shall think no more about
it at this present time,' Mrs Shere said firmly. 'Now, my
dears, we must go down. We have not allowed ourselves much time to dine, and Lord Heston will be here
at eight.'

Again Miranda felt slight panic, but she crushed it
firmly. Why should she be afraid of Heston? The
afternoon had given her time for reflection, and all that
was necessary was to treat him with the civility due to
his position. Sadly, he had the most unfortunate habit
of throwing her off balance with a word or the lift of
an eyebrow. His spurious tenderness in the company of
others was hateful to her. She knew his true opinion of
her character.

He might have made a fortune on the boards, she
thought scornfully. His acting rivalled that of Edmund
Kean.

When he arrived she looked at him askance, though
honesty compelled her to admit that no fault could be
found with his appearance. He was dressed *de rigueur*
in a black swallow-tailed coat and satin knee-breeches
with silk stockings. A splendid waistcoat of watered
silk softened the severity of his garb, but apparently he

had no other modish leanings. The bosom of his shirt was unadorned by a frill.

Miranda stiffened as he bent to salute her cheek. She turned away, but he stayed her with a hand upon her arm.

'My darling, this betrothal gift is unworthy of your beauty, but I beg that you will accept it.' He handed her a long flat box.

Miranda did not attempt to open it, so he took it from her and threw back the lid to reveal a fine string of perfectly matched pearls.

Mrs Shere gasped and Fanny's eyes grew round.

'I trust the necklace pleases you,' his lordship murmured. 'Will you wear it tonight?'

Miranda looked at the gleaming pearls. Their sheen was such that they seemed like living things, sending her a warning.

Chapter Four

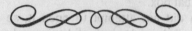

Miranda closed the lid of the box with a snap.

'My lord, you are most generous,' she said smoothly. 'But I cannot wear the pearls. We are not yet officially betrothed. My mama has not given her consent.'

'Dearest, you must not refine too much upon the matter.' Mrs Shere looked startled. 'Nothing is more certain than that she will give you her blessing. . .'

'Even so. . .' Miranda would not be swayed.

'Try them at least,' his lordship pleaded. 'Here, let me clasp them about your neck.' He caught up the necklace and led her to a mirror, turning her to face it, his hands resting lightly on her shoulders.

'There!' He fastened the clasp, his fingers lingering upon her skin.

Miranda flushed as she looked at his dark face beside her own. Although his hands were cool they seemed to burn her flesh. She shuddered. There was a curious expression in his heavy-lidded eyes, and it turned her knees to water. She caught her breath.

'Very pretty!' To her relief her voice sounded calm. 'Another time perhaps, my lord?'

'As you wish, my dear.' Heston returned the pearls to their box and laid it on the sofa-table.

He did not speak to her again until they reached the theatre, reserving his attention for her aunt. That lady answered him politely, but she was quick to admonish Miranda when his lordship spoke to Fanny, careful of her comfort as he led her to a seat with a good view of the stage.

'Dearest, that was not well done of you to refuse to wear his lordship's gift.' Mrs Shere sounded reproachful as she drew Miranda aside.

'I'm sorry, Aunt, but I could not think it right. It must have given rise to comment, and all eyes are upon us as it is.'

Miranda spoke no more than the truth. The appearance of the twins with their aunt in Lord Heston's box had resulted in a buzz of speculation from all parts of the theatre. They were the cynosure of all eyes, and she felt ready to sink with embarrassment as lorgnettes were raised and quizzing glasses levelled in their direction.

Lord Heston seated himself beside her. In her opinion he was much too close, and for one awful moment she thought he intended to lay a casual arm along the back of her chair. Surely he could not be so lost to all sense of propriety?

'My darling, I trust that you are perfectly comfortable?' he enquired in a solicitous tone, which did not deceive her for a second.

A sharp retort rose to Miranda's lips, but she bit back the angry words, aware that her aunt must overhear her.

Heston smiled, knowing that he could taunt her with impunity, and that she was powerless to reply.

She turned her attention to the stage, but later she could recall neither the title of the piece, nor the names of the players. The presence of the man beside her filled her mind to the exclusion of all else. What had she done?

It was all very well to promise herself that she would pay him back for all his insults, but his reaction to her attempt to worst him had been both swift and unexpected.

What could he hope to gain by taking her at her word? She stole a glance at him to find his eyes upon her. His sardonic gaze held her own and she felt her colour rising.

'Puzzled, my dear?' he said gently.

'Not at all, my lord. The piece has a simple plot.' She pretended to misunderstand him, but she saw the flash of white teeth in the semi-darkness as he laughed.

'Has it? You must tell me about it later. . .it is not perfectly clear to me.' He lapsed into silence once more, leaving Miranda to her own thoughts.

They were not pleasant. Not for the first time she felt a stab of panic. Matters had gone much further than she had intended. It had not occurred to her that Heston would be so quick to call her bluff, but who could have supposed that this haughty creature would insist on a betrothal, however false his intentions? And then to appear with her in public, and to offer distinguishing attention to her sister and her aunt? It was not to be borne, but for the moment she could see no way to extricate herself from her predicament.

During the interval, her composure was severely tried as Heston's friends descended upon the box. Miranda knew one or two of them by sight, and also by reputation, but neither she nor her sister had been introduced to them.

His lordship was quick to remedy the omission, and Miranda found herself the subject of a number of speculative glances, especially from the ladies.

'Is she Heston's latest flirt, do you suppose?' The play was about to resume, and Miranda heard the careless words as the door to the box was closing.

Fiery colour stained her cheeks, and she felt ready to sink with embarrassment. The reply did nothing to restore her composure.

'What else? Heston isn't the marrying kind, and even he would not present a bird of paradise to you, my dear.'

Miranda pressed her hands to her burning face. Thankfully, Heston was speaking to her aunt and had not heard the muttered exchange.

'Forgive me, ma'am, but are you quite well? May I bring you a glass of wine?'

Miranda looked up to find that she was being addressed by a gentleman in a military uniform which she did not recognise. There was a slight but attractive foreign accent in his voice.

Realising that she had been too preoccupied to notice him earlier in the press of introduction, she bent her gaze upon him, striving in vain to remember his name.

The young man brought his heels together and bowed.

'Alexei Toumanov at your service, Miss Gaysford. You may not have caught my name. I am with the Tsar of Russia's entourage. May I be of service to you?' A pair of gentle brown eyes looked down at her with an expression of concern.

'You are very kind, but it is nothing,' Miranda said quickly. 'I found the heat a little oppressive, that is all, Count Toumanov.' She sipped gratefully at the proffered glass of wine, thankful that she had at least remembered his title.

As the curtain went up once more, he slipped into a chair beside her after a questioning look at Heston.

His lordship chuckled. 'Alexei, you are a complete hand. Was it your intention to usurp my place?'

'Not at all, my dear Adam, though you did invite me to join you.'

'So I did! Now, was it a mistake, I wonder?' Heston threw a pointed look at Miranda, which she ignored.

She found herself wondering at their obvious friendship. It was clear that the two men were on easy terms, and it puzzled her. In the Count's presence Heston had dropped his supercilious manner, and for the first time she saw something of his charm.

As the play resumed he stopped his banter and took a chair behind her, slightly to her left.

Miranda felt indignant. Did he intend to spy upon her? The look he had given her when he found the Count beside her had spoken volumes. Did he imagine that she intended to try her wiles upon his friend? It was apparent that she was not to be allowed to indulge in any conversation which he might not hear.

During the next interval she was glad to have the opportunity to confound him.

'Do you ladies care to walk about the corridor?' the Count enquired. 'I believe that you would find it cooler there...'

Miranda rose at once and laid her hand upon his arm. With a mischievous smile at Heston the Count took Fanny upon his other side and left the box.

Mrs Shere had no opportunity to do more than look a little dismayed, for Heston was drawing back her chair and offering to escort her.

The crush in the passageway was excessive, but the Count was quick to lead them to a seat in a deserted alcove from where they were able to watch the fashionable crowd about them.

'I doubt if I have ever seen so many people,' Fanny exclaimed. 'Where have they all come from?'

'Many are foreigners, as I am myself,' Count Toumanov explained. 'The Allies intend to celebrate their victory over Napoleon in extravagant style. It is a little hard upon the inhabitants of this city.'

'Oh, no, they will enjoy it, Count. There is not a seat to be had along the processional route, you know.' Miranda gave him her enchanting smile.

'But you, at least, will see it, will you not? I cannot believe that Heston has not made arrangements.'

'He has not told us of them,' Miranda said demurely.

'Then you must allow me. There will be no difficulty, I assure you.'

'Quite unnecessary, Alexei!' Heston had come up to them with Mrs Shere upon his arm. 'You have spoilt my surprise, you villain!'

Unperturbed by Heston's reproof, the Count grinned at him. 'You will not blame me for trying, Adam?'

'Not at all, but you will have enough to do, my friend, upon the great occasion. We shall look down upon you from the comfort of our seats as you clatter along behind your master's carriage. I shall feel for you, of course. It cannot be comfortable to wear all your finery for any length of time.'

'You are speaking to a man of iron, my dear sir.

Later I hope to dance the night away. Ladies, may I beg that you will partner me?'

Fanny was thrown into confusion. 'I do not know, Count Toumanov.'

'As yet our plans are undecided,' Miranda broke in firmly.

'Then I must beg Adam to decide them for you.' The Count's enthusiasm was infectious. 'Come, Adam, what do you say? May we not make up a party?'

'I see that I shall have no choice,' his lordship murmured. 'Leave it with me, and I shall get in touch with you.'

With that the irrepressible Alexei had to be contented. With great good humour he led the ladies back to their box and stayed with them until the play was over.

'You are well acquainted with the Count, my lord?' Mrs Shere enquired as the carriage took them home.

'A boyhood friend, ma'am. We lived in Russia for some time. My father was attached to the Tsar's court.'

'I see.' Mrs Shere looked thoughtful, but she did not pursue the subject, although Miranda suspected that she was disturbed by the young man's evident admiration for the twins.

Her suspicions were confirmed when Mrs Shere made a point of leaving her alone with Heston when they reached the house.

Fanny was inclined to linger by her sister's side, unwilling to abandon her to his lordship's less-than-tender mercies, but Mrs Shere would have none of it. She took Fanny by the hand and led her from the room.

'Well, my dear, another triumph for you! Count Toumanov was smitten to the heart.' Heston gave

Miranda a lazy look. 'I wish you might have heard his raptures when we were alone. . .something about eyes that a man could drown in. . . He cannot decide if they are blue or violet.'

Miranda gave him an angry look.

'He was right, of course,' his lordship continued. 'For my own part, I am sure that they are violet. They darken when you are furious, did you know it? A pity that Alexei cannot see beneath that innocent appearance to the heart beneath.'

'I wonder that you dared to expose him to my evil influence,' Miranda retorted.

'I intend to dare much more than that.' Heston moved to stand in front of her. 'Now, my love, may I claim what is due to your prospective husband?'

Before she could protest he caught her to his chest and his mouth came down on hers. Miranda felt a dizzying sensation. His lips were soft, warm, and most insistent as they found her own.

She had vowed earlier that if he ever tried to kiss her again she would not struggle. Her strength was useless against his own, and she had no wish to find herself once more covered in bruises. She let herself grow limp and unresponsive in his arms.

Heston held her away from him. 'New tactics?' he said in a soft voice. 'They will not serve, my dear. Let us try again. . .' He picked her up and carried her to a sofa. 'I see that you demand finesse.'

Miranda found herself upon his knee. 'The servants. . .' she gasped. 'Have you no sense of propriety, sir?'

'None whatever,' he said equably. He lifted her hand to his lips, turned it over and kissed the palm. Then his mouth travelled upwards along the inside of her arm.

Miranda found the butterfly kisses strangely disturbing, and a new sensation possessed her as he began to caress the back of her neck with the fingers of one hand.

'Please!' She tried to push him away.

'Please what? You must tell me how to delight you, dearest.'

To Miranda's horror his hand travelled from her waist until it cupped her breast. She tried to strike out at him and found herself helpless as both her wrists were gripped.

'No, no, my little termagant!' he reproved. 'Pray do not struggle. To enjoy love, it is necessary to relax.'

'Love?' she spat at him. 'You call this love? How dare you insult me so? I might be no better than one of those creatures who were peddling their wares at the Opera House tonight!'

'You recognised them, did you? It was only to be expected. Tell me, my dear, how do their ambitions differ from your own?'

Miranda looked at the mocking face. If he kissed her again, she would bite through his upper lip. Sadly, he seemed to have no such intention. He set her upon her feet, and rose to take his leave.

'A word of warning, Miss Gaysford! Count Toumanov is not for you. In future, I must beg of you to save your charms for me.'

He was gone before she could reply, but her anger knew no bounds.

Her temper was not improved when she was confronted by her aunt. Mrs Shere took one look at her face, and tried to heal the breach.

'You could not expect Lord Heston to be pleased, my love,' she murmured. 'Count Toumanov was most particular in his attentions. It was not wise to encourage him.'

'I did not encourage him,' Miranda snapped. 'Heston invited him. You would not expect me to be less than civil to his friend.'

'There are degrees of civility, dearest, and the young man seems volatile. . .'

'He was very kind to me and, Aunt, I am not yet betrothed, whatever you may think.'

'Very well, I shall not interfere, but do take care. This is a splendid match for you. You must do nothing to overturn it.'

Miranda kissed her aunt goodnight and sought the sanctuary of her bedchamber. There she found Fanny waiting for her.

'What is Heston about?' her twin demanded. 'Did you see aunt Emma's face when she saw the pearls? They must be worth a fortune!'

Miranda glared at her. 'Do you suppose their cost would weigh with him? Doubtless he hands out similar trinkets to his lightskirts every week.'

'That is hardly fair,' her sister protested. 'I have never seen him in the company of a woman, and nor have you. That is why our appearance in his box tonight created such a stir.'

'Of course we have not seen him with a woman. The type of female he prefers would hardly be thought suitable to hang upon his arm at the Opera.'

'You mean. . .you think he is a libertine? Oh, love, that can't be true. He is thought to be a cold fish.'

'I assure you he is not.' The colour rose to Miranda's cheeks. 'And if he had kissed you you would know it.'

'Oh, dear! I had not thought that he would press his attentions on you in that way. . .'

'Why not? He intends to punish me for daring to stand up to him. What better way than to take advantage of the fact that we are supposed to be betrothed?'

'That is not the action of a gentleman.'

'Great heavens, Fanny, what kind of person do you suppose that we are dealing with? Heston is under the impression that he can walk on water, and I intend to disabuse him of that idea.'

'You are grown very hard,' Fanny ventured.

'Is it surprising? Heston would bring out the worst in anyone. He misses no opportunity to give me a setdown. Do you know that he actually warned me... warned me not to encourage Count Toumanov?'

'But, love, the Count was very attentive to you.'

'To both of us, Fanny, and he meant no harm. It was a pleasure to speak to such a gentle and entertaining person. There was no need to keep up one's guard, as I am forced to do with Heston.'

'It would be hard to find two people less alike than his lordship and the Count,' her twin agreed. 'Their friendship is surprising.'

'Monsters are few and far between, thank goodness! There cannot be another such as Heston. Beside him anyone must seem charming.'

'But he did give you the pearls, Miranda. Why would he do that if he dislikes you so?'

'It was simply another attempt to put me out of countenance. To frighten me, he will carry this deception as far as he dare go.'

Fanny hesitated, twisting her handkerchief between her fingers. 'And how far will he go?'

She looked so pale that Miranda stared at her.

'What do you mean?'

'I am afraid of him,' Fanny said simply. Slow tears

rolled down her cheeks. 'Do you think that he intends to marry you? I could not bear it.'

Miranda went to sit beside her and slipped an arm about her sister's waist. 'What nonsense!' she said in a rallying tone. 'Would his lordship wed a nonentity? He would not give the idea a moment's consideration. Oh, I know he thinks his position unassailable, but he would not care for the humiliation. He has no such thought in mind. In any case, not even he could marry without his bride's consent.'

'I hope you may be right.' Fanny dabbed at her eyes. 'But I fear you are mistaken in him. He does not care for the opinion of the world, else he would not have spoken to Uncle, or agreed to the announcement being made.'

'There is that, of course.' Miranda looked thoughtful. 'But he thinks himself safe enough. He knows that I shall cry off, but I shan't do it yet. This is a test of nerves, my love, and I intend to win it.'

Fanny shuddered. 'Heston is playing some deep game, I know it. Suppose you have misjudged him? He must intend to marry before he is much older. . .there is the question of an heir, you know. For all we are aware, he may decide to wed you simply for that purpose.'

'Stuff!' Miranda was out of all patience. 'Have I not explained that he cannot force me into marriage?'

'He thinks that he need not do so. Does he not believe that you want a title and his fortune? How will he guess that you plan to cry off?'

Miranda felt dismayed as the truth of her sister's words came home to her, but she forced herself to smile.

'He must intend to cry off himself, possibly at the

last moment. Come, Fanny, in your wildest dreams you can't think that he would care to wed me. Mutual dislike is no basis for marriage. His life would be hell, and he must know it.'

'So would yours,' her sister said dolefully. 'He could shut you away in the country, and I should never see you again.' She began to wail.

'For heaven's sake, do stop!' Miranda cried. 'What would you have me do? Am I to confess the whole and take the consequences?'

Fanny raised her head. She looked shamefaced. 'I'm sorry,' she murmured. 'I must suppose that you know what you are doing, and Harry and I are so grateful for your help. Perhaps it will all work out as you would wish.'

'Of course it will! Now, Fanny, we must go to bed. It's very late and I have no wish to look hagged tomorrow. Heston must not think that he is robbing me of my sleep.'

It was a sensible suggestion, but sleep did not come as easily as Miranda hoped. Fanny's words had disturbed her more than she would admit, and it was not only her sister's remark about being shut away in the country, which echoed Heston's threats, made earlier in the day.

What was it Fanny had said? Something about his lordship playing a deep game? Try as she might she could not guess what it might be. Fanny must surely be mistaken, and yet a tiny doubt remained.

What had started as a simple hoax had now turned into something very different, and not only her sister and herself were involved in it. Their mama, their aunt and uncle, Harry Lakenham and Heston himself were all entangled in the deception.

Miranda's face burned. She could never lift her head again when the truth came out. She must have been mad to let matters go so far, but it was no use repining or wishing the events of the last few days undone. There was no going back. The only time she might have told the truth was at the end of that first ugly interview with Heston, and that would have put the cat among the pigeons with a vengeance.

She must go on, but how was she to support this dreadful farce for what might be several months? Her only hope lay in Fanny's volatile temperament. Fickle in her affections, it was more than likely that her twin would discover a passion for someone who pleased her more than Lakenham, before that young man attained his majority.

London was crowded for the coming celebrations, and Heston had made it clear that they were to mingle in the highest circles. Surely there was someone who might take her sister's fancy. With that hopeful thought, Miranda fell asleep.

The following day she was tempted to plead exhaustion as a means of keeping to her room, but Heston's taunt of cowardice had stung. He should never be allowed to think that of her. She dressed quickly and accompanied Fanny to the breakfast-room.

As she sat down she cast an anxious look at the pile of letters beside her uncle's plate. It was only when he had finished reading them that she allowed herself a sigh of relief.

'Uncle, is there nothing from Mama?' she murmured.

'Nay, love, we cannot hope for an answer yet. It is too soon, but do not be fretting yourself. Your match

with Heston must be all that she has hoped for. . .more,
in fact. You will have her blessing, I am sure of it.'

Miranda gave him a feeble smile, feeling relieved
that she was to be spared from the announcement for
one more day. Her hopes were not to be realised. Later
that morning her uncle burst into the room, with a
young man close behind him. He was waving a missive,
and as she looked at him her heart sank. His beaming
face confirmed her worst fears.

'There now! You may set your mind at rest, my dear.
Here is your mother's letter, brought to us by your
brother's friend.'

Miranda nodded to Richard Young, wishing him still
in Yorkshire. He was a neighbour and she knew him
well, but what was he doing in London? It was sheer
bad luck that he had been on hand to act as her
mother's messenger.

'How kind!' The irony in her tone was not lost upon
her twin and Fanny threw Miranda a warning glance as
she moved to greet their visitor.

'It was indeed! Very civil, sir, I must admit,' said
Alderman Shere. 'Now you shall meet my wife, and
you will join us, I hope, for luncheon?'

Richard blushed, but he was easily persuaded. He
came towards Miranda and handed her another billet.

'This one is for you, Miss Gaysford.' He looked from
one twin to the other, an anxious frown upon his face.
'I have it right, I hope?'

'Thank you, Richard.' Miranda held out her hand for
the letter. It was not mere courtesy which stopped her
from begging leave to read it there and then. She could
guess what it contained, and the thought of her
mother's inevitable raptures filled her with despair.

Her aunt was quick to urge her not to stand on

ceremony. 'Mr Richard Young will excuse us if your uncle tells us what your mother has to say. He must be in her confidence already.' She smiled and nodded at the young man. 'We are so excited, my dear sir. Who could have hoped for such a match for Fanny?'

Richard smiled and bowed. 'Ma'am, you are right. Mrs Gaysford is delighted for her daughter.'

All eyes were on Miranda as she opened the letter. The single sheet of paper was covered on both sides with her mother's untidy scrawl, but she could not make out a word of it. The letter had been crossed and re-crossed so many times that it was indecipherable. Mrs Gaysford must have written it with the intention of sending it by the mails.

'I'm sorry, but it is a little difficult to read.' She handed it to her uncle, who raised his eyebrows and gave it to her aunt.

'Now isn't that just like Letty?' Mrs Shere exclaimed. 'She was hoping to save you money, George. What does she say to you?'

The Alderman's eyes twinkled. 'Mine was written in less haste. Shall I read it to you?'

They sat in silence as he began to do so. Mrs Gaysford had been so overcome by the prospect of her elder daughter's brilliant match that the page was filled with superlatives. Her tears of happiness had blotted out several words, but he was able to assure Miranda that all the blessings in the world were called down upon her head.

Miranda squirmed inwardly, and her dismay increased tenfold when Lord Heston was announced.

'My lord, we have splendid news for you!' The Alderman hastened to greet him. 'We have heard from my sister-in-law, who sends you every good wish for your future happiness. She has given her consent to your betrothal.'

'Splendid news indeed!' Heston gripped the older man's hand, but his eyes were on Miranda's face. In their grey depths she detected a look of triumph. It was no more than the impression of a moment. Then he turned as Richard Young was introduced to him.

'My dear sir, we have much to thank you for. We had not hoped for such an early reply. My darling, your cup of happiness must be full.' With an outstretched hand, he drew Miranda to his side.

As his lean fingers gripped her own, Miranda longed to draw away. He sensed it, and his grasp tightened.

'At last!' he murmured tenderly. 'Now the announcement may be made, and the world shall know of our joy.'

Chapter Five

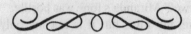

Miranda coloured and her uncle began to tease her. He could not know that her rosy blush was due to anger rather than embarrassment. As Heston slipped an arm about her waist, kissing her hand before saluting her cheek, her rage increased.

'Now, now, there is no cause to be shy, my girl! We all understand his lordship's feelings, and we'll have no ceremony here. You will join us for luncheon, my lord? Quite informal, you know, and Mr Young is to join us.'

'Sadly, I have another engagement,' Heston told him smoothly. 'I came merely to ask if Miss Gaysford will drive with me this afternoon?'

There was no way that Miranda could refuse, though she threw a desperate glance at Fanny.

'Aunt, were we not to drive along the processional route to the Guildhall?' Fanny broke in swiftly.

Mrs Shere looked startled. 'No, no, you are mistaken. I cannot recall that I mentioned such a thing. . .'

'Nevertheless, it is a splendid idea! Perhaps the Elgin marbles first, and a drive through the city later? You will all accompany us, I hope.'

'My lord, you cannot wish for such a large party on

your drive?' Mrs Shere shook her head, but she was pleased.

Heston chuckled. 'You are all consideration, ma'am, but lovers do not expect always to be alone—that is, until they are married.'

'Then, if you are sure. . .?'

'Did you not tell me that your phaeton takes no more than two?' Miranda's tone was hostile.

'Very true, my love, but it is not my only carriage. You will be comfortable in the barouche.'

Miranda did not argue further. Naturally, Heston would have more than one carriage. Most probably he has six, she thought bitterly.

'Shall we say four o'clock, then?' Heston was all courtesy as he consulted Mrs Shere.

Mrs Shere smiled her assent, but when he had gone she drew Miranda aside.

'My dear, you must try to be a little more amenable. Gentlemen prefer to see a smiling face, you know. Now I do not mean to scold. Let us go in to luncheon.'

The reproof was gentle but Miranda felt disturbed. She had allowed her dislike of Heston to betray her into incivility. More worrying than that was her mother's swift acceptance of her supposed betrothal. She groaned inwardly, yet what else had she expected? A feeling of depression seized her, but she forced herself to take part in the conversation of the others, hoping that her low spirits would pass unnoticed.

As always her aunt had provided an excellent meal. Conscious of Mrs Shere's anxious scrutiny she took a little of the asparagus in butter sauce, and a slice or two of a fine York ham.

As one course followed another, she pushed the food

about her plate, hiding it as best she could beneath an Italian salad.

Fanny was chattering happily to Richard Young, and from their conversation Miranda learned that her mother and her brothers and sisters were in good health, and looking forward to her marriage.

'Shall you be wed in Yorkshire?' Richard asked. 'Your mother wishes to know.'

'I have no idea,' Miranda told him helplessly.

'Of course not!' The Alderman broke in at once. 'How could that be? Lord Heston will wish the ceremony to take place in London, as befits his consequence. My sister-in-law will come to us, together with her family.'

'We have not yet decided on a date,' Miranda faltered.

'If I don't misjudge his lordship, it will be sooner rather than later.' Alderman Shere gave his niece a mischievous smile. 'Heston is head over heels in love with you, my dear, and he does not strike me as a man who is prepared to wait for his happiness.'

Miranda felt an uncomfortable churning in the pit of her stomach. 'There is no hurry,' she protested.

'Perhaps not for you, my dear child, but gentlemen have different ideas...' He left it there, but her aunt was not so tactful.

When the meal was over and Richard Young had left them she came into the drawing-room. A glance sent Fanny hurrying away.

'Now, dearest, I must speak to you,' Mrs Shere said firmly. 'You have surprised me. One might think that you did not care to fix Lord Heston's interest. The match is not distasteful to you, is it?'

Miranda hesitated. She longed to tell her aunt of her

deception, but the words would not come. She shook her head.

'Very well, then. You know us well enough, I hope, to believe that we should not wish you to engage yourself to someone you dislike. Is that not so?'

Too stricken to speak, Miranda nodded.

'My dear, you are very young, and you have led a sheltered life in Yorkshire. I doubt if you understand the full extent of your good fortune. Heston is the finest catch in London...' She paused as Miranda frowned.

'Well, perhaps that is an unfortunate expression. I should not wish you to think me mercenary, dearest, but the comfort of a fortune is not to be denied.'

Miranda looked at her with swimming eyes.

'There now, you shall not be distressed, but we must face the facts. Consider your mama, my love. She was cast off by her family, as I was myself, for marrying beneath her.'

'Papa was not beneath her. He was a scholar...'

'Of course, but he had no money. I was more fortunate. George is comfortable, if not wealthy. However, that is not what I intended to say. Do you not see that if you do not go on with this betrothal...if you were so foolish as to give Lord Heston a dislike of you...well then...you would face a second Season?'

'We could not ask that of uncle,' Miranda muttered.

'He would do it gladly, but it rarely serves. There is a certain stigma attached to young women who do not "take", as the saying goes. Too many hopeful maidens are keen to step into their shoes.'

Miranda felt unable to reply.

'Well, there it is.' A comforting arm stole about Miranda's shoulders. 'Do not take my words amiss, my child. I think only of your happiness, and I would a thousand times see you shy rather than unbecomingly bold, but perhaps you should be a little kinder to his lordship.'

Miranda promised to do her best. She dressed with care that afternoon, in an effort to please her aunt.

When Heston arrived she greeted him with every appearance of pleasure which, though assumed, caused him to regard her with suspicion.

She dimpled at him, realising suddenly that to play the part of a loving bride-to-be would baffle him more than covert hostility. If he could play the fond lover, so could she. She would beat him at his own game.

As they drove towards Bloomsbury, Miranda hung upon his lordship's every word, simpering and smiling in what she hoped was a perfect imitation of a shy but excited maiden charmed by the attentions of her lover.

Fanny's face was a study in perplexity, but Mrs Shere looked with approval at Miranda, pleased to think that her words of censure had been heeded.

With the easy address of a man of fashion Heston drew both Fanny and her aunt into conversation. He seemed to know everyone of note in London, including the Prince Regent.

'Have you visited Carlton House?' he asked.

Miranda suspected him of offering them a setdown. He knew as well as she did that an invitation from the Prince would be unlikely to reach the home of Alderman Shere.

'Alas, we do not move in such exalted circles,' she said demurely. 'Nor have we been to Almack's.'

It was an effort to forestall what she imagined would

be his next question, and she would not have her aunt distressed.

Mrs Shere had suffered a bitter disappointment when she was informed that not even Lady Medlicott could obtain the coveted vouchers for her nieces. The high-born Patronesses of that august establishment had not looked kindly upon the hopes of her penniless relations, without even a title to recommend them.

'You haven't missed much,' Heston said indifferently. 'It's a barn of a place without a shred of comfort. Why everyone flocks to King Street to eat stale bread and butter and drink orgeat and lemonade, I can't imagine.'

Mrs Shere could have told him. Almack's was the recognised marriage mart for members of the *haut ton*. Lord Heston might despise it, but for lesser mortals the possession of an entry voucher was prized more than gold. Those unfortunates who were excluded might only consider themselves upon the fringes of society.

'Is it true that they dance only country dances?' Fanny murmured.

'They are moving with the times at last,' his lordship said with heavy irony. 'Quadrilles and waltzes have been approved, so I understand.'

'But that would not affect you, my lord.' Miranda gave him her most enchanting smile. 'You do not dance, I think?'

The heavy-lidded eyes looked down at her, and then his harsh face softened into an expression of what she recognised as spurious tenderness.

'Dearest, I could be persuaded to waltz,' he told her in a sentimental tone. 'The thought of holding you in my arms. . .'

'La, sir, you will put me to the blush.' Miranda

opened her fan and hid behind it. 'We are not alone.'
She was careful to avoid Fanny's eye.

It was not until they were standing amidst the
statuary brought from Greece a few years earlier that
Fanny managed a word alone with her.

'Sister, what are you about?' she asked. 'You are so
unlike yourself that even Aunt must notice, and as for
Heston. . .'

'I'm trying to annoy him,' Miranda chuckled. 'At
least he is confused.'

'So am I. You will give him a strange impression,
and Aunt must wonder at your odd behaviour.'

'Aunt will be pleased. She told me only this morning
that I should be more. . .er. . .forthcoming.'

'Oh, you make me so cross!'

'Do I, love? You must try to bear it. I'd planned to
spray myself with the cheapest, most obnoxious per-
fume I could find, but sadly there wasn't anything
suitable in the house.'

Fanny threw up her eyes to heaven and went to join
the others.

Heston was pointing out the features of the sculp-
tures to her aunt, and in spite of herself Miranda was
drawn to listen to his story of the difficulties involved
in bringing them to England.

'And they were shipwrecked, do you say? Lord Elgin
must have been distraught. We heard that he gave an
enormous sum for them.'

'Something in the region of seventy-four thousand
pounds, ma'am, but look at the craftsmanship. These
wine-bearers are from the north frieze of the Parthenon
in Athens. They are the work of Pheidias.'

Miranda was enthralled as they strolled from one
group of figures to another.

'They are very fine, are they not?'

She had moved away from the others, and was startled to find that Heston was beside her.

'They are quite wonderful,' she breathed. 'The marble almost looks like living flesh, and see how the draperies flow about the figures. Pheidias must have been the finest sculptor in the world.'

'They are not all his work, so it is believed.' The grey eyes gave her a penetrating glance. 'Other splendid artists worked upon the Parthenon and the temple of Nike Apteros, but their names are lost to us.'

'It seems such a pity that they should have been torn away from their original sites. . .'

'You think it wanton destruction?'

She nodded.

'So do I.' For once the mocking note was absent from his voice. 'But since we have them here, we must make the most of the pleasure that they give us. There is some talk of buying them for the nation.'

'Will that happen, do you suppose? I do hope so. At least they would be preserved.'

'I am happy to hear that you approve.' His eyes were warm as he looked at her, and Miranda gave him an answering smile before she remembered that she was acting out of character for the part which she intended to play.

'La, sir, I can have no opinion on the subject,' she simpered.

Heston took her arm and led her behind an enormous group of charioteers.

'Let us have no more of that,' he chided softly. 'You are so much more entrancing when you are yourself, Miss Gaysford. For a time you had me believing that your mother's blessing had brought about a change of heart, but I realise that it is not so.'

Miranda crimsoned, too mortified to answer him, and furious when she heard a low laugh.

'A good try, but unconvincing,' he announced. 'To play a part successfully, one must be consistent.'

'As you would know, my lord.'

'You think I am playing a part,' he said in mock surprise. 'Dearest, my heart is at your feet. . .'

She was spared the need to answer when Fanny came to find them.

'Aunt is a little tired of standing, Lord Heston. She is sorry. . .'

'Not at all! It is I who should apologise. I have been remiss in not considering the length of time we have been here.' He went at once to order the barouche.

'Shall you wish to go directly home, ma'am?' he asked when they were seated in the carriage. 'We may take our drive on another day, you know.'

'No, no, I would not spoil your pleasure for the world,' Mrs Shere protested. 'It is just that my feet are inclined to swell. . .' She paused, uncomfortably aware that the great Lord Heston could have no possible interest in her complaints.

'That can be a trial, ma'am. My own mother suffered in a similar way. She found that lying flat, with her feet raised at an angle, was of the greatest help to her.'

Miranda was astounded. Clearly there was an unsuspected side to his lordship's character. She could not have supposed it possible that he could be so kind in his concern for her aunt. She was forced to admit that his sympathy was unfeigned. What a mystery he was. This man who was said to have no interests other than in horses and in gaming had also surprised her that day with his love of art, and his knowledge of history.

As they drove through the Park, she was conscious once again of the unwelcome interest of the fashionable exquisites who strolled along the footpath arm in arm. Other carriages slowed at their approach and she saw avid curiosity on the faces of their occupants. She shrank back into one corner of the barouche, praying that the ordeal would soon be over.

'I have never before seen such crowds in London,' Mrs Shere said brightly. 'But it was only to be expected. The end of the war with France is certainly a cause for celebration.'

'Let us hope that the celebrations are not premature, ma'am.' Heston's face was grim.

'What can you mean, my lord?' Miranda was startled into speech. 'Napoleon has abdicated and is in exile.'

'On Elba?' Heston laughed. 'If you suppose that the man who has conquered most of Europe will relinquish power so easily, you are more of an optimist than I.'

'But what can he do? He was stripped of everything. His titles, his possessions, his armies. . .'

'The man is a genius. . .a magician, if you like. He was an idol to his men. He has only to land in France again, and the Little Corporal will have an army at his back.'

'Pray do not say so!' Mrs Shere grew pale. 'My eldest son is with Wellington, my lord. I could not bear to think of him in danger yet again.'

'Aunt, it will not come to that.' Miranda threw an angry look at Heston. 'Napoleon is well guarded. How could he escape?'

Her words of comfort cheered her aunt a little and

she began to draw Fanny's attention to the passing parade of fashion. Miranda seized the opportunity to speak to Heston.

'Pray do not frighten my aunt with your ridiculous notions,' she said in a cool tone. 'How could you be so tactless?'

He gave her a penetrating look in which there was more than a hint of sadness.

'Tactless, perhaps,' he said in a quiet voice, 'but the notion of an escape is not ridiculous, my dear. Elba is close to the southern coast of France, and the Emperor still has many adherents. For twenty years, as you know, he was accounted the saviour of his country.'

'I can't think why,' she retorted sharply. 'Unless it is considered admirable to lose so many men in battle.'

'Have you forgotten the Napoleonic Code?'

'No, I have not.' Miranda was about to launch into a spirited discussion when she caught her aunt's eye and subsided.

'An interesting subject,' Heston observed. 'Perhaps we might continue with it later?'

Miranda nodded, though the look of astonishment on Mrs Shere's face was mingled with disapproval. In her view, ladies left all discussions of political matters to their menfolk, who were so much better able to understand them.

It was some comfort to think that Heston had not patronised her. He had not told her not to bother her pretty head about such things, which was the usual reaction from the gentlemen she knew. But then, he was no gentleman. Her lips curved in a tiny smile. For once she found herself in charity with him. He had seemed to be quite interested in her point of view.

* * *

This did not save her from another lecture from her aunt later that day.

'My dear, I did not like to see you pick up Lord Heston in that hey-go-mad way when he spoke of Napoleon,' she scolded. 'Such matters are not for ladies to understand. You would not have him think you a blue-stocking?'

'I doubt if he thinks that, Aunt Emma.'

'He cannot have been pleased to hear you speaking out so boldly. I thought he must have given you a setdown, and you would have deserved it.'

'He seemed quite interested in my views,' Miranda told her mildly. 'But I shall not speak of such things again unless he should desire it.' She changed the subject with a coaxing smile. 'In any case, I do not think he will attend the Grand Masquerade at Vauxhall. We were to go with Lady Medlicott, if you recall.'

'But not without a male escort, my love.' Mrs Shere looked shocked. 'You must give up that plan. I can't think that his lordship would approve.'

Miranda was tempted to announce that his lordship did not own her, but she bit back the hasty words.

'Richard Young has offered to accompany us. He is come to London to see the sights, Aunt, and we have known him all our lives. Mama would not object. . .'

Mrs Shere shook her head. 'It is to be hoped that you know what you are doing, dearest.' It was a dismal echo of Fanny's words. 'I cannot like your manner with Lord Heston. You do not appear to realise the extent of your good fortune.'

Miranda kissed her cheek. 'Lord Heston is not an ordinary man,' she said with perfect truth. 'I am learning to understand him. Believe me, he will not cry off.' She crossed her fingers behind her back.

'You may be right, but it is easy to push good nature too far.' Mrs Shere sighed, and then a thought struck her. 'Your mama approves of Richard Young, you say? Has she hopes of him for your sister? What is his background?'

'Richard is just a country gentleman. He is the eldest son of the local squire and our good neighbour.' She smiled. 'But you shall not raise your hopes, Aunt Emma. Mama aims higher than Richard for my twin.'

'Your sister makes no push to fix any gentleman's interest,' Mrs Shere said sadly. 'And, with the Season well advanced, most of the eligible gentlemen are committed. Will you have a word with her, my dear? Any advice would come better from you and be more readily acceptable. As I say, a second Season is never so successful. The novelty of a new face is gone, and other girls are more admired.'

'I'll do my best,' Miranda promised.

'That's right, my love. You, at least, have exceeded your mother's fondest hopes.'

Miranda went to fetch her twin, thankful that she had escaped with only the mildest of scoldings. To hear Heston described as good-natured had shaken her a little, but she could not deny that he had been charming to her aunt.

'Thank heavens you had the sense to ask Richard to escort us to the Masquerade,' she told Fanny. 'Aunt was about to forbid us to go. Of course, Lady Medlicott must accompany us.'

'Even that will be better than today.' Fanny's face was sullen. 'I can't think what possessed Heston to drag us off to look at a heap of broken stones. I thought I must die of boredom. . . How Harry would have stared to see us there!'

'I expect he would. Sculpture is not to everyone's taste, but I enjoyed the visit.'

'Did you? I thought that you were still acting for Heston's benefit. I thought I should burst out laughing.'

Miranda was silent.

'And then all that dreary talk about Napoleon! So dull! In Heston's company you have more to bear than I imagined. He has no conversation. . .'

'He doesn't gossip, Fanny, if that's what you mean. I suppose if he had entertained us with the latest crim. cons. you would have approved?'

'He moves in the Regent's circles. He might have told us the truth about the Princess Charlotte's broken engagement to the Prince of Orange, or if the Regent really is a bigamist. I confess I'd like to know if he had married Maria Fitzherbert before he was wed to Caroline of Brunswick.'

'You put me out of patience with you, Fanny. It would be most improper of Heston to discuss such matters when he is in a privileged position to know the truth of them.'

Fanny stared at her. 'I thought you hated him? Why do you defend him now?'

'I am not defending him. I am defending the principle that it is wrong to discuss confidential matters, especially when they refer to a friend.'

Fanny was not satisfied. 'Are you beginning to think better of him? I didn't think you'd change your mind so quickly. Have you forgot his insults?'

'No, I have not! For heaven's sake, Fanny, let it rest! I have enough to trouble me. I can't think what I am to do if the announcement should appear in the *Gazette* tomorrow. . .' Her words served to silence Fanny.

*   *   *

But the next edition of the *Gazette* did not carry the news of the supposed betrothal, and Miranda could not disguise her relief. The announcement must have arrived too late to be included, but Mrs Shere was disappointed.

'Perhaps it is for the best,' Miranda soothed. 'Now there can be no objection to our going to the Masquerade with Richard.'

Her aunt looked doubtful. 'Dearest, I am persuaded that his lordship would not like it. You should ask his permission first.'

Miranda kept her opinion of this suggestion to herself.

'Lord Heston is at Carlton House today,' she pointed out. 'And, Aunt, we shall wear our dominoes as well as our velvet masks. No one will recognise us.'

'Very well then.' Mrs Shere gave her permission for the outing with some reluctance. 'But you must not stay too long.'

'We shall be home by midnight,' Miranda promised. 'And with Richard to take care of us, we cannot come to any harm.'

This prophetic statement proved to be untrue. The crowds at the Vauxhall Gardens were immense and it was difficult for the four members of their party to stay together. Lady Medlicott, an incorrigible gossip, insisted upon chatting to those persons whom she recognised, whilst Richard was diverted by the Grand Display of Fireworks.

'Oh, there is Harry!' Fanny cried out in delight. 'Will he know me, do you think?'

Miranda threw her a glance filled with deep suspicion and Fanny pouted.

'I did not know he would be here,' she insisted. 'Don't glare at me, Miranda! This is a chance meeting.'

'Obviously!' Miranda looked at Harry's companions. In addition to one or two gentlemen, there were a couple of well-known Incognitas.

Fanny's face grew pale. She had been about to rush over to her lover, but the sight of the high-flyers had stopped her instantly. A hand flew to her mouth.

'Oh no, he could not. . .' she whispered. Then she swayed and seemed about to faint.

'Don't you dare!' Miranda hissed. 'Do you wish to make a spectacle of yourself and me? Those women may have nothing to do with Harry. You must forget that you have seen him in their company.'

'How could I? Miranda, I must know.' Before Miranda could stop her, she rushed to Harry's side.

It was the height of folly, but worse was to come. Fanny tore off her mask and confronted her lover with accusing eyes. His look of surprise changed to one of dismay, and he led her away from the others into a side turning, off the main promenade.

Miranda plunged after them, but the impetus of the crowd carried her far beyond the little group as it surged towards the Water Spectacle which was about to begin.

'All alone, little lady? You must not lose your footing.' To Miranda's horror, an arm slid about her waist, and she caught a glimpse of gleaming teeth beneath a mask.

'Let me go!' she cried. 'How dare you?'

'Unhand the lady, sir!' Suddenly Richard was by her side. His face was flushed, and his eyes were bright with anger.

'Out of it, stripling! This prize is mine.' Her captor

shouldered Richard aside as he tightened his grip upon
Miranda's waist. Then he swung round. Richard had
gripped his shoulder, and a bunched fist gave notice of
his intentions. Next moment a blow from her attacker's
cane felled Richard to the ground.

'Now let me see your face, my pretty!' A rough hand
swept Miranda's hood from her hair and began to untie
the strings of her mask.

As she fought him, Richard shook his spinning head,
gathered himself and launched another attack upon the
man who held her.

This time he was tripped and landed on his back.
Miranda screamed as she saw the flash of light upon a
gleaming blade. The innocent-looking cane was a
swordstick and its tip was now against Richard's throat.

'You are in need of a lesson, my friend. A scar upon
each cheek will remind you of this night —'

'He is unarmed!' Miranda cried wildly.

A circle had cleared about them as the crowd moved
back. For a frozen moment Miranda stared at the
spectators.

'Will no one help me?' she begged. A murmur of
disgust was the only reply. No one was prepared to
face the swordsman, much as they disapproved of his
actions. She could see Fanny's ashen face on the
outskirts of the group, and beside her Lady Medlicott
was on the verge of collapse.

'Cowards, all of you!' Miranda shrieked. She took a
step backwards and kicked her attacker sharply behind
the knee. Her silken sandals were too soft to injure
him, but he swung round with a curse.

'Hell-cat!' he growled. Then his face changed as his
raised arm was caught in a bone-crushing grip. He gave

a yelp of agony, and the weapon clattered to the ground.

'You! I might have known!' The contempt in Heston's voice brought an ugly flush to the man's face. He scurried away, helped along by a kick to the seat of his breeches.

Chapter Six

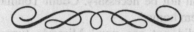

Heston looked at Miranda. 'All right?' he asked.

Miranda nodded. She was shaking so violently that she thought her legs would not support her, and she felt incapable of speech.

Heston reached down to help Richard to his feet.

'My lord, I'm sorry!' The younger man was white to the lips. 'What must you think of me? I made the poorest showing as an escort for the ladies.'

'You did very well.' Heston's harsh, dark face softened for a moment as he smiled. 'An unarmed man has no defence against a weapon such as this.' He picked up the discarded sword, and then he turned to Miranda.

'I think we should leave, my dear,' he said mildly. 'We have provided quite enough entertainment for these bystanders. Where is your sister?'

'I saw her over there with Lady Medlicott.' Miranda pointed with a trembling finger.

'Ah, yes!' His lordship took her arm and led her through the rapidly dispersing crowd.

Lady Medlicott had been supported to a nearby seat.

She looked very ill. Fanny was chafing her hands, but there was no sign of Harry Lakenham.

'Mr Young, will you be good enough to take her ladyship home? I will bring her to the carriage. . .'

'A pleasure, sir!' Richard was eager to make amends for his previous failure to take care of them. 'Shall I take Fanny and Miranda, too?'

'That will not be necessary. Count Toumanov and I will see them home.'

'Oh, I did not see you.' Miranda turned to find Alexei Toumanov by her side.

'Hardly surprising, ma'am. You had more than enough to occupy you.' The Count smiled, but Miranda felt ashamed. What must Heston and his friend think of her? To be discovered in such circumstances was the outside of enough. She looked up at Heston, but his face was inscrutable.

'How. . .how did you find us, my lord?' she murmured.

Heston took her arm and led her ahead of the others, supporting Lady Medlicott upon one arm.

'Later, my love.' With exquisite courtesy he handed her ladyship into the carriage with his wishes for her swift recovery, and the express hope that she would soon forget the ugly incident.

Lady Medlicott was no fool. She nodded, aware of his wish that she should not speak of it.

Fanny had regained her colour. As the carriage drove away, she smiled up prettily at Heston.

'How fortunate that you were here tonight,' she cried. 'I had not supposed you to like masquerades, my lord.'

His penetrating eyes scanned her face. 'I don't,' he

told her bluntly. 'Mrs Shere advised us that you were come to the Vauxhall Gardens.'

'We had thought you occupied at Carlton House,' Miranda faltered. 'I did not expect that you would call on us this evening.'

'Obviously not!' It was clear that he was furious. 'Have you no sense, madam? How came you to be separated from your party?'

'Don't speak to me in that tone, if you please! If you must know, I was carried along in the crush.'

'Really? Without your sister?' Miranda knew that he did not believe her. 'On our way in we passed Lakenham. Had you an assignation with him?'

'No, I had not! I am surprised that you could think it. He knows of our…of our betrothal.' She was speaking the truth, but a blush rose to her cheeks.

'Don't play games with me, my dear. If I find that you have been deceiving me, you will regret it. You asked how I found you? It was simple. When we saw the disturbance, I guessed that you would be at the centre of it.'

'No, no, Adam, that is coming it too strong! Ignore him, Miss Gaysford! Adam is so tall. He looked above the crowd and saw your hair.' Count Toumanov had come up to them and was attempting to heal the breach. 'He is angry because you were in danger.'

Heston glared at him, and then he began to laugh. 'There is some truth in that,' he admitted ruefully. 'But I meant what I said. Trouble has an unerring way of finding you, my love. It is a sobering thought.'

Miranda would not be mollified. She turned to the Count. 'I hope we have not spoiled your evening,' she said. 'This has all been most unpleasant for you. It will give you a sad opinion of London.'

'Not at all!' Alexei bowed. 'Our only disappointment was in not finding you at home. That is one reason for Adam's sour expression. We had hoped to take you to the Piazza for some supper.'

'Famous!' Fanny clapped her hands. 'I should like that above anything.'

'But you cannot wish to go after such an experience?' Heston's eyes were on Miranda. 'I believe we should take you home. It must have been a shock. . .?'

'It was, but I am quite recovered.' Blue eyes locked with grey. 'You need have no fears for me, my lord. I do not plan to faint.'

'As you wish.' His tone was casual, but she saw the spark of something like admiration in his look. 'The carriage is by the gates.' Again he took her arm and led the way, leaving Fanny and the Count to follow.

'Tell me, where did you learn your street-fighting, dearest? It came as a surprise to me, though I have always been aware that you have unsuspected talents.'

'I can't think what you mean.' Miranda said stiffly.

'Must I explain?' He looked down at her dainty silken sandals. 'Let me give you a word of advice. That kick to the back of the knee is more effective when you are wearing stouter shoes, but it served its purpose. Foolish, of course. If he had struck you, you might have been badly injured. I think I must teach you rather better. Your previous tutor left much to be desired. . .'

'My brother did not think that I should ever be in such a situation,' she cried hotly.

'Then I must suppose that he does not know you very well. Personally I have no such sanguine hopes.'

Miranda did not trouble to reply to this gibe. A thought had struck her.

'That man. You know him, do you not?'

'I know of him,' he corrected. 'An ugly customer, my dear, with a string of scandals behind him. It was no surprise to find him here, hoping to find a companion for the night.'

Miranda flushed to the roots of her hair.

'Surely he could not imagine that I. . .that I. . .?'

'That you were available? Why not? You were apparently unattended and he saw his chance. Men are not saints, you know, and you are a prize worth the taking. Your face is likely to be your downfall, madam, unless you take more care.'

'I did not know that such things could happen,' she protested. 'No gentleman would thrust his attention upon a woman in that brutal way.'

She heard an ugly laugh. 'What an innocent you are! Do you know nothing of the reputation of this place? These gatherings in the Vauxhall Gardens offer opportunities for many a lightskirt to find a rich protector. Your aunt should have forbidden this expedition.'

'How dare you criticise her? She could not have known the truth of what you say, and I. . .well, I insisted upon coming here.'

'That does not surprise me in the least. I hope you have learned your lesson.'

'I have learned what cowards people are. Not a man in the crowd would lift a finger to help us.'

'You forget. . .the man was armed. Courage is of little use against a sword.'

'It did not stop you, my lord.' Miranda spoke without thinking. Then she coloured a little.

'Ah, yes, but then, you see, I took your assailant by surprise. You had diverted his attention.'

'Even so, it was a brave thing to do, and I thank you

for it. It was unforgivable to draw on Richard as he
did. . .he threatened to scar his face, you know.'

'He would have done so without a second thought.
Stroud has something of a reputation as a sadist. Not
only was he blackballed at Brooks and White's, but he
is barred from many. . .er. . .houses of ill repute. A girl
was killed upon one occasion, so I understand.'

Miranda shuddered.

'Now I have shocked you. You must forgive me, but
I wished to make the danger clear to you.'

'It is clear enough, my lord. I shall not visit this place
again,' Miranda said firmly, forgetting for the moment
that had he forbidden her to do so she would most
certainly have defied him. 'It is hateful.'

'Not altogether. The concerts and the entertainments
can be delightful if one is in a party, and uses a little
common sense.'

Miranda flushed again, but she did not argue,
although it was not entirely her fault that she had found
herself isolated from the others.

'Even so, I hope that you will accept my thanks,' she
murmured.

'I could do no less for my beloved.' The mocking
note was back in his voice as he handed her into the
carriage.

His lordship did not appear to notice her annoyance.
He chatted amicably to Fanny and the Count as the
carriage bore them towards the Piazza, and Alexei was
quick to extol the excellence of the food.

Then Miranda's ears pricked up.

'Mr Richard Young is an old friend of yours?'
Heston's question was apparently casual, but there was
something in his tone which warned her of his interest.

'He is a neighbour of ours in Yorkshire, and an old friend of my brother,' she said shortly.

'We have known him all our lives,' Fanny intervened. 'He is come to London for the celebrations.'

'You are fortunate in your friend. He does not lack courage. Do you suppose that he would care to join us to see the Regent's procession?'

'That would be kind.' Miranda turned to him, her face alight with pleasure, and surprised something in his expression which she had not expected to see there. She blinked, feeling that she must have been mistaken. It was almost a look of tenderness.

The twins had not previously visited the Piazza, and they were suitably impressed. Their supper was all that the Count had promised but, though Miranda joined in the light-hearted conversation, she felt troubled. The incident in the Vauxhall Gardens had shaken her, but it was not that.

Heston was beginning to fill her mind to the exclusion of all else. She strove in vain to remember how much she had disliked him, but honestly compelled her to admit that she might have been mistaken in his character.

A teasing remark from the Count recalled her wandering thoughts. Knowing of her impending betrothal he was accusing her of daydreaming and being lost in love.

'Adam, you are a lucky dog!' he announced. 'You have captured the heart of one of the two most beautiful girls in London.' As he spoke, he took Fanny's hand and raised it to his lips. His smile was full of mischief. 'I must pin my hopes upon capturing the other.'

Fanny coloured, but she was not displeased by the young Russian's evident admiration.

Miranda's spirits sank. Heston could only be annoyed by this flirtation, innocent though it was. To her surprise, his face was bland as he looked at the other couple.

'You may find it more difficult than you imagine,' he said softly.

A moment of panic seized Miranda. It was a strange remark. Her discomfort was increased by the level look his lordship gave her. How much did he know? Surely he could not have guessed at the deception? It was impossible.

Later that night she tossed and turned as she lay in bed, unable to sleep. Heston did not trust her. He had made that clear. Yet he had warned her not to encourage the Count.

Why had he brought his friend along on that particular evening? Perhaps he imagined that Harry Lakenham would transfer his attentions to her sister. Alexei Toumanov must have been invited as a diversion, but she could not be sure. Suddenly she was tired of the whole ignominious business. She should never have become involved.

Heston was not the monster she had thought him. Common sense told her that. After all, it was not so dreadful for a man to wish to rescue a friend from a designing female. If the truth were to be told, it was admirable.

As for his insults, well, she had brought most of those upon herself. Not for the first time, she bemoaned her hasty tongue.

She was not entirely to blame, although she had been

persuaded into this stupid hoax against her better judgement. The fact that she had sought to protect her sister was no excuse.

Lord Heston had been hasty, too. He had misjudged her from the start. Sadly, that was no comfort now. Somehow it seemed important that he should think better of her as their acquaintance grew.

In this last day or two she had seen him in a different light. He had been kind to her aunt and also to Lady Medlicott. She had been surprised, too, by the wide range of his interests. His conversation was stimulating, and on more than one occasion she had forgotten her dislike of him as they discussed particular topics.

Miranda tossed off her coverlet and turned her pillow, pressing her cheek against the cool linen. Yet still sleep would not come. Something deeper was disturbing her and at last she was forced to face the unpalatable truth. Tonight at the Vauxhall Gardens, her heart had jumped when she found that massive figure by her side, and it was not simply the fact that he had rescued both herself and Richard.

Later, as they supped at the Piazza, she had been aware of no one else. She could recall neither Count Toumanov's conversation nor that of her sister, and the other diners were merely a blur.

Only one thing stood out clearly in her mind, and that was the harsh, dark face of Adam Heston as his heavy-lidded eyes gazed down at her. She knew every detail of those features, the black brows, the acquiline nose, the clean line of his jaw, and the curve of his lips.

Her face grew hot as she recalled his kisses. His mouth had been warm upon her own as he held her to him, and the remembered scent of soap, sweet clean linen and the outdoors came back to haunt her.

She closed her eyes, pressing her palms against them as if by doing so she could shut him out of her mind. It was ridiculous. The last thing she needed was to fall in love with that formidable creature. He despised her. She must remember that, holding on to the thought as if it were some kind of talisman.

All she needed was the firm resolution to keep him at a distance, but in her present situation that was impossible. If only Fanny would fall out of love with Harry Lakenham she might manage to extricate herself from her predicament. She could then announce that she had mistaken her own heart and cry off from her supposed betrothal.

She had meant to chide Fanny for leaving her to run to Harry's side in the Gardens. Now she realised that her sister had said nothing of that meeting. It was strange. In the usual way Fanny was so open.

Miranda had expected tears and sulks. Fanny, she knew, had been shocked to see her lover in the company of such birds of paradise, yet later she had not even seemed subdued. Her enjoyment of the rest of the evening had been obvious.

Miranda looked at the sleeping figure beside her with a mixture of love and exasperation. Then she sighed. Perhaps it was as well that her twin could sleep so soundly, untroubled by the chaotic state of their affairs. She would make a few discreet enquiries in the morning. Upon that thought she fell asleep herself.

She had no opportunity to carry out her plan to question Fanny. The arrival of their aunt with the *Gazette* drove any such idea out of Miranda's mind.

'See, my love. The announcement is here in black

and white!' She brandished the paper under her niece's nose.

Miranda took it from her with a shaking hand. She had expected it, but somehow the words leapt out at her, larger, blacker, and more final than she could have dreamed. Heston had been given all his titles, but it was her own name which burned into her mind.

'Now at last we can make plans,' Mrs Shere announced happily. 'You must dress at once, my dearest. His lordship is sure to call within the hour. I'll send your maid. Will you wear the French sprigged muslin?'

Miranda nodded, but her heart was thumping in a most alarming way, and she felt a little sick. With an effort she controlled her nausea and slipped out of bed.

The news had awakened Fanny. As their aunt left the room she looked across at her twin.

'Are you all right?' she whispered. 'You look so pale. . .'

Miranda took refuge in a sharp retort. 'Why did you leave me in the Gardens?' she demanded. 'You should not have gone to Harry, and well you know it. If you'd had any sense at all, you'd have pretended not to see him.'

'I could not do it, Miranda. I had to know what he was doing with those awful women. You need not scold. You would have done the same yourself.' Fanny began to sulk.

'No, I should not. We all know that gentlemen have convenients in their keeping, but we need not recognise them.'

'I didn't speak to them. Harry took me away. . .he wished to explain that the. . .er. . .lightskirts were with his friends.'

'That may be true, but you need not have taxed him with it there and then. Suppose Lord Heston had seen you? He did meet Harry later.'

'But not when he was with me,' Fanny told her in an injured tone.

'Even so, he asked if I had arranged an assignation. I said not, but I doubt if he believed me.'

'Does it matter? You were with Richard when Heston found you.'

'I was, indeed! And what he must have thought I can't imagine, with Richard lying on the ground and a swordsman standing over him.'

'That was not my fault,' Fanny pouted.

'You can't escape all blame. Had our party stayed together, the man would not have dared approach me.'

'It seems I can do nothing right. Perhaps you have forgot that Lady Medlicott stayed behind, chatting to her friends, and Richard was watching the fireworks?'

'That isn't the point,' Miranda cried impatiently. 'The whole thing might have been avoided if you had shown a little more conduct.'

Fanny shrugged her shoulders as she sipped her morning chocolate. 'We came to no harm.' Her face brightened. 'Was it not splendid at the Piazza? I am so glad that the Count and Heston came to find us. I did enjoy our supper, and I was even in charity with his lordship. He was not angry, was he?'

'He was furious,' Miranda told her shortly. 'And with good reason.'

'Why should you care?' Fanny gave her sister a curious glance. 'Was it not your intention to annoy him?'

'Not by risking Richard's neck, and making a spectacle of myself.'

'Don't be such a crosspatch!' Fanny nibbled at a roll. 'Alexei Toumanov is a character, isn't he? Do you like him?'

Miranda swung round on her.

'For heaven's sake, don't set your sights on him,' she cried. 'Heston has already warned me not to encourage the Count.'

'Naturally, you may not, but the same cannot apply to me. They came to invite us both to supper. That was an odd start in Heston if he did not wish his friend to know us.'

Miranda had thought much the same herself, but she was not prepared to discuss the matter.

'What of Harry?' she demanded. 'Is your affection for him fading already?'

'Of course not!' Fanny looked uncomfortable. 'Yet I may not see him. You said as much yourself, and I won't wear the willow else Aunt would notice my low spirits.'

It was the most transparent of excuses for Fanny's clear delight in the Count's obvious admiration.

'Stuff!' her twin said rudely. 'Fanny, if you bring more trouble down upon our heads, I shall wash my hands of you.' With that threat she swept out of the room.

For the rest of the morning the knocker went incessantly as notes were delivered to her uncle's door by hand. All bore good wishes for her future happiness.

Miranda was leafing through a pile of cards and invitations from members of the *ton* who had not previously acknowledged her existence when Heston was announced.

'You, too?' He grinned at her as he looked at the

scattered pieces of pasteboard on the table. 'Today we are the most popular pair of lovers in London.'

Miranda turned her head away. Her lips were trembling, and for some unaccountable reason she was on the verge of tears.

'Come for a drive with me,' his lordship suggested gently. 'The air will do you good.'

Miranda shook her head. Then his hand cupped her chin and forced her to look up at him.

'Courage, my love! Yesterday you faced a swordsman. You will not tell me now that you cannot bear the scrutiny of the Polite World?'

The great blue eyes looked too large for her pale face, and Heston dropped a kiss upon her nose.

'Get your bonnet!' he insisted. 'My devotion will wear thin if you keep my horses waiting.'

His teasing restored her spirits a little.

'Don't worry,' he promised. 'I shall not throw you to the wolves. All you need do is smile and bow and look delightfully as you always do. I will take care of the rest.'

His kindness brought fresh tears to her eyes as she hurried away. She would never understand him. At one moment he could be hard and ruthless, so secure in his pride and arrogance that she found it easy to detest him. His concern to help her through the coming ordeal was far more difficult to bear. Fanny had suspected him of playing some deep game, but what it was she could not begin to guess, and nor could Fanny.

As she settled a gay little hat upon her copper curls, she began to regain her composure.

'Charming!' he announced as she rejoined him. 'I like the jaunty feather.'

Miranda felt far from jaunty as they drove into Hyde

Park. Their appearance was the signal for a crowd to surround their carriage, and she found herself the centre of a large group of well-wishers.

Astonishment was plain on many faces, and she fell prey to acute embarrassment. Most probably these people imagined that Heston had run mad to offer for a bride so far beneath him.

'Cheer up, my love!' he whispered. 'No one will say it to my face, but they are all happy to see a confirmed bachelor caught by the foot at last.'

That was not true of all his lordship's acquaintance.

'We have not met before, I think.' A matron in an ornate turban signalled to her coachman to pull up. She eyed Miranda with undisguised hostility. 'Where have you been hiding your betrothed, my dear Heston?'

Miranda flushed to the ears. The cold words had made it sound as if there were something shameful in her which Heston had been at pains to hide.

The girl beside her was as scarlet as Miranda. She held out her hand. 'I hope you will be very happy,' she murmured in a voice choked with mortification.

'Thank you.' Miranda smiled. 'Is this your first Season?'

'It is!' The matron answered for her daughter, as she tried to stare Miranda down. 'We do not see you at Almack's, Miss. . .er. . . Miss. . .?'

'Miss Gaysford,' his lordship supplied helpfully. 'My apologies, ma'am. I should have spoken more clearly. I had forgot your difficulty in hearing well.'

It was a crushing setdown, and it had the result which Heston had intended. An alarming purple flush stained the woman's face, and her several chins began to wobble as she sought for a reply. Words failed her. She poked her coachman in the back with the tip of her parasol, and with a last dagger-look at Heston she was borne away.

Miranda had difficulty in keeping her countenance. Her shoulders were shaking as she made an unsuccessful attempt to turn a chuckle into a cough.

'Something amuses you, my dear?' Her companion looked down at her. His expression was as bland as usual but his eyes were twinkling.

'I fear you have made an enemy for life, sir. The lady will not soon recover from such a snub.'

'You may be right. It is a lowering thought, but I shall try to bear it. It would not do to fall into a fit of the dismals. . .'

His words were too much for Miranda, but she made a last attempt to hide her amusement.

'You were not kind,' she reproached.

'Neither was she. An ill-natured creature, Lady Eddington, and well known for her vicious tongue.'

'I liked her daughter,' Miranda ventured.

'Amabel?' his lordship shrugged. 'A pleasant girl with a heavy cross to bear in such a mother. I pity her future husband with a dragon for a mother-in-law.'

Miranda was silent, but his next words filled her with dismay.

'Tell me about your own mama,' he said. 'Is she like you or like your sister?'

'My lord?'

'I wished merely to know what I am to expect, my dearest.' His smile filled her with acute foreboding. He could not be serious. He intended no more than she to go through with the marriage. Miranda stiffened. It was just another attempt to frighten her.

'I don't quite understand you,' she replied in a cool tone.

'I think you do. You and your sister are so unlike, are you not?'

Panic seized Miranda. Was Heston beginning to suspect that he had been deceived?

'We are thought to be identical,' she babbled. 'Few people can tell us one from the other.'

'How odd!' he mused. 'I do not find the slightest difficulty in doing so. It is something about the eyes, I think.'

This was dangerous ground. Miranda cast about wildly in her mind for some way to change the subject.

'You have not answered my original question,' he reminded her.

'Oh, you mean in her nature?' Miranda made a quick recover. 'Mama is more like Fa—like my favourite sister.'

Heston did not appear to have noticed the slip, but Miranda's blood ran cold. She had come so close to giving herself away.

'Then I have nothing to worry about.' Her companion did not look at her, but his lips twitched.

'Do you mean that as an insult, sir? It is unworthy of you.' Miranda spoke with some heat, hoping that a quarrel would divert his lordship's attention from this perilous topic.

Heston would not be drawn.

'It was meant as a compliment,' he told her smoothly. 'Your sister is of a sanguine temperament, I believe.'

'You don't mean that at all! You think her silly and frivolous and flighty!' Miranda stopped in dismay. Swift in defence of her twin, she had allowed her annoyance to lead her into saying more than she intended.

'Don't you?' he asked mildly.

'How dare you! You do not know her in the least.'

'Then I crave your pardon. I must get to know her better. . .' He stopped as a cavalier on horseback came up to their carriage to offer his congratulations.

Miranda sank back thankfully against the cushioned seat. She had been reprieved, but for how long? Was Heston playing with her as a cat might play with a mouse before the kill?

That morning he had almost trapped her into betraying herself, and she found his veiled remarks deeply disturbing. If he should carry out his promise to get to know Fanny better, she could place no reliance upon her twin's ability to deceive him. If he pushed Fanny far enough, the result might be a hysterical outburst in which everything would be revealed.

Her face showed nothing of her inner emotions. She smiled prettily at the compliments offered to her, and by the time the horseman moved away she had regained much of her composure.

'Do you dine at Carlton House tonight, my lord?' she asked.

'Unfortunately, yes. The Prince is giving a dinner for the Tsar and the King of Prussia. To refuse the invitation would be to give offence.'

'You do not enjoy these gatherings, it would seem.'

'The food is beyond reproach, and the music excellent.' There was a cynical note in Heston's voice. 'That is, if one enjoys a "descent into hell".'

'My lord?'

'A favourite saying of the Prince's guests, my dear. The heat throughout the house is suffocating.'

'I had heard that the Prince is afraid of draughts, but surely the interior is very fine? A friend described one of the chandeliers as looking like a shower of diamonds.'

'It was probably almost as costly. You will go there, naturally, and you may see for yourself. The Regent will wish to meet my bride-to-be.'

Miranda heard his words with dread. This was the worst blow of all. How could she appear at Carlton House under false pretences? It would likely be considered treason and she would end up in the Tower.

A shaky laugh escaped her lips.

'I like the idea of going there no more than you do,' she protested.

'You will find that you have no alternative,' he told her lightly.

Chapter Seven

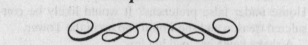

The thought of deceiving the heir to the throne effectively destroyed the last traces of Miranda's peace of mind. Her face whitened to the lips and she could not speak.

'Come now, pray do not look as if you have seen a ghost! Prinny is no ghost, in fact very much the opposite. You will find him charming. It is his greatest gift.' Heston took her hand and raised it to his lips.

In the ordinary way Miranda would have snatched it away, but now she left it in his grasp, her fingers tightening instinctively. He responded to the pressure, and then he released her to take up the reins once more.

'Chin up!' he said. 'All is not yet lost, I assure you.'

It was an odd remark, and it struck her forcibly. Distraught though she was, she could not let it go unchallenged.

'You speak in riddles, sir.' She gave him a look of deep suspicion.

'Hedgehog!' he reproved. 'I meant merely that you will enjoy a meeting with the Regent and his friends.

He is a cultivated man, and a great patron of the arts, the best since Charles I.'

As he had intended, Miranda's attention was diverted.

'But he is hissed and booed by the public whenever he appears, my lord.'

'Are you surprised? The English distrust an intellectual. In the public mind, hunting is more to be admired than sculpture, gaming rather than an interest in literature, and the work of the finest artists is not to be compared with an afternoon at the races.'

'But the Prince does all those things,' Miranda pointed out.

'He did. He has not hunted for some years, and he was never more popular than when his colours appeared on the racetrack. The scandal was unfortunate. . .he gave up racing on the spot.'

'Scandal? I had not heard of it.'

'It happened more than twenty years ago. His horse, Escape, was said to be the finest on the turf. It failed one day at Newmarket, and the odds against it shortened to five to one. Next day it won with ease, and both the Prince and his jockey, Chifney, were thought to have made large sums of money. The Prince was told that if Chifney rode for him again, no gentleman would start against him.'

'But surely it was not true? The Prince would not stoop to cheating?'

'Of course not! It was just malicious gossip. Chifney published a vindication some time later, but the Prince had vowed that he would not race again.'

Miranda gave him a curious glance. 'You like him, don't you?'

'I do. Admittedly, he is his own worst enemy. The

public sees him preoccupied with expensive trivia, his dress, his passion for building and redecoration, but how else is he to spend his time? He is excluded from the serious business of governing the country.'

'He has a good friend in you, I think.' Miranda smiled at her companion, quite forgetting her previous fears.

'I can give him little else but friendship,' Heston murmured. 'So much has gone amiss for him.'

Miranda was silent. It would have been presumptuous to comment upon matters of which she knew so little.

'Much of it is due to his disastrous marriage to the Princess Caroline.' Heston seemed to be speaking more to himself than to her. 'One could wish that Mrs Fitzherbert had been born a Protestant princess.'

'But the people sympathise with the Princess of Wales,' Miranda protested. 'She is cheered when the Prince is hissed and booed.'

'The public do not know her.' Heston's face was sombre. 'Few of them can have considered what it must be like for a cultured and fastidious man to be wed to a hoyden who is not even clean in her person, and whose way of life is such that not even the most liberal-minded can condone it.'

'She may not be entirely to blame,' Miranda ventured. 'It is said that she loved someone else before she was married to the Prince.'

'So did he!' Heston looked down at her then, with a strange expression in his eyes. 'What deep pits we dig for ourselves when in the grip of strong emotion. It is as well to guard oneself against such follies.' His mocking tone annoyed her.

'You can be in no such danger, sir,' she told him coolly.

'Very true, my dear. The more tender emotions are not quite in my style, or in yours, I believe.'

'How well you are getting to know me, sir. You have expressed my feelings perfectly.' She turned away, so that he would not see the glitter in her eyes. He thought her hard and mercenary and she could not bear it.

'I'm happy to know that you won't suffer because I am forced to leave you for a day or two,' Heston said lightly. 'The Prince is to go to Oxford to receive a loyal address and I am invited to form part of his entourage.'

Miranda looked her surprise.

'He has earned it,' Heston replied to her unspoken question. 'He is an honorary Doctor of Civil Law, and has founded two university readerships, among other things.'

'How long will you be away?' Miranda's first feeling of relief was tempered by a sense of disappointment, which she did not care to examine too closely.

'Am I to suppose that you will miss me?' Heston's smile did not reach his eyes. 'How touching!'

'I doubt if I shall go into a decline, my lord.'

'I doubt it, too. Until our next meeting, then?' He had drawn up before her uncle's house, and sprang down from the phaeton to help her to alight.

She turned to bid him farewell, but he took her arm and accompanied her indoors.

'I must pay my respects to your aunt,' he said.

That lady was descending the staircase as they entered the hall, and Heston greeted her with the utmost courtesy, explaining as he did so that he would be out of London for a day or two.

'I expect that you would like to take your leave of

each other in private,' Mrs Shere said kindly. 'There is no one in the salon at this present time. . .'

Heston's eyes sparkled with amusement, but Miranda had no alternative but to accompany him. She stalked ahead of him and tossed aside her hat.

'That's right,' he murmured. 'Delightful confection though it is, the veil is something of an obstacle.'

Next moment she was in his arms and his mouth came down on hers.

Miranda had promised herself that the next time he kissed her she would not respond. If she stood quite still, this demanding creature would soon grow tired of making love to a statue.

It was easier said than done. The touch of those warm lips was producing a most alarming sensation in the pit of her stomach and turning her limbs to jelly. Insensibly she relaxed within his arms.

'Let us sit down,' he said. He slipped an arm about her waist and led her to a sofa. Miranda stiffened as he took a seat beside her. Then she turned her face away.

'Shy, my love? That will not do. . .' His lips grazed her cheek. 'What a tease you are!' He began to kiss her eyelids, and then he pressed his mouth against the hollow of her neck. 'Must you be so cold?'

'Please, my lord. . .you really must not. . .' She tried to fight a sudden urge to throw her arms about his neck and hold him to her. She wanted to press her cheek to his, to trace the curve of those smiling lips, and to stroke that thick dark hair.

Then he found her mouth again and the world was lost. Her pleasure was such that she felt powerless to resist him. She found herself responding with a passion that startled her.

When he released her, she could not look at him.

Nothing in her experience had prepared her for the emotions which now threatened to overwhelm her.

She was trembling and made no effort to resist when he took her in his arms once more.

'So there is fire beneath the ice?' he murmured. 'I had suspected it.' There was no trace of mockery in his voice as he turned her face to his. 'Blushing, my love? There is no need. It is nothing to be ashamed of, rather to be delighted in.'

'Please go!' Miranda choked out the words. She felt ready to sink with mortification.

It was not until later when she was alone that his curious reaction struck her. It seemed that he had understood that this was her first experience of true passion. Yet that could not be true. Heston despised her as a mere adventuress. . .a fortune hunter. Was it likely that in that role she would be unversed in the ways of love?

She was still lost in thought when her aunt came to find her.

'Don't look so sad, my dear. Lord Heston will not be gone for long.' Mrs Shere patted her hand.

Miranda managed a reluctant smile. 'It is not that,' she said.

'What then? Has something happened to disturb you?'

'Oh, Aunt, I feel so worried. Heston says that he will present me to the Regent.'

'Is that all? Love, I must imagine, has driven all thought of protocol from his lordship's mind.'

'What do you mean?'

'Dearest, you cannot appear in the presence of

royalty before you have been formally presented at Court.'

Her aunt's words went some way towards restoring Miranda's peace of mind, but it was quickly shattered.

'I have been considering the matter,' Mrs Shere said thoughtfully. 'Lady Medlicott is not quite the person to sponsor you. Perhaps we should consult his lordship. . .'

'Yes, let us do it.' Miranda was anxious to change the subject. 'Richard has promised to call on us tomorrow. He has promised to take us to see the Balloon Ascent in Hyde Park. . .'

'Should you be going about so much without Lord Heston? I cannot think he would approve. If you had but seen his face when he called here last night and found you had gone to the Vauxhall Gardens. . .'

'His lordship can have no wish that I should stay indoors, Aunt Emma. In any case, I should not heed him if he had.'

'My dear girl, think what you are saying!' Mrs Shere was scandalised. 'In a few weeks time you will promise to obey him. . .'

'But not yet! In any case, he has not forbidden it. A pleasure outing in an afternoon is unexceptionable.'

'Oh, dear, I suppose so, though I could wish that you were not so headstrong, dearest. You speak out so freely, and the way you take decisions in such a determined way is not quite—'

'Ladylike?' Miranda kissed the older woman with a rueful smile. 'Aunt, I have had to make decisions all my life. Mama will not do so.'

'I know it. Your mama is lost without a husband to guide her. She has had to rely so much upon her children, but now all will be changed. What a comfort it will be to her to be able to ask our dear Lord Heston for advice. Such a sensible man, and most good-natured, too!'

It was clear that his lordship had won the heart of at least one of Miranda's relatives.

'Do you think so?' she murmured.

'Of course, my love, and your uncle is much taken with him. Perhaps I should not say so, but we had heard that he was excessively proud and disagreeable. We both feared that you would find him so, and not even the prospect of a splendid match could be allowed to weigh against your future happiness.'

Miranda was silent.

'You can't think what a relief it was to find that gossip had lied,' her aunt continued. 'I am persuaded that jealousy has much to do with it. His lordship's manner is charming. . .so courteous! He must be a model for any gentleman. Only the most depraved could take against him!'

A smile touched the corner of Miranda's mouth. She had not previously considered herself a monster of depravity, and she had most certainly taken against him.

'Aunt Emma, I must believe that you think Lord Heston perfect,' she teased.

'Don't you, my love?' Mrs Shere saw the amusement in Miranda's expression and she returned the smile. 'Well, perhaps not perfect,' she admitted. 'A saint would be difficult to live with, but one can't fail to admire his character.' She looked steadily at her niece. 'You don't know him well, as yet, my love. I don't expect transports of affection, but you think well of him, I hope?'

'He puzzles me,' Miranda said with perfect truth. 'I wonder if anyone would grow to know him well.' She saw her aunt's troubled expression and hastened to amend her words. 'You are right, of course, the more I am in his lordship's company the more I realise that much of what is said of him is unjustified. He is not a mere gamester, with no interests beyond his horses.'

Her aunt kissed her. 'You are growing up, my dear. You will not take it amiss if I tell you that at first I thought you much more frivolous than your sister? Now I see that I was mistaken. . .' She patted Miranda's cheek. 'Enjoy your outing with your friend.'

Left alone, Miranda's thoughts were troubled. It was becoming more and more difficult to play the part of Fanny. The twins were so different in character, and Mrs Shere had noticed it. She herself had spoken without thinking when she had mentioned the need to make decisions for her mother. Fanny had never done so. She must make an effort to indulge in charming nonsense, to giggle, and to be light-hearted. She had never felt less like indulging in such behaviour.

A sense of relief swept over her as she stepped into the carriage the next day. Fanny knew the truth. There would be no need to dissemble with her twin.

As for Richard, he was too excited by the prospect of seeing his first Balloon Ascent to notice that Miranda was not her usual self.

'I have never enjoyed myself so much in all my life,' he announced happily. 'I wish you had been with me yesterday. . .the city was ablaze with light. It is the illuminations, you know. . .at night it looks a different place. . .'

'And so wonderful!' Fanny told him earnestly. 'I could not go back to live in Yorkshire ever again.

When one has lived in the capital the rest of England seems so. . .so provincial!'

'It's all very well to be here for a celebration,' Richard said defensively. 'But, Fanny, it does smell vile, and I can't say that I care much for the crowds.'

'It isn't always like this.' Fanny was in the mood to quarrel. 'The foreigners are everywhere. . .'

'They won't be here for ever,' Miranda intervened. 'Richard, you are looking very fine today. . .quite the town beau, in fact.'

'This rig?' Richard glanced down at his yellow pantaloons with assumed indifference. His brocade waistcoat was so brightly patterned that it was dazzling to the eye. Above it, his stiffly starched shirt-points rose almost to the middle of his cheeks, making it difficult for him to turn his head to left or right.

'It don't do to look the country cousin,' he explained defensively. 'I'd stand out like a sore thumb here in London.'

'Whereas in that waistcoat you are all but invisible,' Fanny giggled.

Richard's face fell. 'Do you think it too much?' he asked anxiously. 'M'father said I might buy what I chose.'

'It looks very well.' Miranda frowned at her sister. 'Quite the latest thing, in fact. I'm sure you looked about you to see what others are wearing before you visited the tailor.'

'Oh, I did, and he told me that it was all the crack, you know.'

'Then you may be easy in your mind.' Miranda smiled at him. His garments were expensive, and she felt sure that he had been persuaded into parting with a great deal of money in his efforts to become a gentleman of fashion. She would not spoil his pleasure for the world, although she felt sure that the shirt-points in particular were causing him discomfort.

'Well, it would not do for Yorkshire.' He grinned at her a little consciously. 'But one must be in the correct way of things.'

Miranda nodded her agreement. She had always been fond of him. Good-natured to a fault, he, more than any of her brother's friends, had been the one to take the twins' part in any of their scrapes. Scorned by the other boys, who refused to have mere females take part in their adventures, Richard had raised no objections. He bore the expostulations of his friends with great good humour, but he would not be swayed.

She looked at him with renewed affection. He was hung about with fobs and an expensive tie-pin gleamed in the folds of his cravat, but he did not quite achieve the appearance of a dandy, which was clearly his intention.

Miranda suspected that he had chosen his present rig knowing that he was to escort them, and wishing to do them credit.

'Are any of your friends in London?' she asked kindly.

'No, but I am putting up at Grillon's, and I made a new acquaintance. He is a famous fellow. We went to see the wild beasts in the Tower, and to Astley's Ampitheatre. . .' He did not think it prudent to mention the cock-fights to which his new friend had taken him, nor his visit to Gentleman Jackson's saloon to watch that gentleman sparring with other devotees of The Fancy. Ladies were not interested in such exciting sports.

He saw her worried look and smiled at her. 'He is

not an ivory-turner. You may have no fears on that
score.'

Miranda felt relieved. In the short time she had spent
in London, she had heard stories of the men who lay in
wait for gullible boys, leading them to ruin in the many
gaming hells which had sprung up in the capital.

At that moment she was hailed by Charlotte Fairfax.

'Do you go to the Ascent?' her friend called out.

The twins nodded in unison.

'Then may we go together? We must walk from here,
you know, and I want to talk to you.' Charlotte's face
was alive with curiosity as she dismissed her brother.

Young Fairfax needed no urging to be relieved of his
charge. He handed his sister down from their carriage
and, with a bow to Miranda's party, he went off to find
his friends.

'Wretched boy!' Charlotte said with feeling. 'I wish
you might have heard the fuss he made when Mamma
said that he must bring me.'

'Brothers are all the same,' Fanny agreed. 'It was
only Richard here who would ever allow us to go about
with him when we were children.'

Charlotte looked at their escort, a question in her
eyes. 'This gentleman is not your brother? I had
supposed. . .'

'Richard is a family friend.' Miranda made the
necessary introductions. Under the cover of the ensuing
civilities, Fanny tugged at her elbow.

'You will not fly into the boughs if we see Harry, I
hope? He is quite likely to be here today.'

'Of course not! We can't prevent him from going
wherever he wishes, but pray do not slip away with
him. It is a different thing if you meet him in company.'

'You two are the outside of enough!' Charlotte

teased. 'Now which of you am I to congratulate upon
your betrothal?' She turned to Richard. 'Do you find
the same difficulty, sir? If you have known Fanny and
Miranda from childhood, perhaps you can tell them
apart?'

Miranda froze, and beside her she felt her sister
stiffen. It was true that Richard knew them as well as
their own family.

She should have thought of it before. It was no more
likely that they could deceive Richard than that they
could deceive their own brother. Yet he had handed
her the letter from her mother with no more than a
moment's hesitation, clearly believing that she was
Fanny. It was that which had lulled her into a sense of
false security. She held her breath, waiting for the blow
to fall.

'We have not been much in each other's company
for these past few years,' Richard said easily. 'I was at
Oxford, Miss Fairfax. Meantime, the twins have grown
even more alike. Sometimes they confuse me, too.'

Miranda looked at him with gratitude in her eyes.
He met her own with a level gaze and only the faintest
of smiles. It was enough. He knew of the deception,
she was convinced of it.

Fanny took her arm. 'You must wish my sister happy,
Charlotte. She is the fortunate bride-to-be.'

Charlotte threw her arms about Miranda. 'Sly creature!' she chaffed. 'We had not the least idea. . .why, I
almost fainted when I read the announcement. I would
not believe it! Lord Heston of all people! I thought it
must be some mistake when you had both taken him in
such dislike.'

Miranda gave her an ironic look, and Charlotte's

hand flew to her mouth. 'Oh, my stupid tongue again. . .
I should not have said that. Indeed, I wish you happy.'

'I know you do.' Miranda rescued her from her
confusion. 'We had best go, or we shall miss the ascent.'

As they strolled through the crowds to get a better
view, Miranda allowed Fanny and Charlotte to go
ahead. She fell into step with Richard.

'Thank you,' she said simply.

'For what?'

'I think you know quite well. When did you guess?'

'When I brought the letters.'

'But you gave Mama's letter to me, and it was
addressed to Fanny.'

'Your uncle made it clear that he thought that you
were Fanny. It was not up to me to correct him.'

'You must be wondering. . .!'

'I wondered if you were in a scrape again. It wouldn't
be the first time. . .'

She heard a low chuckle.

'This time it isn't so amusing, and it is all my fault. If
I hadn't lost my temper and said things which I now
regret, we should not be in this situation.'

'You will not tell me that Fanny had no hand in it? I
should not believe you.'

Miranda hesitated.

'You need not tell me if you don't wish, you know,
but if there is anything I can do. . .?'

'There is nothing anyone can do, I fear. Sometimes I
long to turn tail and run back home.'

'That isn't like you. You were always the one with
the lion heart. Can you not think of a way to put
matters right?'

'I wish I could. Meantime, I feel wretched to be

deceiving everyone in this way. Oh, Richard, I should not—'

'You should not worry so. Neither you nor Fanny would do anything really bad. I know you well enough for that. It will all come right, you'll see. . .'

With these words of comfort he took her arm and caught up with the others.

They had found a vantage point beside the roped-off enclosure from which the balloon ascent was to be made. The silken globe was already tugging at its moorings in the breeze, the brilliant colours gleaming in the sunlight. At each corner men held tightly to the mooring rope, whilst some argument seemed to be taking place beside the wicker basket which was to hold the occupants.

'How many will it hold?' asked Charlotte.

'Two, or possibly three, I should imagine.' Richard eyed the proceedings with interest.

'Oh, no!' Fanny's eyes were upon one of the men at the centre of the argument. He was muffled to the eyes, but she had no difficulty in recognising Harry Lakenham. 'He cannot be planning to go with them.'

'I fear he does. Fanny, please.' Miranda gripped her sister's arm. 'You must not go to him.'

'I will! I will! He is sure to be killed. . . I know it. . .' Fanny's voice had risen to a shriek and several people turned to look at her.

'Don't worry, they will not take him if he is inexperienced. Is he a friend of yours?' It was a casual question, but something in Richard's tone caused Miranda to throw him a sharp glance. His eyes were on Fanny's face, and in that moment he betrayed himself.

Miranda groaned inwardly. This was yet another complication and one which she could well do without.

She could not doubt that Richard was in love with Fanny, and he could not fail to be hurt. Suddenly she felt fiercely protective towards him.

'Pull yourself together, Fanny!' she urged. 'See, they have turned Harry away. . .'

It was true. As she watched, the two intrepid flyers climbed into the basket and signalled to their assistants. Harry had been motioned to one side with a couple of stalwarts between himself and the balloon. They jumped out of the way as the ballast was thrown out and the wind filled the silken dome. As it began to rise, Harry saw his chance. He dodged the men and leapt for the basket, catching at a trailing rope, already high in the air.

As the crowds watched in horror, Fanny crumpled at Miranda's feet. She fell to her knees beside her sister, but Richard was there before her. He lifted Fanny tenderly in his arms.

'We must get her home at once,' he said.

Miranda nodded dumbly, but she could not take her eyes from the struggle taking place above her head. As she watched, Harry gained the rim of the basket, causing it to sway alarmingly. Then he was pulled to safety inside. Next moment he was on his feet again, waving cheerfully to the onlookers below.

Miranda heard a murmur of disgust from those beside her.

'Doubtless he did it for a wager,' one man said. 'But he might have killed them all. I have no patience with such folly.'

Miranda was in complete agreement with his sentiments, but Fanny was her more immediate concern. She followed Richard through the press of people with Charlotte by her side.

'You will come home with us?' she asked Charlotte. 'We shall never find your brother in these crowds, and we cannot leave you here alone.'

Charlotte herself was pale and trembling. 'I feel quite faint myself,' she admitted. 'If Lord Lakenham had fallen. . . It does not bear thinking about.'

'Then don't think about it. It was the most stupid thing I have ever seen, and I don't propose to give myself a fit of the dismals over Harry Lakenham's idiocy. It would have served him right if he had fallen and broken a leg.'

'He was more likely to have broken his neck.' Charlotte shuddered and was still trembling as their carriage reached its destination.

'You are back early,' Mrs Shere began as Miranda stepped into the hall. Then she saw Richard with Fanny in his arms. 'What is it? What has happened?'

'My sister fainted, and Charlotte is not well. There was an accident during the Ascent, but no one has been hurt. . .'

'Bring her in here and put her on the sofa, poor child. Miss Fairfax, do sit down! You shall take a glass of brandy.'

Charlotte took a glass from Richard's hand, sipping at the spirit with a small moue of distaste. It soon restored her, and she cast an anxious look at Fanny, who lay inert upon the couch.

'Here, my love!' Mrs Shere forced a little of the brandy between her niece's pallid lips. 'This will make you feel better.'

Fanny had recovered consciousness in the carriage, but she had not uttered a word since her collapse. Now her eyes met Miranda's in a heart-rending plea for reassurance.

'Tell me the worst,' she murmured at last. 'I must know. . .even if he is dead.'

'Lakenham is not dead, though he deserves to be,' Miranda told her sharply. 'I know that his stupid action was a shock for you, as it was for all of us. Charlotte almost fainted too.' She looked a warning at her sister as she spoke. In her present state of near-hysteria, Fanny was only too likely to betray herself. 'Let me take you to your room. . .you should have rest and quiet.'

'That will be best,' Mrs Shere agreed. 'If Mr Young will be good enough to see Charlotte home? My dears, I can't believe such folly! Apart from all else, it has quite ruined your outing.'

Miranda caught Richard's eye. With his usual courtesy he had agreed at once to escort Charlotte home, but his normally cheerful expression had disappeared and she knew the reason why. Fanny's outburst had convinced him that she was in love with Harry Lakenham.

Miranda was quick to caution Fanny when they were alone.

'I know that you could not help fainting. It was a terrifying experience, but, Fanny, do take care what you say. Aunt Emma must have wondered. . .'

'I could not help it. I was sure that Harry must have been killed. You would not lie to me? He is really safe?'

'The last time I saw him he was waving to the crowd with all the effrontery in the world, and it did not make him popular. Everyone realised that he might have killed others beside himself.'

'It was just a high-spirited prank,' Fanny pouted.

'You did not think so at the time, and I doubt if it would have seem so to the widows of the men he might have destroyed.'

'You never make allowances for him. He is young. . .'

'He is, indeed, and, in my opinion, far too light-minded to think of getting wed. I'm not surprised that his grandfather is against it. Had you been a duchess, with the largest dowry in the world, Lord Rudyard must have been of the same opinion.'

Slow tears rolled down Fanny's cheeks. 'I love him. . .' she said brokenly.

'Well, I don't admire your choice. If you married him, you would not have a moment's peace of mind. A handsome face is no substitute for common sense.'

'I don't expect you to understand. You have never fallen in love. . .'

'When I do, it won't be with a man like Harry Lakenham.'

'Then I'm surprised you didn't take that fat old creature who offered for you when we first came here. Surely he was staid enough for you?'

'Mr Norton?' Miranda smiled. 'He was a little too staid, even for me. Oh, Fanny, I don't mean to criticise. No one can tell where their heart will lead them. . .'

She grew silent. For some reason the memory of a harsh, dark face swam into her mind. Heston would be a rock, a man upon whom any sensible woman might rely. It was strange how that penetrating gaze could soften into a smile which had the oddest way of making her heart turn over. She brushed the treacherous thought aside. How could she reproach Fanny further when her own fancies were just as wayward?

'Won't you rest?' she begged. 'Richard had promised to return this evening to see how you go on.'

'I won't come down. If he wishes, he may call again tomorrow.' Fanny turned her face away. 'I wish that life were not so dull at present. You have forbidden me to see Harry, and Count Toumanov is away at Oxford.'

'Haven't you had enough excitement for one day?' Miranda teased gently. 'Would you like me to sit with you this evening? I could read to you, or we might play cribbage?'

'You need not! I don't care to listen to any more lectures.'

'As you wish.' Miranda was losing patience. She changed quickly and left the room before she was tempted to utter words which she might regret. It was useless to argue further. She would abandon Fanny to her sulks.

During supper she was obliged to relate the day's events again for the benefit of her uncle.

The Alderman's face grew dark with anger. 'That young man needs taking in hand,' he announced. 'Such folly! When Lord Rudyard gets to hear of this escapade the lad will be sent to the country on a repairing lease, and high time too.'

'It was very bad,' Mrs Shere agreed. 'But I fear that young Lakenham has been indulged too much by his grandfather. His mother and father are both dead—'

'That is no excuse! How true is the old adage "to spare the rod and spoil the child".'

'He is a charming boy,' Aunt Emma ventured.

'Too charming!' came the gruff reply. 'That has been his undoing... Now let us speak no more of it. It will ruin my digestion.'

This dire prediction did not affect his appetite and he made an excellent meal. As usual, Mrs Shere left him to his port and led Miranda through into the salon.

She was playing a favourite song upon the spinet when Richard was announced. Miranda closed the instrument at once, and walked towards him.

'Your patient is better, I trust?' He bowed to both ladies as his eyes searched their faces.

'My sister is much recovered from her fright, though she is tired. She will not come down this evening, but she will be glad to see you in the morning.'

Richard hid his disappointment with a good grace. He did not refer to the incident again, confining himself to an exchange of pleasantries, and a remark about the mock battle on the Serpentine which was to take place during the following week.

It was not until Mrs Shere was called out of the room that he spoke of the subject closest to his heart.

'I have no right to ask,' he told Miranda. 'Do not answer me if you think it indiscreet, but has Fanny formed an attachment for Lord Lakenham?'

'Mere calf-love,' Miranda said briskly. 'I suspect that it is a youthful infatuation on both sides. If I am not mistaken, it will come to nothing.'

'I must hope that you are right.' His eager look dismayed Miranda. 'I do not ask from a mere vulgar curiosity. The thing is...well... I have always been fond of her, even when we were children. I felt that she needed protecting, you see.'

'You are right,' Miranda told him drily. 'And more from herself than from any outside influence.'

He smiled at that. 'You were always the strong one, Miranda. It's hard to believe that you are twins.'

'Fanny has many qualities that I lack.'

'I doubt if that is so.' He coloured to the roots of his hair. 'Seeing her again after so long...well... I won't deny my feelings. I had hoped to ask her to become my wife.'

'Dear Richard, how good you are! Fanny is a lucky girl, if she did but know it.'

'But she must not know of my wishes, at least for the moment. I would not have her feel awkward with me, or obliged to say. . .to say. . .'

'To refuse you? No, you are quite right. Let her get over this youthful passion. If I know her, it will not take long.'

'You think your mama would not object to my offering for Fanny? She seems to believe that both of you should marry well.'

'How could she object, my dear Richard? You are the son of one of her oldest friends. As to marrying well. . .in my opinion, Fanny could not do better than to wed a man with such a loving heart as yours. Mama will be satisfied with the thought of my own match.' Miranda looked a little conscious as she spoke, but Richard did not notice.

'Indeed, I wish you happy, Miranda. I cannot doubt it. Lord Heston is such a splendid fellow, isn't he?'

Miranda gave him a mechanical smile. She nodded, thinking as she did so that Richard might be the answer to her prayers. If he and Fanny were to make a match of it, she would be free to cry off from her own supposed betrothal. The prospect should have cheered her, but she found it unaccountably depressing.

Chapter Eight

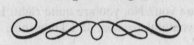

Richard was an early visitor on the following morning and Fanny greeted him with unaffected pleasure. She had recovered from her fright and was disposed to regard with a kindly eye any visitor who promised an opportunity to chatter and make plans for the coming week.

Now she dimpled as she welcomed him, drawing him aside to sit with her by the window.

Miranda regarded them with some anxiety. To flirt with any personable young man, even a childhood friend, was as natural to Fanny as breathing. Thank heavens Richard understood her. It would be cruel to raise his hopes by leading him on in that careless way she had.

Richard caught Miranda's eye, and a faint smile curved his lips. Inwardly, Miranda blessed him. His face betrayed nothing of his inner turmoil. To all appearances he was his usual amiable self. He knew very well that Fanny's lively manner did not indicate a change in her feelings for him.

'More visitors!' Fanny jumped to her feet and looked out of the window. 'Why, it is Charlotte and her brother! Now we shall be gay!'

She abandoned Richard and hurried to greet her friends.

'Are you recovered, Charlotte? What a fright we had! I thought that I should die of terror!'

'So did I!' Charlotte's manner was still subdued. 'I cannot forget the sight. Last night I could not sleep. Mama is furious. She had intended to write to Lakenham's grandfather, but now she says that she will speak to Lord Heston instead, rather than worry the old man.'

'Lord Heston?' Miranda was surprised. 'What can he do?'

'He acts in some way as Harry's guardian. He is not, of course, but there is a connection. Heston is Lord Rudyard's godson. You did not know of it?'

Miranda shook her head.

'Heston keeps an eye on Harry to oblige his grandfather. Lord Rudyard is said to be a martyr to gout. He can no longer get about as he was used to do.'

'I see.' Miranda grew thoughtful. Much that she had not understood before was now becoming clear to her. She had wondered why Heston should take so keen an interest in Harry's affairs. His concern had seemed to her to go far beyond the claims of friendship.

She sighed. Even had Heston been in London on the previous day, she doubted if he would have been drawn to attend a Balloon Ascent. In any case, Harry was no longer a child. Heston could not be expected to watch over him as if he were still in leading-strings.

Her irritation grew. Harry Lakenham, like her sister, sailed through life with little regard for the peace of mind of those about them. When she next saw him, she would give him a piece of her mind.

The opportunity came at once. They had not been

sitting for more than a few moments when the door was opened cautiously and Harry's laughing face appeared.

'Must I throw my hat in, Mrs Shere?' he cried.

'Come in, you wicked creature!' Mrs Shere strove to preserve a stern expression, but Harry was a favourite of hers. She was not proof against his charm. 'I should send you about your business. It is certainly what you deserve. . .frightening us as you did!'

Miranda was furious. Harry must be mad to come here. She could not look at him. Instead, her eyes flew to Fanny's face, and was dismayed by what she saw there. Fanny's heart was in her eyes. In another moment she must betray herself.

Miranda stepped in front of her twin and greeted Harry with cold civility.

'Are you very angry with me?' he said penitently. 'You look so severe, Miss Gaysford. I confess I am quaking in my boots. . .'

'That I must doubt, my lord!' Miranda stepped aside and allowed him to make his bow to Charlotte and her brother.

Then he moved to Fanny's side. 'Helmsley tells me that you are the person who suffered most from my ill-judged behaviour,' he said softly. 'Indeed, I am sorry for it. Will this make amends?' He handed her a small parcel.

Fanny could not answer him. Her hands were shaking as she busied herself with the wrappings.

'Let me!' He took the packet from her and opened it to reveal a book of poems. 'They are by George Byron,' he explained. 'I remembered that you liked his work.'

'Thank you.' Fanny's reply was almost inaudible.

'You feel more yourself, I hope?' Harry continued

eagerly. 'I should have called last evening to see how you did, but we landed far out in the country and I did not see Helmsley until midnight.'

'Then you were not injured?' Fanny murmured. 'Oh, if you only knew how much I have suffered!'

'It was the sudden shock which overcame your nerves,' Miranda broke in quickly. 'Charlotte was in much the same case and so were many others. . .' She picked up the book of poems. 'I had not imagined that you were a lover of poetry, Lord Lakenham.' It was a desperate effort to change the subject.

Harry grinned at her. 'I'm not,' he said frankly. 'Can't understand what the women see in the fellow. All these romantic vapourings. . . He's naught but a poseur. . .sleeps with his hair in curling papers.'

'That can't be true,' Mrs Shere protested. She, too, was an admirer of the noble lord. 'It is simply malicious gossip.'

'Upon my word, it is the truth. M'friend called on him one morning and saw it. Byron admitted that he was as vain of his ringlets as a girl. Begged Scrope Davies not to speak of it, of course, but the joke was too good to keep it to himself.'

'You will ruin my niece's pleasure in her book,' Mrs Shere reproached. 'No matter what is said of Lord Byron, there is still his poetry, which I find most uplifting.'

'Are you an admirer of his work?' Richard addressed Miranda in an effort to keep the conversation away from dangerous subjects. He had supported his introduction to Harry Lakenham with perfect civility, but there was an indefinable air of tension in the room.

'He is not quite in my style, though the fault must lie with me, I fear.' Miranda smiled at him. Byron had spoken to her on one occasion, drawn by her beauty and clearly expecting to be met with the same adulation which he regarded as his due from the female sex. She had been unimpressed, finding this lion of London society so self-centred as to be a bore. He had soon moved away in search of a more appreciative audience.

'Have you missed Heston? He is at Oxford with the Prince, I hear. . .' Harry's eyes danced with mischief as he teased her.

Miranda resolved to pay him back in his own coin.

'Lord Heston returns to town today, so I understand. Doubtless he will wish to seek you out without delay.'

'I expect so, if only to give me a roasting. . .' Harry pulled a comical face. Then, undeterred by this warning of Heston's displeasure, he grinned. 'He'll be full of stories. The Prince is a wit, you know.'

'We heard that the Regent has a humorous turn of phrase,' Mrs Shere agreed.

'It's clever, but not always kind.' Harry began to laugh. 'He described the Marquess of Wellesley as a Spanish grandee grafted on to an Irish potato. The Wellesleys are of Irish stock, as you know. It was so apt. Richard Wellesley is a stiff old stick.'

'Yet the Duke of Wellington thinks highly of his brother, I believe. It is said that the Marquess is the cleverer of the two.' Richard spoke quietly, but Harry Lakenham looked up.

'My dear sir, you sound like Adam Heston. . .' He was smiling, but there was a challenge in his eyes. His careless gossip had not met with universal approval and it did not please him.

Miranda turned to Charlotte. 'Shall you watch the procession to the Guildhall?' she asked quickly. 'Heston has promised that we are to go. . .' The rest of her words died upon her lips when the door opened and the subject of her conversation walked into the room.

At the sight of his tall figure, Miranda's heart began to pound. She could not decide if this disturbing sensation had arisen from joy or fright.

As always, Heston's face was impassive, but by now she knew him well enough to realise that he was very angry. She rose and went towards him.

'I am glad to see you, my lord,' she said with perfect truth. It was strange, but there was something so dependable about him.

'Are you, my dear? I am glad to hear it.' He kissed her hand and then her cheek.

'We did not expect you this morning,' she continued brightly. 'Here you find us talking about the procession to the Guildhall. . .' She prayed to heaven that he would not give full vent to his displeasure in the presence of her aunt.

'I see.' His indifferent gaze roved from one face to another as he greeted the assembled company with his usual civility, albeit with some reserve.

It was enough to persuade Charlotte and her brother to take their leave. Richard was about to follow them when Heston stopped him.

'Mr Young, you have not forgot that you are to join our party?'

'Your lordship is very kind. I had not forgot—indeed, I am looking forward to it.' Richard bowed and walked towards the door.

'Wait, I will go with you. . .' Harry made as if to join him.

'Must you rush away so soon?' Heston's gentle words stopped Harry in his tracks.

'I have just remembered an appointment.' Harry's face was the picture of guilt.

'An urgent appointment, I am sure. . . Will you wait upon me, say, at six o'clock? I shall be expecting you.' Heston's tone made it impossible for Harry to refuse. He gulped, nodded, and hurried away.

'My lord, you will not be too hard on him?' Mrs Shere pleaded. 'It was just a boy's trick. Lord Lakenham did not think that it might have serious consequences.'

'You are too generous, ma'am.' Heston gave her a faint smile. Then his frown returned. 'That is Harry's problem. . .he never considers the consequences of his actions until it is too late. I have been at fault. I should not have agreed to his coming to London, but that is easily remedied.'

'What do you mean?' Fanny spoke so sharply that Mrs Shere shot her a quick look of reproof.

Heston bent his penetrating gaze on Fanny. 'Harry must return to his grandfather,' he announced. 'I had thought him grown to manhood, but he is still a thoughtless child, In the country he may fall out of trees and into the river without harming others.'

Fanny gasped and burst into tears. Then she fled from the room.

'Oh, dear! My lord, you must forgive my niece. Her nerves are on edge since yesterday. Poor child. . .such a shock. I must go to her. . .'

Heston waited until the door had closed behind her.

'And how are your nerves, my dear?' he said smoothly. 'I heard that you had fainted in the Park.'

'No, I did not!' Miranda snapped. 'It was my sister who was overcome. . .'

'Curious! But then I expect that you are made of stronger stuff. . . I won't say I'm surprised.'

Miranda did not answer him.

'What does surprise me, however, is to find Lakenham here this morning. . . No doubt you will tell me the reason?'

'He. . .he came to apologise,' Miranda stammered. 'My sister and Charlotte Fairfax and many other ladies felt ill when they saw Lord Lakenham in danger of his life.'

'Touching! But then, you have such tender hearts, have you not? It has always been a source of some amazement to me that you ladies form such attachments for gentlemen with rakish tendencies.'

'Harry is not a rake,' Miranda cried hotly.

'He is well on the way to being so. Harry is a lightweight, and well you know it.'

'Do I?'

'I think so. I have never imagined you to be a fool. You think me hard, perhaps? Let me assure you that if Harry stays in London, not satisfied with forming an unfortunate attachment, he will also fall into the hands of ivory-turners and will lose his patrimony as soon as he comes of age.'

'That must be a source of anxiety to you,' Miranda said with a touch of irony.

'It is.' Heston ignored the sarcasm. 'I have known men die before the age of thirty, ruined by drink and gaming.' There was no trace of mockery in his voice and Miranda felt ashamed of her outburst.

'I know that it can happen,' she agreed.

'Well then, my love, we are in charity with each other once again, I hope? I have some news for you.

My mother longs to meet you. Next week she will come here from Warwickshire. . .'

'Your. . .your mother?' Miranda eyed him with dread.

'Of course. Why should you be surprised? I have a mother, you know. I did not spring to life fully formed, like some character of old.'

'You have not mentioned meeting her before,' Miranda said faintly.

'I was not sure that she would come to London. She is an artist, and painting is her life. I thought perhaps a quiet dinner in Brook Street, to include your aunt and uncle and your sister, if that would please you?'

Stunned by this news, Miranda could only acquiesce.

'It will give you an opportunity to see your new home. You may like to make some changes to the furnishings, but I will leave that in your hands. . .'

Miranda looked at him in desperation. 'My lord. . .'

'No, don't talk! We have been parted for too long.' He drew her to him and sought her lips.

'Please, you must not!' she protested.

'But I must! Kiss me, dearest! I have thought of you each waking moment since I saw you last.'

'Humbug!' she cried fiercely.

A quiver of emotion disturbed the calm of Heston's expression, and his shoulders began to shake.

'How unkind!' he reproached in a bland tone. 'At our first meeting you struck me. Now you throw my words of love back in my face. . . I am beginning to believe that I am betrothed to a termagant.'

Miranda was strongly tempted to inform him that he was not betrothed to anyone, but she bit back the angry words.

'I am aware that you find our situation amusing,' she retorted.

'Oh, I do, my dear, I do! I haven't been so entertained in years. You are a constant joy to me. I had begun to believe that there wasn't a woman in London possessed of any spirit. . .and you have always some surprise in store for me.'

'I shall try not to disappoint you in that respect.' Miranda spoke with feeling. She had a number of surprises in store for this self-assured creature. Her eyes began to sparkle. Then she recalled how quick he was to sense her every mood. She stole a glance at him, but he was regarding her with that false expression of tenderness which she disliked so much.

'I doubt if you could ever disappoint me, even if you would,' he murmured in sentimental tones as he slid an arm about her waist. He drew her to him, and then his hand stole up her spine. As he began to stroke her neck, little shivers of delight swept over her. He bent his head and kissed her beneath her ear.

'Must you always stiffen when I touch you?' he whispered. 'Relax, my love. You will enjoy it more.' He took the small pink lobe between his teeth and nibbled at it gently.

Miranda did not pull away from him. Insensibly she was losing the power to resist his caresses, but she made a last determined effort. There was something she had to say.

'My lord, may I ask you something?'

'Anything, my dearest!'

'I have been thinking. Would it be wise to send Lord Lakenham out of London in disgrace? He is high-spirited. It may persuade him to do something foolish.'

Heston released her and rose to his feet. There was a curious glitter in his eyes.

'You think that he might yet elope? How could that be, my dear, when you are promised to me? Or do you still have a tendre for him?'

'Of course not! I was never in love with Harry—' Miranda's hand flew to her mouth. She had betrayed herself at last. Now she waited for the explosion of wrath and demands for explanations which must be sure to follow her outburst.

'I did not think you were. . .not for a moment. On your part it was a business arrangement, was it not? My hope that you will not cry off from our engagement must lie in the fact that my fortune is greater than his.'

The cruel words struck Miranda like a blow to the heart. Tears stung her eyes, and her mouth was trembling.

'You may believe what you will,' she whispered.

'What else can I believe? You made your position very clear. You shrink from my caresses and you answer my attempts at tenderness with insults.'

'Tenderness? From you? Sir, you shall not think me a fool. I know very well what you are about.'

'I wish that I could say the same, my love.'

His words were casual enough, but they filled Miranda with dread. How much did he suspect? She hardly dared to look at him, but when she did so he appeared to be absorbed in studying the intricate pattern carved into the lid of his snuff-box.

'You speak in riddles, my lord. I do not understand you. . .'

'You will come to do so, I suspect, though it may take a lifetime. You do not find it a lowering thought to consider the trials ahead of you?'

Miranda had recovered her composure. She gave him her most enchanting smile. 'I shall do my best to bear them,' she said sweetly.

'You do not lack courage, as I have observed before. Will it carry you through an evening at Almack's?' He produced two of the coveted vouchers and laid them upon a table.

'You wish me to make an appearance there? Well, I suppose that I must do so. You will not wish me to be exposed to further insults from your friends.'

Heston looked mystified and then he laughed. 'You are referring to Lady Eddington? She is no friend of mine. I thought merely that you might like to satisfy your curiosity about the place, and Alexei finds it amusing.'

'You will invite Count Toumanov?'

'Only if you do not object. I believe you find him entertaining. . .' His voice was bland.

'I find him charming.' Miranda gave her tormentor a hostile look. 'He is so kind.'

'A worthy trait of character! Would that I could lay claim to it. . .sadly, I am irredeemable.'

'In that, at least, we are in agreement, sir. When is this visit to Almack's to take place?'

'If Alexei is to join us, it must be tonight. Those hallowed portals are open only on Wednesdays, and by next week he will be gone.'

'He returns to Russia?'

'Unless his master gives him leave to stay. It is unlikely.' Heston looked at his watch. 'Much as it distresses me, my love, I must tear myself away from your side for the moment.'

'I will try to bear it, sir.'

Heston grinned at her. 'Always the hard word, my

dearest? Until this evening, then. . .shall we say at nine?'

Miranda walked to the door and opened it a trifle. He would not attempt to kiss her again in full view of the servants. When she looked up at him she saw his mocking smile.

'Minx!' he chided. 'That would not stop me, but you may have your way. Don't worry about Harry Lakenham, by the way. I could not send him out of London, even had I wished to do so. I am not his guardian, but I'll give him a dressing-down he won't forget. What his grandfather may decide is something else.'

Miranda was thoughtful as she made her way upstairs to Fanny. Heston was the most extraordinary creature she had ever met. She needed time to think. . .to understand her own emotions. . .

In the course of the last hour her feelings had fluctuated wildly. At the sight of his tall figure she had experienced an unguarded moment of joy. It had been followed almost at once by dread of his reaction to the sight of Harry in her company.

Then she recalled the words which had hurt her so. She closed her eyes in agony. Heston had made his opinion of her only too clear. He considered her a fortune-hunter, no better than the expensive Incognitas who swarmed about the capital.

He had not made the best of bargains, either. At least those harpies gave value for money, and it was not unreasonable of him to expect the same from her.

Her face burned. If he only knew how she had longed to melt into his arms, to return his kisses, to trace the curve of that mobile mouth. . . She dared not.

It was much too dangerous. Only by keeping him at arm's length could she hope to carry out her plan.

But what was that plan? With every day that passed her motives grew more hazy. Her own honesty compelled her to admit that Heston was right in his judgment of Harry's character. She herself had given him no reason to think well of her; in fact, she had been at pains to do the opposite. Why should she object when he accused her of being what she had claimed to be?

She entered the bedchamber to find Fanny staring at the ceiling.

'Has Heston gone?' her twin demanded.

Miranda nodded.

'Of all the rude, arrogant, overbearing men in the world, he must be the worst,' Fanny cried. 'How dare he speak of Harry so?'

'He had some justification,' Miranda pointed out.

'I don't know how you can defend him. Harry was right. . .he needs a setdown. To threaten to send my darling away as if he were a naughty child? I tell you— Harry will not go.'

'Lord Heston is not his guardian. He has no power to banish him from London, so he tells me.'

'He did not give me that impression.' Fanny sulked. 'Did you get round him, then?'

'There was no need. The decision rests with Harry's grandfather. Heston will speak to Harry, of course, as someone must do.'

'Pompous creature! One might suppose that he had never been young. Lord Rudyard, I suppose, will get a full report from him?'

'I doubt it, Fanny. Heston, whatever his faults, does

not strike me as a tattle-tale. Others will be ready enough to put Lord Rudyard in possession of the story.'

'It must come to the same thing,' Fanny mourned. 'Harry will be sent away and we shall never see each other more.'

'You still feel the same about him?'

'Of course I do. I know you think me fickle, but yesterday, when I thought Harry dead, I knew I could not live without him.'

'Luckily he is still alive and so are you. Now do cheer up. Heston has obtained two vouchers for Almack's for us.'

'You are not serious?' Fanny brightened up at once.

'Indeed I am. We are to go this evening. Heston has asked Count Toumanov to make up our party. That is, if you feel well enough. . .?'

'I would not miss it for the world!' Fanny jumped out of bed, a beaming smile upon her face. 'We must tell Aunt Emma. She will be so pleased.'

'You feel you can bear Lord Heston's company, then?' Miranda asked wickedly.

'I shall ignore him. The Count is so charming. I shall leave you to put up with Heston's rudeness and sarcastic comments.'

'Thank you so much! It promises to be a very pleasant evening. . .'

Fanny regarded her twin. 'You seem to deal together,' she said. 'He never takes his eyes off you.'

'I hope you are mistaken. He worries me, I will admit. I am beginning to wonder if he suspects.'

'Nonsense! How could he?' Fanny waved the suggestion aside. 'What are we to wear tonight?'

Her final decision required more than an hour of

serious consideration, but at last she settled upon a gown of spider-gauze, with ribbon braces.

'Our zephyr cloaks will go well with this toilette,' she announced. 'Do you think them suitable?'

Miranda nodded absent-mindedly. She had taken little interest in the selection of gowns which Fanny had paraded for her approval. Heston filled her mind to the exclusion of all else.

Was he playing some deep game? It was becoming more and more impossible to doubt it. He had taken her so far along the road to matrimony that she could see no escape.

Yet he could not mean to go ahead with it. A fortune hunter, tainted by the smell of trade, and penniless into the bargain? No, it was impossible. He was planning some hideous retribution. Perhaps he intended to leave her at the altar, the butt of the Polite World. Or at best he might jilt her even earlier, and go abroad.

In her own heart she did not believe him capable of either of those actions, but the alternative might be worse. Surely he could not intend to marry her and punish her for the rest of her life? She pushed the thought aside. She was allowing her overwrought imagination to overcome her common sense.

She went to find her aunt.

To her surprise, that lady found herself unable to give the proposed visit to Almack's her unqualified approval.

'Your sister should rest,' she announced. 'She is not yet recovered from the shock of her experience yesterday.'

'The invitation has raised her spirits, ma'am.'

'Well, of course, we must all be delighted by the vouchers, but. . .' Mrs Shere hesitated '. . .my dear, I cannot think it right that you should appear there in the company of two young men, and without a chaperon. Lady Medlicott does not have the entrée. She could not go with you.'

'Heston did not mention the matter, and, Aunt, as you well know, he is a law unto himself. . .'

'Not at Almack's, dearest. Why, Willis turned away Wellington himself because he was wearing pantaloons instead of knee breeches. . .the rules are very strict.'

'It is not quite the same thing. Heston is my. . .er. . . betrothed. That must make all perfectly respectable.' Miranda looked a little self-conscious as she spoke, but her embarrassment went unnoticed.

'I don't know, I'm sure. Still, dear Lord Heston will always behave with propriety. You and your sister may go, my dear, though I believe that I should mention it to him.'

In the event, there was no need for Mrs Shere to undertake this duty. When Heston appeared, resplend-ent in black coat, satin knee-breeches, silk stockings and buckled shoes, he was quick to assure her that Alexei's sister, the Princess Chaliapine, would be happy to undertake the role of chaperon.

'Her husband will be with her, ma'am,' Alexei told her with a smile. 'Between us, we shall take good care of the young ladies.'

Mrs Shere beamed at him. She had a soft spot for a handsome young man, and Alexei was a dazzling figure in his dress regimentals.

Even so, there was no comparison between the two men, Miranda thought to herself. Heston lacked Alexei's classical features, and he was so large that he might have appeared clumsy. Yet he did not. There was some quality about him. . .an air of physical grace, perhaps?

Above all, a certain air of authority in his bearing drew all eyes, making the man beside him seem insignificant.

Chapter Nine

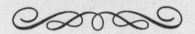

When they reached King Street, the guardian of
Almack's, the great Willis himself came forward to
greet them.

'Welcome, my lord!' He made a low obeisance. 'This
is an unexpected pleasure. . .'

Heston nodded an acknowledgement, chatting ami-
ably as the ladies removed their cloaks.

'Is my sister arrived yet?' Alexei enquired. 'She is
the Princess Chaliapine.'

Willis bowed again. 'I believe that you will find the
Princess in the ballroom, sir. May I take you through?'

'Great heavens! We'll never find her in this crush.'
Alexei gazed about the crowded ballroom.

Yet their arrival had not gone unnoticed, and a
laughing girl soon appeared at his side. She was accompanied by a burly man much older than herself. He was
dressed in Russian military uniform, and Miranda
guessed from his insignia that he must be a high-
ranking officer.

'Xenia, may I present the Misses Gaysford to you
and the General?' Alexei took his sister's hand and
kissed it. 'You have heard me speak of them, I know.'

'Very often!' the Princess teased. Then she turned to his companions and held out both her hands.

'How delightful! And I am to be your chaperon? I could not wish for prettier charges, and I shall not be too strict, I promise.'

Even the General smiled at that. It was clear that he was devoted to his lovely wife. So slender as to seem ethereal, the Princess yet bore a strong resemblance to her brother with the same clear ivory complexion, a full mouth which revealed perfect teeth when she laughed, and large almond-shaped hazel eyes. Her gown of creamy silk was cut with the simplicity which showed the hand of a master couturier, and it formed an ideal background for a necklace of the largest diamonds Miranda had ever seen. The overall effect was that of some exotic creature from another world.

In the face of such splendour Miranda felt ill at ease, but the Princess was quick to banish her shyness. She was perfectly unaffected and natural in her manner, and her charm was such that Miranda warmed to her at once.

'Adam, you are the luckiest man in London,' the Princess announced. 'I might have guessed that you would steal away one of these two beauties for yourself. There is no need to wish you happy, my dear friend. You cannot fail to be so.' She took Miranda's hand.

'I am so glad to meet you,' she went on. 'Alexei has spoken often of the lovely Gaysford twins. I see now that he did not exaggerate.'

'Princess, you are too kind,' Miranda murmured.

'Not at all! It is quite true. Have you met the Patronesses yet? They are quite formidable. Such *grandes dames*! But you must not be afraid of them.'

'I do feel nervous at the thought of meeting them,' Miranda admitted.

'But you have brought Adam here. That must most certainly be a mark in your favour. In the ordinary way he shuns the place, and they do not care to be ignored, you know. Now here comes Lady Castlereagh. See if she does not make a fuss of him.'

Miranda looked up as the wife of the Foreign Secretary bore down upon them. This high-ranking lady was not only married to the leader of the House of Commons, she was the second daughter of the Earl of Buckingham, and centuries of authority showed in her bearing.

'So, Heston, you have deigned to visit us at last?' Her mock severity left his lordship undisturbed.

'As you see, Emily. May I present to you my bride-to-be and her sister?'

Both girls made their curtsies, and were rewarded by a bow from her ladyship.

'Charming!' she murmured. 'Heston, you never cease to astonish me!'

A quiver of emotion disturbed the calm of his lordship's expression. 'You flatter me, ma'am. I had not thought it possible.'

'Wicked creature! Do you think to put me out of countenance?'

'I should not dare to attempt such a thing. It would be useless.'

Lady Castlereagh smiled. Then she turned to Prince Chaliapine and his wife, keeping them in conversation for some minutes.

Alexei had moved aside with Fanny, and Miranda found herself alone with Adam Heston.

'Well, is this temple of fashion all that you expected?' He looked down at her with a question in his eyes.

Miranda gazed about her. The room was crowded and both men and women were ablaze with jewels which caught the light and dazzled the onlookers. Toilettes of great magnificence adorned the persons of the ladies, showing to advantage against the regulation costumes of such gentlemen as were present.

'Everyone looks very fine,' she admitted cautiously. 'But I had not expected such a crush.'

His lip curled. 'My dear, this place is considered the seventh heaven of the beau monde. To receive an invitation is to achieve the peak of happiness, whilst to be excluded can only mean despair.'

'I wonder why?' Miranda murmured, half to herself.

'I have wondered too. There is a desire to mix in "select" company, as some would have it. One must dance and gossip in the best company, after all, and it is a recognised marriage mart.'

She look up sharply. Was this yet another gibe? She would never know, for Heston's attention was fixed upon the doorway. Following his gaze, she saw Harry Lakenham in the middle of a group of friends.

Her companion uttered a low exclamation beneath his breath. 'Damn the boy!' he said savagely. 'He did not say a word to me. Did you tell him of our visit here?'

'No, I did not!' Miranda snapped. 'We have not seen him since we knew that we were to come to Almack's. What is more, my lord, you will please not to use that tone with me!'

He was about to reply when Princess Chaliapine rejoined them.

'Do you like to dance?' she asked Miranda. 'It is my

passion, but they have strange notions here. The quadrille is not yet allowed, although I hear that Lady Jersey is considering it. We must be satisfied with the old English country-dances, and those energetic Scottish reels. It is a pity, as I so love to waltz.'

'Would you cause a scandal, Xenia?' The harsh, dark face softened as Heston smiled down at her.

'I shall not have the opportunity, my dear. I doubt if the musicians have ever heard of it.' She allowed herself to be led away by the gallant who had come to claim her hand.

'Shall you care to join them?' Heston asked.

'I think we are too late, my lord. The sets are made up.'

'Good evening, Miss Gaysford.'

Miranda turned to find Harry Lakenham at her elbow. She recognised the man beside him as Heston's cousin, Thomas Frant.

'Ma'am, I'm happy to see you again,' said Thomas. 'I shall hope for a dance this evening—that is, if Adam will allow it.'

'Mr Frant, I shall be happy to partner you,' Miranda replied.

Thomas looked startled by this evidence of independence, but he took her card and marked it for a Scottish reel.

Miranda did not glance at Heston. He did not own her, she thought fiercely, and she would dance with whom she chose. She half-expected some caustic remark, but his lordship was addressing Harry.

'Is not Almack's a little tame for you?' he said. 'I had not thought to see you here tonight.'

'We came for the gaming.' Unconcerned, Harry grinned at him.

'You may have done so,' Thomas announced, 'but I intend to dance. Some fine-looking women here tonight, saving your presence, ma'am. Who is that gorgeous creature over there. . .the one with the diamonds worth a ransom?'

'That is the Princess Chaliapine,' Heston informed him in repressive tones. 'The General standing by the wall is her husband.'

Thomas sighed. 'Ain't it always the way? The beauties are snapped up before you can say "knife". Will you introduce me, Adam? The General won't object if I ask her for a dance. . .'

'Ain't she a little above your touch, old boy? Dancing ain't your thing, you know. You caper like a farmer's boy,' Harry told him frankly.

'Good of you to say so!' Thomas had stiffened. 'You ain't much of a hand at it yourself.'

Heston sighed. 'Come, my dear, let us leave these two young cockerels to their quarrelling.'

He led her through the throng and into the supper-room. There he found her a seat in a secluded corner.

'May I bring you something to drink?' he asked. 'Sadly, I fear it is a choice between orgeat and lemonade.'

'I should like some lemonade, my lord.'

'Very wise! Are you hungry?' There was mischief in his eyes as he asked the question.

Miranda shook her head, but when he returned he carried a plate which he set before her with an air of triumph.

'Positively Lucullan!' he announced as he inspected the food through his quizzing-glass. 'Do pray note the interesting way in which this bread and butter has curled at the edges. It must be concern for the health of the patrons here. Fresh bread is thought to be so bad for the digestion.'

Miranda's sense of humour got the better of her. She looked up at him with laughter in her eyes.

'You did warn me,' she admitted.

'I could not be sure that you believed me. Now, my dear, you must not be shy. I shall not blame you if you fall upon this feast with ravenous appetite.'

'My lord, you are a most complete hand. Suppose one of the Patronesses should hear you?'

'I should be banished at once, and thereby cast into obscurity.'

Miranda giggled in spite of herself as she pushed the plate away. Then she remembered. She must not allow herself to be charmed into being in charity with this formidable creature, even though his wit amused her.

'We should rejoin the others,' she murmured. 'My sister will be wondering what has become of me.'

'Will she? I had supposed that perhaps Alexei might divert her thoughts from more pressing problems.'

Miranda shot a suspicious glance at him, but his expression was bland.

'Well, I should like to dance,' she said hastily. She was on dangerous ground and she was anxious to change the subject. Heston would be unable to speak to her throughout the country dance.

'And so you shall, my love.' He held out his arm and she had perforce to take it.

They took their places in the next set, and once again her companion succeeded in surprising her. He moved through the figures with a grace peculiarly his own.

'You told me that you did not care to dance,' she accused as they joined hands.

'That depends upon my partner.' He looked down

smiling at her upturned face, and something in his eyes made her heart turn over. In her confusion she missed a step.

'Careful!' he whispered. 'We are the cynosure of all eyes.'

'I beg your pardon, sir. I was not attending. . .' Her eye fell upon the couples in the adjoining set. Surely that was Fanny with Alexei, and this must be her second dance with the same young man.

As the music stopped, she moved to her sister's side. 'Pray don't dance with the Count again,' she whispered in a low tone. 'It must give rise to comment.'

'Don't be such a prude, Miranda! You are become as stuffy as Heston himself. I may not speak to Harry, and now I may not dance again with Alexei. Do you intend to make my life a misery?'

'Of course not, but you will not wish to lose your voucher. The Contess Lieven has been watching you. . .'

Fanny looked dismayed. 'I meant no harm,' she sulked.

'I know it, but you must choose from another of your beaux. There are enough of them, if I am not mistaken. . .'

Fanny brightened. 'I did dance with Mr Frant, but he trod upon my toes, and Alexei is such a perfect dancer.'

'He is not the only one. Why not give your hand to Mr Rushton? He has been hovering about you for this age.'

Fanny smiled prettily upon the gallant who had pursued her from their entry into the ballroom, and crowned his happiness by giving him her card.

Satisfied that a crisis of ill humour had been averted, Miranda turned her attention to the dancers.

The Princess Chaliapine was so graceful, she thought in admiration. Light on her feet, she executed entre-chats with consummate grace as Thomas Frant endeavoured to keep up with her.

Inspired by her example, Thomas sprang into the air, determined to be a credit to his partner, and to emulate her performance. It was then that disaster struck. Thomas landed in a heap upon the ballroom floor. He made a quick recover, but his face was scarlet as the music ended.

Beside her Miranda was aware of Harry Lakenham, convulsed with laughter.

'Shouldn't have tried it, dear old boy,' he choked out as Thomas came towards him. 'You ain't the build. Getting fat as a flawn.'

A picture of injured dignity, Thomas did not take this chaffing in good part.

'Lakenham, you will apologise for that remark,' he said stiffly. 'Otherwise you may name your friends.'

'For laughing because you landed on your rump? Come off it, Thomas. . .'

'I don't like your tone, and you may not speak such words to me. I take it you ain't afraid to meet me?'

Harry's face changed. 'Do you accuse me of coward-ice?' he said quietly.

Miranda gasped. She could not believe what she was hearing. What had started as a simple joke had turned into a quarrel and now into something much more serious. Desperate to avoid what promised to turn into a duel, she threw a glance of appeal at Heston.

Her plea was just too late. He had already stepped between the combatants.

'Stop this, you idiots!' he said in icy tones. 'Will you make yourselves the laughing-stock of London? Harry, you would do well to keep a still tongue in your head. And Thomas, as for you, if you cannot take a joke against yourself, it is a poor business. You had best shake hands and forget this nonsense. For one thing, you embarrass the ladies.'

For a full minute Harry continued to glare at his challenger. Then he laughed and stuck out his hand.

'My fault entirely, Thomas. Shouldn't have liked it if you'd said the same to me. I need to have my head examined. . . Will you forgive me and accept my apology?'

Thomas took the proffered hand. 'My fault too, old thing. I must have looked like a grounded whale. Can't blame you for laughing. . .thing is, I felt a fool.'

'I expect you turned your ankle, sir,' Miranda broke in swiftly. 'It is easily done, and very painful. I did the same myself on one occasion. . .'

'Did you, Miss Gaysford?' Thomas brightened. He had felt the humiliation keenly, but now Miranda's words in some way restored his dignity. 'That must have been it. I'll take care not to slip again.'

'Then you may beg pardon of these ladies, both of you. Take yourselves off to the gaming rooms, for heaven's sake. We've seen enough of you for one evening.'

This command was enough to quell any argument, and with Heston's severe gaze fixed upon them both young men made their apologies and disappeared.

Behind her Miranda heard a tired sigh. Fanny's face was drained of all colour, and she was clutching at Alexei's arm.

'Will you excuse us?' she asked. 'I find I have torn a flounce. My sister will help me pin it up.'

Heston gave her an ironic look, but he made no

comment as she seized Fanny's hand and led her through the crowd to the nearest retiring-room.

Once there, she swung round upon her twin.

'Do pull yourself together,' she urged. 'If you are to faint whenever Harry takes one of his odd starts, your secret will soon be common knowledge.'

'I didn't faint,' her twin protested in a low voice.

'You were on the verge of doing so. Take care, or you will betray us both. As for Harry, I am out of all patience with him. I could box his ears. How you can bear. . .?'

'I can't.' Fanny turned her face away.

'Oh, love, I'm sorry, but his behaviour is too bad.'

'I know it. It is so lowering, to be always on pins, wondering what he will do next.'

Miranda was surprised. She had expected the usual fierce defence from Fanny, coupled with excuses for Harry's folly. A tiny flicker of hope stirred in her heart. Perhaps Fanny was beginning to grow out of her infatuation. She picked up her sister's card and studied it.

'We should go back to the others,' she said quietly. 'Your next partner will be searching for you, and I'm sure you don't want the suicide of a disappointed beau upon your conscience.'

Unresisting, Fanny allowed herself to be led back to the ballroom.

As Miranda had predicted, her next partner was waiting to claim her twin, but Heston was quick to intervene.

'My dear sir, will you excuse Miss Gaysford?' he said mildly. 'She has the headache. . . I expect it is the heat.'

Overcome by being noticed by the famous

Corinthian, the young man murmured a wish that Fanny might soon recover, and bowed himself away.

Miranda looked at Fanny, but her sister was too dispirited to take exception to the summary dismissal of her partner.

'Do you wish to go home?' his lordship asked. His tone was gentle, and Miranda threw him a look of gratitude.

Fanny shook her head. 'I am quite well, my lord, but if we might sit down...'

'Of course.' Heston led them to a vacant sofa by the wall. 'You will perhaps like to watch the dancing for a time.'

The Count was dancing with his sister, his skill clearly matching her own.

'They make a handsome couple, don't they?' Miranda was anxious to draw Heston's attention from her sister's woebegone expression.

'Indeed they do. Looking at Alexei now, one could not guess less than two years ago he was with Platoff's Cossacks, driving the French from Russia.'

Fanny's ears pricked up.

'He never speaks of it, my lord.'

'No, he would not. No one who took part in that terrible campaign cares to recall the horrors witnessed by both sides, but Alexei was decorated more than once.'

Miranda shuddered. Even in Yorkshire they had learned of that fearful winter of 1812, when the French armies, which had conquered most of Europe, had been defeated by the Russian snows and the bravery of the men who were determined to defend their homeland.

The Cossacks, she knew, had appeared as avenging

hordes from the wide and icy wastes, falling upon the starving and retreating French to wreak appalling havoc. Then, ghostlike, they had disappeared, only to return when least expected.

'The Count looks too young to have seen such sights,' she murmured half to herself.

'It changed him, as such experiences must do...' Heston rose to greet two of his acquaintances who came to offer their congratulations on his betrothal. They were among the many to whom Miranda had been introduced that evening.

'I shall never remember half their names,' she whispered to Fanny.

Her sister was not attending. Alexei had returned to her side, and there was hero-worship in her eyes.

'Tell me about Russia,' she begged. 'Oh, I do not mean to remind you of the war, but the cities must be very fine.'

'You would like St Petersburg, Miss Gaysford.' He began to speak of the wonders of that city, and Fanny hung upon his every word.

'Do you care to dance again, my dear?' Heston's eyes rested upon Fanny and the Count, and then returned to Miranda.

She consulted her card. 'The next dance is to be a Scottish reel, I believe. I am promised to Mr Frant.'

Heston laughed. 'Do you think he will venture upon the floor again after his mishap? If he does, I must commend his courage, and your own.'

'His courage is not in question,' Miranda replied. 'Here he comes...'

Thomas looked a little self-conscious as he stood before her. 'Perhaps you will not care to partner me?' he ventured shyly. 'I shall understand—'

'Nonsense, I am looking forward to our dance.' Miranda allowed him to lead her out. 'You will not trip again, you know. It happens very rarely.'

Thus encouraged, Thomas began the reel with great enthusiasm, bounding high in the air, but without attempting the more intricate flourishes. He acquitted himself well and, when the dance was over, he was flushed with pride.

'There, you see! Did I not tell you? I knew you would enjoy it.'

'I had a splendid partner, Miss Gaysford. I say, you really are a brick! Adam is a lucky dog, and I shall tell him so.'

When he took her back to Heston, it was to find that the Princess Chaliapine had rejoined their little group.

'Adam, can you spare Alexei?' the Princess asked. 'Chaliapine is called away, and I need an escort home.'

'We, too, should be going.' Heston looked a question at Miranda and she nodded her assent. 'Don't worry, I will see the ladies home.'

'But I fear I have broken up your party.' The Princess looked so penitent that Miranda smiled and shook her head. 'You are quite sure? I promise to make it up to you when we meet again.' With that, she took her brother's arm and went in search of her carriage.

'She does not care to see me in Alexei's company,' Fanny murmured in an undertone.

'Hush!' Miranda felt uncomfortable. She looked at Heston, but he was engaged in conversation with a friend. 'Is that so wonderful? You should not have danced with him so much. It cannot have gone unnoticed.'

Miranda was quite sure that it had not, but the

Princess had been too well bred to comment upon this social gaffe.

Such criticism was enough to send Fanny into the sulks and she was silent on the journey home. Once indoors, she excused herself with a plea of exhaustion, leaving Miranda to explain away this uncivil behaviour. She was about to speak when Heston forestalled her.

'Your sister is not herself tonight?'

'Lord Lakenham has given her another shock, I fear. She was frightened, as I was myself, when he quarrelled with Mr Frant. I could not believe that they would call each other out over such a trivial matter.'

'Men have fought for less,' Heston said indifferently. 'Once the actual challenge has been made, it is almost impossible to draw back.'

'But that is ridiculous!' Miranda began to pace the room. 'There can be no need to accept a challenge. . .a man of good sense would let it go unheeded.'

'And be accused of cowardice? I see you have not heard of General Thornton, who was excessively fond of the dance. Theodore Hook gave him the title of "The Waltzing General", to which Thornton took exception. When they quarrelled Hook insulted him further, but Thornton did not call him out. He was accused of cowardice and asked to resign from his regiment.'

'What nonsense! At least you, my lord, put a stop to the quarrel tonight before it could go further. . . I was so thankful.'

'Were you, my dear?' Heston took her hands and drew her to sit beside him. 'I am delighted to hear that I have won your approval at last.'

Miranda was silent.

'It may surprise you to hear that I am entirely of

your own opinion in this matter. Too many men have lost their lives over incidents of little consequence.'

She looked up at him then. 'It does surprise me,' she told him frankly. 'I doubt if I shall ever understand you.'

'Did I not tell you it would take a lifetime?' He dropped a kiss upon her nose. 'Now what is it in particular that you do not understand?'

'I don't know. It's hard to explain. You mix in the highest circles, and yet you do not seem to share the opinions of Polite Society.'

'Because I do not care for Almack's, and I disapprove of duelling? It's true... I may yet become a social outcast...it is a lowering thought.'

Miranda could not repress a smile. 'You are impossible!'

'So I'm told. Now I must go, my love. It is late and you are looking tired.'

'Thank you so much, my lord. There is nothing more heartening than to be told that one is looking hagged.'

'I did not say that.' He wound a finger around a copper curl and tugged it gently. 'You could not look other than beautiful, but must you always be as prickly as a porcupine?' He began to stroke her cheek.

Miranda jumped to her feet. 'Sir, will you take a glass of wine?' she asked hastily.

'That would be delightful.' His face was bland. 'I confess to feeling parched. Those fearsome liquids which were served tonight are sufficient to decimate the population. You will join me, I hope?'

Obediently she filled two glasses and took a seat as far away from him as possible.

'Tell me about your sister,' he said suddenly. 'Her nerves are sadly on edge, I fear.'

Miranda eyed him nervously. What was the reason for this sudden interest in Fanny? Was he too afraid that she would become involved with Alexei Toumanov?

'She. . .she is sometimes a little high-strung, my lord. She was delicate as a child. Mama was always afraid that she would lose her.'

'I see. Yet nowadays she looks the picture of health.'

'Oh, yes, she is quite recovered. She grew out of her childish ailments. . .'

'But old habits die hard, and you continue to indulge her?' Heston gave her a quizzical look.

'Of course not!' she replied hotly. Then she blushed at the lie. 'Well, perhaps we do, a little. . .but, sir, you must not think ill of her. She has a loving heart.'

'And you?' He drew her to her feet. 'What of your own heart?'

Miranda could not answer him. He was so close, and suddenly she felt breathless. Beneath the fine cambric of his shirt she could feel the beating of his heart, and his nearness made her tremble. She hung her head, not daring to look at him. Then a long finger slid beneath her chin and he raised her face to his. His mouth came down on hers and the world was lost.

When he released her she clung to him, afraid that her limbs would no longer hold her upright. He kissed her again, and this time so tenderly that the tears sprang unbidden to her eyes.

'I wish you felt that you could trust me,' he murmured gently.

Miranda stiffened in his arms. 'I don't know what you mean,' she cried in confusion.

'Oh, yes, my dear, I think you do.' With those words he left her.

Chapter Ten

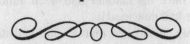

Miranda walked upstairs unsteadily. Coming as they had done at the close of a passionate embrace, Heston's final words had robbed her of all hope of sleep.

She allowed a drowsy Ellen to undress her and dismissed the girl. Then she slipped into a dressing-robe and sat by the window, gazing at the gaily illumi-nated streets with unseeing eyes.

Heston suspected something. He had made that clear when he had invited her to take him into her confi-dence. She longed to do so, but it was impossible. How could she trust him? To divulge her secret would mean that she would lose him for ever.

And that she could not bear. . .not now, when all her happiness lay in his hands. Her own honesty compelled her to admit the truth. She loved him dearly, and would do so for the rest of her life.

She could not think how it had happened. She had hated him so at first. Now the very sight of his tall figure heightened all her senses. In his company the world became a different place, so wonderful that until now she felt she had been blind to all its glories.

Yet it was all so hopeless. A tear rolled down her

cheek. Her deception could not be hidden for ever, and when it came to light he would believe the worst of her.

It was too much to bear, especially as he too seemed to have changed in his attitude towards her. On one or two occasions his gentleness had surprised her, and more than once his manner had been almost tender. Perhaps she had imagined it.

Either way, it did not matter. She had no hope of winning his love. It was true, she did not understand him. Why did he persist in continuing with this mock betrothal? They had gone so far along the road to marriage, but he could not mean to go through with it at the end.

She buried her flushed face in her hands. She knew it now. She longed to be his wife, but a future with a man who held her in contempt could only be a living hell.

A disturbed night left her heavy-eyed and listless and brought a comment from her uncle on the following day.

'You must not overdo it, my dear child,' he reproached. 'Burning the candle at both ends, I fear. I must speak to his lordship.'

'We shall not see him today. His mama arrives from Warwickshire, so he will be engaged. He has asked if we will dine with them in Brook Street as she will wish to meet my family. That is, if you agree.'

'Naturally, my dear. We must not be lacking in observance to her ladyship, but to be correct they should dine here first.'

Miranda summoned up a spurious show of enthusiasm. She would not have her uncle think that she was ashamed of her relations.

'I'll send a note to Brook Street,' the Alderman assured her. 'In the ordinary way I would not suggest it, but Lord Heston ain't in the least top-lofty, in spite of all that's said of him. He makes himself at home here, though I doubt if he's ever set foot in Bloomsbury before.'

'You are mistaken, sir. He knows the Museum well.'

'Is that so? Well, the gentry have their own ideas of entertainment. At least her ladyship need not fear our food. She won't get a better dinner in London. I'll speak to the cook at once.'

'Shall I do that?' Mrs Shere asked anxiously.

'No, Emma, not on this occasion. No expense must be spared.' He went off happily, humming with pleasure as he considered the feast which he intended to lay before his honoured guests.

'My dear, you should have a quiet day.' Mrs Shere patted Miranda's hand. 'Why not read your book? It always takes you out of yourself, as I well know. How many times have I asked you something, and you have not heard me? We shall deny all visitors for this morning.'

'Pray do not do so, ma'am. If Richard calls, I think we shall be glad to see him. He is a restful person.'

'As you wish, my love. Is Fanny still asleep?'

'I believe so. She was very tired when we came home. . .'

'We must take better care of you. Alas, it is always the same at the start of an engagement. . .so many invitations and congratulations, and so much to be done. You have not fixed a wedding-date?'

'Not yet.'

'Well, I must suppose that Heston wishes to consult with his mama. And then, you know, we must make arrangements for your own mother to bring the family up to London for the ceremony. . .'

Suddenly Miranda could bear no more. She excused herself on the thin pretext of searching for her book.

Fanny was still asleep, so she picked up the thick volume and returned to the salon, intending to curl up on the window-seat for the next few hours.

Mrs Shere gave her an anxious look. 'My dear, I have been thinking. If you were to take up tatting, it would help to pass the time. . .'

Miranda chuckled. 'Aunt Emma, you have seen examples of my tatting. You can't believe that I have a gift for it?'

'Well, then, perhaps some tapestry work? You might cover the dining-chairs in your new home.'

'No, no, you cannot wish that upon Lord Heston. Ma'am, we should have no guests. Who would sit on them?'

Her aunt was forced to smile. 'They are suitable occupations for a lady,' she said half-heartedly. 'But there, my love, you had always a lively sense of fun. Perhaps you are right.' She went away to oversee the running of her household, and Miranda was left in peace.

As her aunt had predicted, she was soon lost in her book, and though roused at times by the sound of the front door-knocker, no visitors were allowed to disturb her.

It was time for luncheon before Fanny came to find her. A night's rest had done much to restore the spirits of her twin, and now she sparkled with vivacity.

'I vow I have never laid so long abed,' she cried. 'I

have missed all our morning callers. Tell me, who has been to see us?'

'Aunt is guarding us today.' Miranda smiled. 'No one has been admitted.'

'Oh, how dull! I had wished to see Alexei, that is, if he called, but perhaps I have not missed him. There is still the rest of the day. . .' She stood by the window, gazing along the street.

'I half-expected Richard,' Miranda admitted. 'I asked that aunt Emma should not send him away.'

'Did you?' Fanny's tone was indifferent. 'Well, better his company than none at all, I suppose.'

'How can you say such things? I know quite well that you are as fond of him as I am.'

'Richard is well enough in his way but, when I compare him with Alexei, I confess that he seems dull. Miranda, did you ever hear anything so exciting as the story of the Cossacks when the Russians fought the French? And to be decorated twice? Alexei is a hero.'

'I agree, although there are degrees of heroism, you know. I have felt often that it must be difficult to be a non-combatant, held by other ties of duty.'

'You can't mean that! I don't agree at all!' Fanny's eyes grew dreamy. 'How I should love to visit Russia. . . to see St Petersburg. . .to skate on the frozen lakes. . . and to drive in a troika through the snow, wrapped in wonderful furs.'

'And outrunning the wolves if possible?'

'There you go again! sometimes I think you have no soul. You are always so prosaic.'

'I have a keen imagination, Fanny. Shall we go down to luncheon?'

It was clear that Alexei's heroism had raised him even higher in her sister's estimation. Miranda suspected that Harry Lakenham now appeared to be no more than a foolish boy in Fanny's eyes.

She hoped that it was so. With Fanny cured of her infatuation, all might yet be well. A rueful smile curved her lips. It was a vain hope and she knew it in her heart.

Fanny now showed every sign of transferring her affections to the handsome Count Toumanov, but Miranda doubted if he had thoughts of anything more than a light flirtation. Such protestations of devotion were common currency in Polite Society and were not taken seriously by girls with more experience than her sister.

Fanny, as she knew of old, would build them up in her imagination until she had convinced herself that she and Alexei were in the throes of a *grande passion*.

Miranda could only comfort herself with the thought that the Tsar and his entourage would soon return to Russia. Little harm could come to Fanny in the next two weeks.

She looked across at her twin, and then she thought of Richard. Dear Richard! He was far from being the shining knight on a white charger who appeared in Fanny's dreams. How could he compete with a handsome warrior, resplendent in a military uniform, who had taken part in so many dashing adventures?

If only he could rescue Fanny from a burning building, or snatch her from the path of runaway horses. Miranda's sense of humour bubbled to the surface, and she laughed aloud. There seemed little likelihood that any such desirable events would occur in the near future.

'There, my love, you are much better for the rest, as I knew you would be. I am glad to see you more yourself again. Will you not share the joke with us?' Mrs Shere said fondly.

'It was nothing, Aunt Emma. . .just a silly fancy. . . Do you go out this afternoon?'

'I think not. I have just been saying that I have obtained a copy of Ackermann's *Repository of Fashion*. I thought that we might look at it this afternoon. It will take some time as there are a full four hundred and fifty plates to study if we are to decide upon your bride-clothes.'

Fanny clapped her hands. 'Famous!' she cried. 'We shall like that above anything. . .'

'It can do no harm to look at it.' Miranda threw her twin a warning glance. 'But, Aunt, we have so many gowns. We shall never wear them in a twelvemonth. It would be extravagant to order more.'

'Do not let your uncle hear you say so. Your bride-clothes are to be his present to you.'

Miranda murmured her thanks, but she was determined that the Alderman should not be put to any more expense on her behalf.

This resolution was sorely tried as the ladies examined the coloured plates. Tempting visions of the latest fashions appeared before her eyes. Charming light dresses in both white and coloured sarsnets, chamerry gauzes, muslins and tiffany were all suggestions for the summer. Many of them were trimmed with gold or silver fringe. Most had short puffed sleeves, but all were caught high beneath the bosom with matching or contrasting ribbons.

'Pray look at these dear little hats!' Fanny exclaimed in delight. 'They are so unlike my own poke bonnets. They just sit on the back or the side of the head, and this one, with the plumes of feathers, is the most ravishing of all.'

'I declare! We shall be spoilt for choice. My dears, do examine the shoes. They are charming.'

Obediently Miranda looked at a selection of demi-boots in satin with gilt buttons, black kid shoes with a yellow underlay, and similar versions in a blue and black print.

Fanny was exclaiming over white silk slippers with self-ruching and binding.

'These would be my choice,' she said with longing.

'Of course! They would be just the thing for heavy snow. . .' Miranda teased.

'But, my dear, we shall have no snow before November at the earliest.' Mrs Shere was mystified. 'And it is not yet the end of June.'

'I am just funning, Aunt, but you will agree that white silk is not very practical?'

'It would quickly soil, but that cannot be a consideration when you become Lady Heston. Perhaps this grey silk, with the lower part of black leather, is a better choice? You may not have much time, you know, once your wedding date is set, and nothing is more trying than to be rushing about at the last moment. It quite ruins all one's pleasure.'

Thus pressed, Miranda had an inspiration.

'You will not take it amiss, ma'am, when I tell you that Heston has decided views upon a suitable toilette? Perhaps I should consult him before making a decision?'

'Has he, my dear? I confess you have surprised me. I had not thought that gentlemen took much interest in such matters, preferring only to see the results. Still, his lordship is so elegant himself. I expect that you are right. He will advise you on what is suitable for the life you are to lead.'

Miranda gave an inward sigh of relief. It would be wrong to involve her uncle in spending money upon a wedding which would not take place. Such conduct would be inexcusable.

But so much of her conduct had been inexcusable, she thought sadly. Even if Fanny was in the way of falling out of love with Harry Lakenham, it would not help her own disastrous situation. How could she confess the truth to Heston?

She was roused from such dispiriting thoughts when Richard was announced. He had forsworn his former dress in favour of a blue coat with brass buttons, leather breeches, and immaculately polished top-boots. His shirt-points no longer reached half-way up his cheeks, and he looked much more comfortable.

After the usual civilities had been exchanged he looked at Mrs Shere.

'Ma'am, I was wondering. . . If you do not object to travel in a hackney carriage, you might like to drive out to the Park this afternoon with Fanny and Miranda.'

'My dear boy! What a happy thought! We should enjoy a breath of air, but there is no need for a hackney.' She pulled at the bell-rope and ordered her own coach.

'Off you go, my dears, but put on your pelisses. I think it is not warm enough for just a spencer.'

As Fanny hurried away, Miranda begged to be excused.

'I should like to sit quietly for a time,' she said. 'Will you forgive me if I do not join you?'

Mrs Shere gave her an arch look. 'I understand

perfectly, my love. You will not wish to be abroad in the town if Lord Heston should chance to call.'

Miranda coloured. 'I doubt if he will do so,' she replied. 'He did not speak of it last evening.'

'Well, well, one never knows! In any event, you will not be lonely. You may keep your uncle company. He will soon be home. . .'

They had not been gone above half an hour when the Alderman returned from the city.

'Aha! You have caught me playing truant from my business, my dear.' Mr Shere looked so like the picture of an errant schoolboy that Miranda smiled.

'Let me guess,' she teased. 'You were worried about the plants in your glasshouse.'

'I admit it. In the summer months, you know, they need more care, and some must be watered twice a day. I leave instructions, but John is inclined either to drown them, or to miss one or two.'

Miranda laid aside her book. 'Will you let me help you? I can't tell exactly when the time is right to water them, but if you were to tell me. . .'

'It is just a matter of experience.' He looked doubtfully at her figured muslin gown. 'You will not wish to soil your dress. . .'

'I shall be careful,' she promised.

'Very well, then.' The Alderman removed his coat and followed her into the garden. Once there, his progress to the glasshouse was delayed incessantly as he paused to examine one or other of his extensive collection of exotic plants and shrubs.

'It is a pity the garden is so small,' he sighed. 'I have been thinking. . .perhaps I should buy a villa on the outskirts of the city, with more ground.'

'I suspect that in your heart you are a countryman, sir.' Miranda gave him an affectionate look.

'Your aunt would agree with you. She claims to be a gardening widow as it is. . .but I cannot resist a new plant. They are mighty expensive, though. I heard that the Marquess of Blandford gave five hundred pounds for a rarity.'

'So much?'

The Alderman winked at her. 'I haven't yet fallen so far from grace. Now let us see how we go on in here. . .' He opened the door to his glasshouse. 'Hmm, it is as I thought. Take up this small pot, my dear. Do you feel how light it is? That tells you that it is in need of water. With more experience one may know by simply tapping the pot. . .'

Miranda picked up a watering-can.

'No. . .no. . .not that way. Set it in this bowl of water until the soil darkens. That way you will not get moisture upon the crown.'

He moved about among his treasures, murmuring an occasional instruction to her until he was satisfied that all was well. Then, as they were leaving the glasshouse, his eye fell upon a tangled jasmine by the door.

'Dear me, this will not do! It has fallen away from the support and will come down if we have high winds.' He took a small knife from his pocket and cut some small lengths of twine. Then, with infinite care, he began to tease out the winding tendrils of the plant.

Miranda sat upon a rustic bench and watched him. It had always been a source of amazement to her to find that his chubby hands could be so gentle. Totally absorbed in his task, he had forgotten her for the moment.

She found it soothing just to sit there, not speaking,

yet grateful for his presence. There was something about his solid figure which was comforting, and she could forget her troubles for a time.

Suddenly she was aware of being watched. Looking up, she found to her surprise that Heston was standing not three yards away, his eyes intent upon her.

'My lord, we did not expect you today,' she cried in confusion. She rose to her feet, scattering the knife, the lengths of string, and the ball of twine. Her heart was pounding in the most alarming way.

Heston bent to retrieve the fallen objects, apologising as he did so for telling the servant that there was no need to announce him.

'Quite right, Lord Heston! You need stand on no ceremony with us. . .indeed, I hope that you will not. But now, as you see, you have caught me in all my dirt, so I won't offer to shake hands.' The Alderman looked delighted to see his unexpected visitor.

'I see that you are busy, sir. That is a fine jasmine, and the scent is so powerful, is it not?' Heston put out a long lean hand to examine one of the leaves.

'It is a good variety, my lord. Repton recommends it. . .'

'You know his work? I wonder if you believe, as I do, that he will change the nature of gardening in this country?'

'He has some very fine ideas. I make use of some of them here.'

'So do I, Mr Shere. Perhaps you may care to visit me in Warwickshire, where he did some work for me?'

The Alderman's eyes were bright with interest. Heston had hit upon the subject closest to his heart.

'You are most kind.' He bowed. 'You received my note, Lord Heston?'

'Indeed I did. We shall be honoured to dine with you tomorrow, though I should warn you that my mother is not much accustomed to company. By her own choice she leads a somewhat solitary life. . .'

'She will not object to coming into Bloomsbury?'

'My dear sir, it is quite her favourite part of London. When she visits the capital, which is not often, she spends her days in the Museum. Sometimes I have suggested that she might take up residence there. . .'

The Alderman laughed heartily. 'It would be uncomfortable to live among the antiquities, I should imagine, although I have not seen them. My lord, will you excuse me? I shall get a roasting from my wife if she discovers that I have received you in my present state.' He hurried into the house.

'Your mother is well?' Miranda ventured when she and Heston were alone. 'I trust she did not find the journey trying?'

'I doubt if she noticed it.' Heston grew thoughtful. 'She is not quite in the common way, you know, and she is very shy. To be in company is a torture to her. I think I need not ask, but, my dear, may I beg you to be kind to her?'

'You are quite right. You need not ask that of me,' Miranda answered gently. 'Shyness is an affliction which those who do not suffer from it find hard to understand.'

'Yet you do and I think that you have never been shy in all your life.'

Her enchanting smile peeped out. 'You may have noticed, sir, that I find it difficult to keep a still tongue in my head when I have strong opinions upon a subject.'

'Yes, I had noticed,' he agreed drily. 'On occasion

there can be a certain...er...paralysing frankness about your conversation.'

Miranda flushed to the roots of her hair. Was he referring to that dreadful interview when she had announced herself ready to become his bride? She felt ready to sink with embarrassment, and she would not meet his eyes.

He looked at her bent head and his lips twitched with amusement. 'No answer for me? I can't believe it! I was congratulating myself upon winning for my bride the only girl in London who does not look at me as a terrified rabbit might gaze upon a stoat.'

'Now you are gammoning me,' she murmured. 'That can't be true, my lord.'

'Indeed it is! I have pondered upon the matter. It is so disheartening that on occasion I have been tempted to put a period to my existence...'

Miranda repressed a giggle. 'How astonishing!' she replied in a demure tone. 'There can be no reason for this strange effect you have upon the ladies. After all, sir, your manner is so engaging on first acquaintance.'

'Minx! That's milled me down.' He took a seat beside her and smiled down at her upturned face. Miranda's heart turned over.

'You... I mean...it was good of you to invite my uncle to see Repton's work on your estate,' she said hastily. 'Gardening is his passion.'

'I guessed as much. He and my mother will deal together famously. In her painting she has recorded every flower in the grounds.'

'I wish I had her gift, but I believe it to be inborn.'

'You are right. One can acquire a certain facility, but there can be no comparison with the work of a true artist.' He looked about him. 'All this is very pleasant and comfortable.' He drew her head down to rest upon his shoulder. 'I have a confession to make,' he said.

'Yes, my lord?' Miranda was startled, and she stiffened. Was he about to tell her that he knew of her deception? A moment's reflection convinced her otherwise. Heston would not be sitting here at his ease if that were the case.

'I met your aunt and your sister in the Park. I came here in the hope of finding you alone.'

'I see,' she answered faintly. 'Was there some reason, sir?' She prayed that he would not start to question her or ask her again to trust him.

'Need you ask?' His fingers tickled the back of her neck, and a shiver of pleasure ran down her spine. She ought to pull away from him, to make some excuse to go indoors, but she could not. His caresses were beginning to produce such sensations of delight that she was losing all power to resist him.

'My uncle is pleased that you and your mother have agreed to dine with us tomorrow,' she whispered. It was a last desperate effort to divert his mind from this seductive love-making. 'You seem to have changed your mind about his ill intentions. . .'

Heston held her away from him and looked deep into her eyes. 'In these past few days I have changed my mind about so many things,' he told her. Then his lips found hers and once again she was swept away into a world where only they existed.

When he released her her head was spinning, but his next words brought her back to reality with a jolt.

'May I hope that you too have changed your mind?' he asked. 'Or do you still intend to punish me, my love?'

Miranda stared at him in horror. He must have seen

through all her plans. Racked with despair, she could think of nothing to say to him.

Then providence came to her aid in the shape of Fanny, who came tripping down the path.

She stopped short at the sight of Heston.

'Why, my lord, I did not expect to see you here,' she said. 'I thought you had a pressing engagement. . .'

'I had,' he told her smoothly.

Fanny looked at her sister's face and then at his. What she saw there brought a look of astonishment to her face. It was quickly hidden.

'Then I must beg your pardon for disturbing you,' she faltered.

'Lord Heston was just leaving,' Miranda told her. 'Did you enjoy your drive?'

'Oh, yes. After you left, Count Toumanov stayed on with us, sir. We set him down at the Imperial Hotel in Piccadilly. Is it not strange that the Tsar should choose to stay there, rather than at Carlton House?'

Heston laughed. 'After the cold of the Russian steppes, the Tsar may have found the heat at Carlton House somewhat stifling. The Prince is afraid of draughts, even in the height of summer, and the windows are never opened.'

'But does not the King of Prussia stay there, and General Blücher, too?'

'On their own terms, Miss Gaysford. I hear that they sleep on army cots, rather than in the luxury of canopied beds.'

'How very odd of them!' Fanny was about to question him further when Miranda gave him her hand.

'We shall not detain you further, sir. It was good of you to call in answer to my uncle's note.'

She saw the laughter in his eyes, but he accepted his dismissal with good grace.

'Miranda, you do not fool me for a moment,' Fanny began as soon as he had left. 'I have suspected for some time that you don't dislike Heston as you once did.'

Miranda was silent.

'Why don't you answer me? Surely you cannot have a *tendre* for him?'

'Would it be so strange?' her twin said slowly. 'I believe I have misjudged him. . .'

'Oh, pray don't say so! He means you harm, I know it! To make you fall in love with him. . .what better way to injure you?'

'I don't think that of him.'

'Then you are a fool! You will not tell me that he holds you in regard? Think of the things he said to you.'

'I can't forget them.'

'Then how can you care for him?'

'I don't know, except that he has changed, and so have I.'

'Then you had best go on with this remarkable betrothal, and I wish you joy of him.' Fanny's face grew bitter.

'You need not do so. He will never marry me. How could he when the truth is out?' Her anguish was too deep for tears and she turned away.

Chapter Eleven

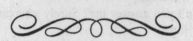

Fanny did not broach the subject again. She was
tempted to do so, but the closed look on Miranda's
face warned her against it.

Instead, she set herself the task of diverting her
sister's thoughts into lighter channels, and Fanny could
be charming when she chose.

'Will you not read aloud to me?' she coaxed. 'I have
finished *The Mysteries of Udolpho*, whilst you are still
reading *Ivanhoe*!'

'But I am halfway through the book. You will not
understand the story.'

'You could tell me the beginning. Perhaps we might
go to the library tomorrow. . .'

'Do you mean to meet Harry Lakenham again?'
Miranda asked.

'Of course not. I have not seen him, so you need not
be suspicious.' Fanny gave her a bright smile.

Miranda was satisfied. Her sister was incapable of
dissembling. It was clear that Harry's star was fading,
or Fanny would not look so cheerful.

'Very well then. In any case, the library will be closed

tomorrow. Have you forgot the Procession to the Guildhall?'

'But that is not until the following day.'

'So it is. I must be dreaming. . .tomorrow is the day when Lady Heston is to dine with us.'

Fanny looked uncomfortable. 'I'm sorry for what I've done, believe me, especially as. . .'

'As you no longer think of marrying Harry Lakenham?' Miranda said steadily.

'Well, you see, I am not sure. . .he has behaved so badly, as you said yourself.'

'Is it not rather late to be convinced of that? I wish you had discovered it before we found ourselves in such a tangle.'

'It's easy to make a mistake,' Fanny pouted. 'You have done the same with Heston.'

'So I have. There is no point in recriminations, is there?'

'At least you are free to cry off from your supposed betrothal, if that is what you wish.'

Miranda lost her temper. 'You think it will be easy? When he is coming here tomorrow with his mother?'

'She may take you in dislike and forbid the match.' Fanny's brow cleared. 'That would be the obvious solution.'

'I intend to make sure that she does not take me in dislike. Heston has asked particularly that we make her welcome, and we shall do so.'

'You are very anxious to oblige him.'

'In this particular case I am, and I expect the same from you. None of your tricks, remember! You will be civil to her, if only for Uncle's sake.'

'I shan't forget my manners,' Fanny sulked.

'Make sure that you don't. I warn you, Fanny, I won't put up with any of your nonsense!'

Fanny grew more conciliatory. When Miranda spoke in that particular tone it was time to retreat.

'Is Lady Heston very *grande dame*?' she asked. 'Did Heston tell you anything about her?'

'Only that she is shy and does not go much into company. . .'

'How odd! I mean, with her position in society and all her wealth, one might suppose. . .'

'She is an artist. . .a gifted painter.'

'Well, that is something. Better a Bohemian than a fearsome dragon like the Countess Lieven. Did you see the high-nosed way she looked at us at Almack's?'

Miranda gave up. 'Do you wish to hear the story of *Ivanhoe* or not?' she snapped.

Fanny subsided. 'More than anything,' she said meekly.

The candles were guttering in their sockets before Miranda laid aside the book. Then Mrs Shere appeared.

'Not abed yet?' she reproached them. 'I saw your light and wondered if aught was amiss.'

'We were reading, Aunt. I beg your pardon. . .we have been wasting the candles.'

'As if that mattered, my dear child. Still, it is late, and we shall have a busy day tomorrow. You will need your rest.'

She kissed the twins and left them to their slumbers, but it was a long time before Miranda fell asleep. The thought of meeting Lady Heston filled her with dismay, and it was long after midnight when she closed her eyes.

* * *

On the following day the household was astir at an early hour. Amid the bustle Miranda sought out her aunt.

'Is there anything we can do to help?' she asked.

'Perhaps the flowers, dearest girl? The cook tells me that we have no milk. . . I might have expected it. Milk has been so difficult to come by with all these people in the city. As for the linen. . .it has not yet been returned. Those washerwomen leave our orders to put those of the foreigners first. I will look out some more just in case. . .' She hurried away.

Miranda decided to leave the flower arrangements until later in the day. They would wilt in the sultry heat.

The day before her stretched out endlessly, and she was glad to accompany Fanny to the library. It would help to pass an hour or two.

Luncheon that day consisted of cold meats and salads and she was glad of it. Her appetite seemed to have deserted her. When it was over, she took Fanny with her and went into a chilly pantry which normally did duty as a flower-room. John had plunged the cut blooms up to their necks in water to keep them fresh.

She and Fanny began upon their task, but even that did not take long. Afterwards the hours seemed to crawl. It was the oddest thing. In Heston's company the time flew by, but without him the hands of the clock refused to move.

'What are we to wear tonight?' Fanny asked. 'I suppose we must be very fine.'

'Your white gowns with the French bead edges would be suitable,' Mrs Shere suggested. 'And perhaps a small wreath of flowers in your hair?'

'I think I'd prefer a ribbon,' Miranda answered

hastily. The flowers would make her look too much like a bride.

'As you wish, my love. The ribbons should match the blue tiffany sashes, and you will wear your pearls tonight, I hope? You would not have his lordship think that you despised his gift, and yet you have not worn it.'

Miranda nodded her assent. There was no way she could refuse. Mild panic seized her as she thought of the woman she was to meet that evening. How many others would be drawn into this deception before it ended? And how she disliked herself for going on with it.

When the twins came down that evening Mrs Shere inspected them with approval. Miranda was wearing her pearls, much against her own inclination. Beautiful though they were, she felt that they must burn her skin and brand her for the trickster which she felt herself to be.

'I have not seen you in better looks, my dears,' Mrs Shere said kindly. 'Now, tell me what you think of the dining-table. . .'

They accompanied her into the panelled room. In the soft candlelight, the huge silver epergne which formed the centrepiece glistened with reflections. Beside it stood small pillars holding wreaths of trailing plants.

Miranda caught her breath. 'How lovely!' she exclaimed. Then something about the table settings caught her eye. 'Aunt, the servants are mistaken. They have laid for eight, and we are only six.'

'Did I not tell you? I vow that today my head has been in such a spin that I forgot. I have invited Count

Toumanov and also Mr Young. Eight is such a comfortable number for a dinner, and we could not have four ladies and two gentlemen.'

Fanny's eyes began to sparkle. 'How clever of you, Aunt!'

'Well, you know, my dears, I thought it might take away any little awkwardness which might occur. Lady Heston is well acquainted with the Count, and she will like to have a friend here. As for Mr Young, he is always welcome, and Lord Heston seems to think well of him.'

'So he should!' Miranda cried warmly. 'Richard need not fear to be in any company.'

'Of course not, dearest!' Mrs Shere patted her hand. 'You must be calm. To meet one's future mother-in-law is always an ordeal, but she cannot fail to love you as Heston does himself.'

There was no time to say more, for at that moment Richard was announced. As he came towards them, Miranda blessed him. Dear Richard, always so calm and pleasant, and so dependable. She gave him her hand.

'How do you go on?' he murmured in an aside. 'This cannot be very pleasant for you.'

'It is hateful,' she replied. 'But I have no choice.'

'There is always a choice, Miranda, though you may not care to make it. . .'

'Oh, don't' she cried in desperation. 'Please don't! If you only knew. . .'

She looked up as the rest of the party was announced, allowing Heston to take her nerveless hand in his. Then he led her forward.

'This is my bride, my dear Mama. I hope you will love her as I do.'

Miranda sank into a deep curtsy, hardly daring to look up at the woman who stood before her.

When she did so, she was reassured. Lady Heston was very tall, but so thin as to make her son seem larger than ever. There was little resemblance between them, except for the raven darkness of their hair and brows. In place of hard grey eyes, her ladyship's were of a blue so dark as to appear violet. What struck Miranda most was the peculiar sweetness of her expression, combined with a certain reserve.

'I am glad to meet you,' Lady Heston murmured in a musical voice. 'Adam is so happy, and I must thank you for it.'

Miranda shot a fleeting glance at Heston, but he was regarding them with an air of benevolence. She could hope for no help from that quarter. She felt a surge of indignation. How dare he claim to love her when both he and she knew that it was untrue? When it came to deception, she was not the only one who had cause for self-reproach.

She felt even worse when Lady Heston took her hands and kissed her, knowing what it had cost this shy and sensitive woman to make such a gesture of affection.

'Ma'am, you are very kind,' she said in a low voice. 'Adam tells me that you are an artist, with an interest in flowers and plants. My uncle shares that interest. You might care to see his collection. . .?'

'Will you show it to me later?'

'It would be my pleasure, Lady Heston, but my uncle is the expert. I have little knowledge, and could not give you the Latin names.'

The Alderman had been listening to their conversation. Now he stepped forward with an offer to take her ladyship into the garden.

Miranda sighed with relief. She had no wish to enter into a private conversation with Lady Heston. Her ladyship might appear to be reserved and even diffident, but loving her son as she did her perception would be keen. She must soon discover that all was not as well as it might appear to the less interested observer.

Fanny was deep in conversation with Count Toumanov and Richard was chatting to her aunt. Miranda stood by the long windows watching Lady Heston as the Alderman trotted beside her down the garden path.

'Did I not say that they would deal famously together?'

She turned to find Heston by her side, and frowned at him.

'Now do not look black at me,' he reproached. 'What have I done to deserve it?'

'You need not have claimed to love me,' she replied with strong feeling. 'We both know that it is not true.'

'You must forgive me,' he told her smoothly. 'It was but a natural desire to set my mother's heart at rest. She disapproves of arranged marriages, with no serious attachment on either side. I fear she regards them as a certain path to disaster.'

'She is quite right,' Miranda said hotly.

'Do you think so, my dear? You have surprised me yet again. . .' He gave her a dangerous smile. 'I had not supposed that your affections were engaged. Am I to hope that you are learning to think of me with kindness?'

The colour rose to Miranda's cheeks, and for the

moment she was robbed of speech. She turned away from him, throwing a pleading glance at Richard as she did so.

He came to her rescue at once, leading Mrs Shere to join them, with the expressed desire to pay his respects to Lord Heston.

His lordship was all civility, but his lips twitched.

'What should we do without our childhood friends?' he murmured to Miranda. Then, in his usual easy manner, he began to speak of the Prince's recent visit to Oxford.

'The Regent was well received there?' Mrs Shere enquired. 'I fear that he is not always treated well in London, and I cannot think it right that the people should behave so ill as to hiss and boo him, when perhaps they do not understand. . .'

Heston bowed. 'The visit was a great success, ma'am. His Royal Highness is popular in that city. In his speech he said all that was gracious.'

'It was a great occasion.' Alexei brought Fanny over to join them. 'Two hundred persons dined at the Radcliffe Camera.' His eyes twinkled. 'There were lighter moments, Mrs Shere, in spite of all the gold plate. General Blücher enjoyed the wine to such an extent that later he got lost in search of his lodgings.'

They all smiled at that.

'And my master insisted upon strolling down the High Street afterwards to see the candles shining a welcome in every window. He may be Tsar of All the Russias, but the spectacle pleased him immensely.'

'He is thought to be extremely handsome, is he not?' Fanny's eyes shone. 'How I look forward to seeing him tomorrow.'

'Where will you be?' Alexei asked eagerly. 'I shan't forget to wave to you as we pass.'

Heston was explaining the exact position of their vantage point when his mother came up to him. Her arms were filled with flowers, and she was smiling.

'See how spoiled I am,' she murmured. 'I feel so guilty. . . Mr Shere has stripped his garden for me.'

'Let me take them, your ladyship.' Richard stepped forward and relieved her of her burden. 'Should they go into water?'

Mrs Shere signalled to a footman, who bore the blooms away. Then the Alderman returned, and Lady Heston went to him at once.

'I have done more damage than a plague of locusts, my dear sir. I must hope that your garden will recover. . .'

The Alderman waved her apologies aside. He was glowing with pride. 'Happy to have pleased you, ma'am. As I say, some of the roses are cuttings from the Empress Josephine's collection at Malmaison. A friend was good enough to bring them over.'

'I have seen them only in paintings by Pierre-Joseph Redouté until today.'

'By next year they will be well established. I shall hope that you will come to see them. The Gallicas, in particular, should be very fine. . .' He was about to launch into a discourse upon his favourite topic when Mrs Shere caught his eye.

'Well, well, I must not be a bore upon this subject,' he said cheerfully.

At that moment the gong sounded and they went in to dine.

In spite of her aunt's efforts, Miranda had feared that the atmosphere at the dining-table must be strained. As she glanced about her, she sensed with some surprise that it was not so.

Seated at the Alderman's right hand, Lady Heston had clearly found a friend. She was chatting to him without the least trace of reserve.

Seated at the other end of the table his wife had Lord Heston by her side, and he at once engaged her in a conversation which touched upon the Prince Regent's courtesy in translating General Blücher's speech in German for the benefit of the General's English audience.

Miranda turned to Richard, who was seated on her right.

His eyes were fixed upon Fanny, who faced him across the table, and was absorbed in listening to the Count.

'Take heart!' she murmured inaudibly. 'She is quite recovered from her previous infatuation.'

'And in the way to falling into another one?' His face was sad. 'How can I compete? I can't appear in a splendid uniform, or tell of my adventures. There isn't much adventure to be found in Yorkshire.'

'The Tsar and his entourage will leave next week,' Miranda told him. 'You have heard of the old saying that out of sight is out of mind?'

Richard brightened visibly. Then his face fell.

'There will be someone else, with more to offer than I.'

'Stuff! You shall not think so poorly of yourself.'

She might have gone on, but the conversation became more general. Peace with France was to be proclaimed on the twentieth of June, and later that week the Fleet was to be reviewed at Portsmouth.

'Shall you go there, my lord?' The Alderman addressed himself to Heston. 'It will be a fine sight.'

'I believe so, sir. I'm not yet sure if I shall accompany the Prince, but Alexei will go, of course.' He glanced across at his friend with a slight smile in his eyes. 'It won't be a favourite occasion for him. He is the worst of sailors.'

'You are right!' the Count shuddered. 'Give me a horse beneath me rather than a rolling deck. The motion of the sea is the worst sensation in the world. Shall you go to Portsmouth, sir?'

The Alderman shook his head and laughed. 'We shall content ourselves with the mock battle on the Serpentine in August.'

'Very wise, if I may say so. Is it not to be a re-creation of the Battle of Trafalgar?'

Fanny clapped her hands. 'Oh yes, and it is to be exact, down to the cannon and the rammings, and the smoke. Someone told me that the crews are to be dwarfs, to make the ships seem larger.'

'The Regent does nothing by halves, ma'am.' Heston turned to Mrs Shere. 'He intends that the celebration of the first centenary of the House of Hanover shall be an unforgettable spectacle.'

'I cannot blame him,' Mrs Shere replied. 'It will be a grand occasion, and the more so because we shall have our feet on dry land. I share your dislike of the motion of the sea, Count Toumanov. I cannot be easy even in harbour.'

'Dry land is much to be preferred,' Alexei agreed. 'Alas, I shall not see the battle. We return to Russia after the Fleet Review.'

Fanny's face fell. 'Oh, no!' she began. Then a sharp

look from Miranda silenced her. Her sister's obvious disappointment went beyond the bounds of propriety.

'You do not stay on?' she asked. 'We shall all be sorry to lose you.'

'It is not for another two weeks or so. Meantime, there is much to see and do. I have not yet visited the Temple of Concord, or the Chinese Pagoda. . .'

A general discussion of these wonders relieved Miranda of the need to speak overmuch herself. She had eaten little of the splendid meal, although the Alderman's cook had lived up to his reputation.

White almond soup with asparagus had been followed by a fine turbot with a side dish of fish quenelles in bouillon, and another of tiny vols-au-vent filled with shrimps, as well as a salver of whiting.

There was something for every taste, from salmis of duckling in wine and epigrammes of chicken to ham braised in Madeira and a baron of beef.

Miranda looked about her. Her own lack of appetite had gone unnoticed due to the Alderman's concern that Lady Heston should eat more. Smiling, that lady shook her head.

'I seldom dine on more than a single course,' she protested. 'But I must compliment you upon your chef. Everything is so delicious. It will put our own man upon his mettle, I assure you.'

Heston was quick to agree with her. He, at least, had done full justice to the meal, as had Alexei and the Alderman himself.

Heston looked at Miranda's plate. 'Have you been influenced by George Byron?' he teased in a low voice.

'I don't understand you, sir.'

'It is one of his little foibles. He dislikes to see

women eat, preferring to think of them as ethereal creatures.'

'What nonsense!' she cried warmly. It was enough to persuade her into accepting a serving of summer fruits in jelly.

'You are not an admirer of the noble lord,' he asked carelessly. 'I thought I saw a book of his upon your table the other day.'

'That belongs to Fa— to my sister. Lord Lakenham gave it to her.' Miranda could not look at her companion. Once again she had come so close to giving herself away.

Apparently he had not noticed the slip. 'Lakenham gave her a book?' He looked incredulous.

'It was a peace-offering,' she explained hastily. 'He was sorry to have caused her to faint at the Balloon Ascent.'

'Very civil of him,' Heston said smoothly. 'If he continues in his present ways, he will be forced to buy up half the books on sale in London. Don't you agree?'

'I have no idea. We have not seen him, sir.' It was a curt reply and she flushed. She had warned Fanny to be civil to their guests, and now she herself was guilty of rudeness.

Heston waved aside the cheeseboard and changed the subject. 'We shall not stay late this evening. Tomorrow we must make an early start if we are to get through the crowds before the procession begins.'

She nodded as Mrs Shere broke in with a question about the arrangements for the following day.

Miranda turned to Richard.

'I believe I shall go back to Yorkshire after the Parade,' he said. He looked so disconsolate that her heart was wrung with pity.

'Pray don't leave just yet,' she begged. 'Your father will spare you for another week or two. . .'

'But will it do any good?' he sighed. 'Fanny does not look at me.'

Miranda frowned a warning at him. Heston had sharp ears. If he heard Fanny's name on Richard's lips, all would be lost.

'Give her time!' she insisted. 'You heard the Count. In two weeks' time he will be gone, and that will be your opportunity.'

'I hope you may be right.' His face cleared a little. 'I'll stay if you feel that I have the slightest chance of winning her.'

'Of course you have,' she encouraged. 'Would that I could discover a monster for you to slay. . .'

She smiled at that, though he looked rueful. 'I know you think her foolish, but I love her so. I would care for her, you know, and she would have all she could desire. Once away from London, she will be different.'

'I agree,' she told him quietly. 'Perhaps it was not the best idea for us to come here. Mama was delighted and Uncle believed that it would be an opportunity for us but things have gone so sadly wrong.'

Richard pressed her hand. 'Are you quite sure of that?' he asked.

'I'm afraid so. I can see no way out of our difficulties that will not hurt the people I love best.'

His face was grave, but he pressed her hand again. 'I believe you to be mistaken, and that all will yet be well for you.'

She was about to deny his words when Mrs Shere rose from the table and the ladies withdrew to the salon.

'Do you like music, your ladyship? Both our girls play so well upon the spinet. . .'

Miranda threw her aunt a glance of gratitude. She had been wondering what on earth she was to say to Lady Heston if they should find themselves tête-à-tête.

A pleasant smile of encouragement sent her to the instrument, with a gloomy-looking Fanny beside her.

On the pretext of searching through the music, she managed to have a private word with Fanny.

'For heaven's sake, smile!' she urged. 'Would you have everyone notice that you dislike the thought of Count Toumanov going away? They may imagine that you have a tendre for him.'

'London will be so dull without him,' Fanny sighed.

'Then we had best go back to Yorkshire.'

This dire prospect startled Fanny. 'You cannot mean it! How can you say such a thing? You cannot leave Heston, can you?'

'No, I can't, and well you know it. Now turn the music, and try to look as if you are enjoying it.'

Subdued, Fanny did as she was bidden and Miranda began to play a favourite piece. As always, she found the music soothing, and it as not until she reached the final bars that she was aware of being watched. She looked up quickly to find Lady Heston's eyes upon her. In their depths she saw a question, or was it her imagination?

Their aunt beckoned to the twins. 'Come and sit down with us,' she said. 'My dear, we have been discussing a date for your marriage.'

Miranda froze. Why had she supposed that matters could not possibly grow any worse? She stared from one face to the other, but it was Fanny who broke the silence.

'Must it be just yet?' she asked in a hollow voice. 'There is so much to be done, and Mama will wish to make arrangements to come to London. . .'

'Naughty girl! You must not put difficulties in your sister's way, my dear child.' Mrs Shere turned to her ladyship. 'You must forgive my niece, ma'am. The twins are so close that they dislike the thought of separation, one from the other.'

'That is perfectly natural,' her ladyship agreed quietly. Her thoughtful gaze rested upon Miranda's face. 'There is a special bond between twins, so I understand, and you are identical, are you not?'

'Yes, your ladyship.' Miranda sat down suddenly, clenching her hands as she waited for the next blow to fall. It came soon enough.

'We have decided upon the first week in September, if Lord Heston agrees. That will give us more than two full months to make our preparations, and allow plenty of time for your mama to come down for the ceremony.'

Fanny dared not argue further, and Miranda could think of nothing to say. To protest would be unthinkable. How could she disgrace her aunt and uncle by announcing her decision to end her betrothal at this moment?

She prayed that something would happen. . .anything to extricate her from her present predicament.

Her prayers were answered briefly when the door opened and the gentlemen came to join them.

Mrs Shere rang for the tea-tray.

'Your ladyship, if you will be kind enough to ask Lord Heston for his views?'

'Upon what, ma'am?'

'We have been speaking of your marriage,' his

mother told him. 'We thought perhaps the first week in September? Is that agreeable to you?'

'Much too far away!' He grinned at her. 'But if it suits my bride, then her wish is my command.'

He sat down beside Miranda and took her hand. 'What do you say, my dear?'

She knew then that she must end this hoax without delay, but this was neither the time nor the place. She kept her eyes fixed firmly upon the carpet.

'It shall be as you wish,' she said.

Chapter Twelve

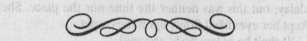

As Heston had promised, the company did not stay
late, but Miranda was only half-aware of their leaving.

She felt that she was drowning in deep water, and
reality no longer had a meaning for her. She was
drifting as though through a dream from which she
must awaken. Even her own voice sounded strange to
her.

Fanny and Richard watched her with concern. They
alone knew how she was suffering. They stood together
in one corner of the room, and Fanny's lips were
trembling.

When they were alone that night, she flung herself
upon the bed and wept as if her heart must break.

'Don't cry!' Miranda told her quietly. 'It can serve
no purpose.'

'But what will you do?' her sister wailed. 'I did not
think it would come to this. . .'

'What did you expect? When one is betrothed,
marriage must follow.'

'But you are not betrothed!'

'Sadly, I am, and everyone knows it.' Miranda felt
like an automaton. She was moving about the room,

taking off her gown and her undergarments and even the ribbon in her hair, but she was not aware of it.

'But you can't marry Heston. . .you can't.'

'No, I can't. I won't cheat him to that extent.' Something in her voice made Fanny look at her, and then she began to weep afresh.

'You love him, don't you?'

'Yes I do. I had not intended it, but there it is.'

'Then, dearest, you must wish to marry him. If you love him, would it not be possible. . .to go ahead with it, I mean?'

Miranda's smile was a ghastly travesty. 'You think I should deceive him further? Sometimes I wonder what you must *think* of me. I won't do it, Fanny. Tomorrow I shall tell him everything.'

Fanny paled to her lips. 'Oh, please, you can't! He will blame me, I know it. If you must cry off, why not start a quarrel? That would give you the excuse. . .and then no one would need to know—'

'Your part in this hoax, or mine? I might take your advice if I thought that it would serve, but it won't.'

'Why not?'

'You don't know Heston as I do. He would see through it in a moment. Sometimes I think that he suspects already.'

'How could he?'

'I don't know. It is the things he says and the way he looks. . .'

'If he loves you, he will not care, and he must do so or he would have taxed you with it.'

'If he loves me?' There was no amusement in Miranda's laugh. 'Fanny, you know what Heston thinks of me. He has made his opinion only too clear.'

'Then I think it wrong of him to pretend to love you,

especially to his mama. He is guilty of deceit, as much as any of us.'

'It really doesn't matter as to who is most to blame. The point is that I must put an end to it. We can't go on like this and I shall tell him so in the morning.'

'Oh, please, you can't! Not tomorrow, I beg of you. . . everyone will be there to see the Procession and I could not face them all. We shall be disgraced and sent back home at once.'

'It can't be helped.'

'Yes, it can! I think you are being very selfish, Miranda. I do not care to be sent away from London. Alexei has only a few more days with us, and you might think of me instead of yourself.'

This remark caused Miranda to gaze at her sister in stupefaction. Words failed her for the moment.

'Besides, you will think of something. . .some other way to free yourself,' her sister announced. 'You spoke of telling Heston that you had mistaken your heart. Would that not be better than to shame us? You must consider Aunt and Uncle.'

Miranda was silent.

'Won't you wait a little while?' Fanny coaxed. 'It is not as if you were to be wed next week. September is a full two months away. . . In the meantime, anything might happen.'

She looked a little conscious as she spoke and Miranda's heart sank. Surely Fanny did not expect an offer from Count Toumanov? It stiffened her resolve to put an end to the hoax without delay, but there was much to consider in her sister's pleas.

She grew thoughtful. A scandal must be avoided if possible. She had been badly shaken to hear that a date was to be set for her wedding, but as her composure returned she knew that it was panic which had over-whelmed her. Her plan to confess everything to Heston had been born of desperation and a feeling of being trapped.

'There may be another way,' she admitted with reluctance. 'I can but try. . .a quarrel might serve.'

On the following day she was given no opportunity to carry out her scheme. The household was astir at an early hour, but the Strand was already crowded as the Alderman's coach bore them towards the building which was their destination. Their progress was slow, but they arrived at the appointed hour.

Heston had used his influence to reserve a series of rooms with long windows which would give them a splendid view of the Procession. Nothing had been neglected for their comfort, from easy chairs to tables laid for a late breakfast.

His mother was already seated by a window, sketch-ing the scene before her and Heston was chatting to Richard Young.

He turned as they entered and came towards them with a smile.

'We shall have some hours to wait,' he said. 'Will you take some refreshment?'

He was the perfect host, apparently casual, but Miranda noticed that his eyes missed nothing which might add to their pleasure in the occasion.

How could she possibly quarrel with him? Miranda thought in despair. He neither did nor said anything which she could take amiss. In any case, this was not the occasion upon which to carry out her plan. She gave up all thought of it for the time being and began to enjoy herself.

Whatever the future held, she would forget her troubles for this one day. It might be the last occasion upon which this man whom she loved so much would look at her, if not with love, certainly with admiration in his eyes.

That she could not mistake. When their meal was over, he came to her and took her hand.

'Unfair, my love!' he murmured softly. 'How can you tease me so?'

'My lord, you speak in riddles. I do not understand.'

'Don't you, my dearest? Can it be possible that you do not know how delicious you look today? It is a severe test of my self-control. I want to take you in my arms and kiss you here and now.'

'Please, my lord. . .someone will hear you.' The colour rose to Miranda's cheeks, but she was glad that she had chosen to wear her new walking-dress of French cambric, with a charming Oldenburg hat. She was not immune to flattery, although it was mortifying to be forced to admit it.

'Now I have made you blush,' he teased. 'Will you always do so?'

Miranda's face grew warm. She did not pretend to misunderstand his meaning.

'Sir, I beg that you will not continue with this conversation. Do you wish to provoke me into quarreling with you?'

He laughed and patted her hand. 'No, I won't do that. Did you think to escape me with a quarrel?'

With these thought-provoking words, he moved away to speak to Mrs Shere.

Miranda stayed where she was, frozen into immobility. It was as she had feared. Heston seemed always to be able to read her mind.

'You are very quiet.' Richard slipped into the seat beside her. 'I can't say that I blame you.'

'No, it is all getting out of hand, and I don't know how to put an end—'

'Do you wish to?'

Miranda looked up in surprise. 'You know that I must. I am so ashamed of all the lies and the deceit.'

'That's understandable, but Fanny tells me—'

'Fanny should not gossip,' she cried in anger.

'She did not tell me anything that I did not already know,' he told her gently.

'Oh, Richard, is it so obvious that I love him?'

'It is to me, but then I've known you since you were a child. What of Lord Heston?'

'He wishes only to punish me. I tricked him into this betrothal, in a way.'

'I doubt if there is a soul alive who could trick him into anything.' Richard looked at her with smiling eyes. 'You misjudge him, my dear.'

'I don't think so. What other reason could he have?'

Richard laughed aloud. 'Neither you nor your sister could claim the prize as the ugliest women in London,' he chaffed.

'There are others with more beauty.'

'But none with the same spirit as your own. Oh, I'll admit that you might have angered him at first, but has it not occurred to you that he might have changed his mind?'

'I wish it might be so,' she faltered. 'But I cannot believe it.'

'Then you must be blind. Do you think him a man of honour?'

She looked at him dumbly. Then she nodded.

'So do I. It would be beneath him to seek to harm

you.' Richard spoke with conviction. 'Don't do anything foolish, I beg of you. In time all will be well.'

'What are you trying to say?'

'If you will have it straight, I believe Lord Heston
loves you.'

For the first time a little flame of hope burned in
Miranda's heart. Then she shook her head.

'That isn't possible, but even if it were true it cannot
help me. How could I accept that love knowing all that
I do? No marriage can be built upon a lie.'

'It might be built upon love, as I hope my own will
be. . . Do you hear the cheering? The Procession must
be close.'

He led her over to the window and settled her in a
chair as the clatter of horses sounded in the distance.

The Procession was a tribute to the Prince Regent's
love of splendour. First came a company of the
Eleventh Light Dragoons in their uniforms of blue and
buff, and they were followed by a number of carriages
bearing the officers of the Prince's household. Then
came those of the foreign generals, and the state
carriages of the Regent's brothers, all of them Royal
Dukes.

It was all a feast for the eye, and the number of
dignitaries seemed endless. All the members of the
Cabinet were there, together with the Speaker, in
splendid isolation in his own coach. Then came a troop
of Horse Guards, their accoutrements glittering in the
sunlight as they preceded the Royal officers of state
and certain of the foreign suites.

The Regent himself looked sullen, and even the
presence of his popular allies did not prevent the crowd
from booing and making cat-calls as his eight cream
horses drew the State Coach past.

'Shame on them!' Mrs Shere cried indignantly. 'Today, at least, they might have honoured him.'

'He does not look as if he is enjoying himself,' Fanny murmured. 'It must be galling to hear the cheering for the others. But, Aunt, he is enormous, positively gross, in fact. What a disappointment!'

'Fanny, remember where you are!' Miranda hissed. 'I hope that Lord Heston did not hear you.'

Fanny was not attending, for at that moment the Tsar's procession came into view.

'At last!' she cried in high excitement. 'Here come the Russians and the Tsar himself.' She clasped her hands in rapture. 'He is everything I had expected. . . tall and slim. . .and so handsome. Some may think him dandified, but I do not agree. . .'

A murmur of amusement went around the room, but Fanny did not notice.

'Where is Count Toumanov? I do not see him, and he promised to ride upon this side.' She leaned out of the window, peering anxiously at the cavaliers below.

'Dearest, do take care,' Mrs Shere pleaded. 'You must not risk a fall.'

Fanny was oblivious of the danger. She leaned out even further. 'There he is!' She began to wave her handkerchief and was rewarded when Alexei looked up briefly and grinned at her. 'Does he not look splendid, and see how well he controls his horse?'

'Yes, yes, my love. Now do pray close the window, or her ladyship may take a chill.'

It was unlikely on that pleasant summer day, but Fanny obeyed her, unconscious of the fact that her conduct had gone beyond the bounds of propriety.

'How I should like to have attended the banquet!'

she cried. 'I wonder that Uncle could not have obtained an invitation for us.'

'He will tell us all about it later!' Miranda was aware of her aunt's dismayed expression. Fanny's present behaviour was the outside of enough. She shuddered to imagine what Lady Heston must think of such a lack of restraint.

Apparently her ladyship had not noticed. She was preoccupied with her sketching and seemed lost to all else.

Heston touched her lightly on the shoulder. 'Do you care to stay here for a while?' he asked. 'I shall not be long, but I must see the ladies home.'

Richard offered at once to perform that office for him, but Heston shook his head.

'Then I shall bear her ladyship company, if she will permit,' Richard said shyly.

'How very kind of you!' Lady Heston had taken a liking to this quiet young man who seemed so diffident. 'Then I shall not mind how long Adam is away. Now tell me, Mr Young, do you feel that I have captured something of the atmosphere today?' She held out her sketchpad to him, and came over to Mrs Shere.

'Will you come to Brook Street with your nieces whilst Adam is in Portsmouth?' she asked. 'We must learn to know each other better, but first I hope that you will bring the Alderman to dine. Shall we say three days from now?'

Mrs Shere thanked her, and the ladies took their leave. Fanny continued to chatter brightly on the journey back to Bloomsbury, but when Heston had left them her aunt took her to task.

'It grieves me to say so, but I was ashamed of you today, my dear. How could you behave so ill? That hoydenish way you leaned out of the window, and called to Count Toumanov? I could not believe my ears.'

Fanny looked startled and dismayed. 'I did not think—'

'Then it is high time that you began to do so. How could you disgrace your sister in that way? What your mama would have said I can't imagine.'

'Pray don't be cross with me.' Fanny's eyes filled. 'I was so excited. . .'

'Well, it will not do. I cannot help but notice that you are either in high alt, or down in the cellars, my dear girl. Such nervous excitement is not good for you. I wonder if I should write to your mama?'

'Please don't!' Fanny began to cry in earnest. 'I didn't mean to be so bad, and I will try to be better.'

As always, the sight of tears had their usual effect upon Mrs Shere's tender heart. She laid a comforting hand on Fanny's arm.

'It is the thought of your sister's marriage which has disturbed you so, I think. But you will grow used to the idea, believe me. Now dry your eyes, my dear one. Lady Heston did not seem to notice your behaviour and for that we must be thankful. Dear me, I must confess that I find her somewhat odd. To be drawing at such a time is most unusual.'

'She has been so kind,' Miranda ventured.

'To be sure she has. You are fortunate in your mother-in-law, my love. I doubt if she will take the trouble to interfere in anything you may wish to do.'

Miranda forced a smile. 'She is devoted to her son, my dear ma'am. His wishes will come first with her.'

'But of course. With his father dead, he is the head

of the household, and so capable. Dear Lord Heston! How very lucky you are, my dear.'

Miranda had reservations upon that point. Luck was the last word she would have used to describe her present situation, but she murmured a feeble assent.

When their aunt had left them, Fanny rounded upon her.

'You might have supported me,' she complained in an injured tone. 'Aunt Emma was so cross and you did not say a word in my defence.'

'If she had not done so, I was about to speak to you myself,' Miranda told her grimly. 'Aunt was right... you embarrassed both of us.'

'Oh, you are grown as high in the instep as Heston himself... I do not know you any more. Are we to sit like statues, unsmiling, and without a word to say? That may be your idea fo fun, but it is not mine.'

'No one asks that of you, but can't you see how you expose yourself to gossip?'

'As if I cared!' Fanny tossed her head. 'Since you have known Heston you are changed. You were used to be light-hearted. Now all you care about is the proprieties—'

'That isn't true! But we aren't children any more. What passed for high spirits long ago in Yorkshire is not acceptable in Polite Society, and you know how tongues can wag.' Miranda sighed. 'Sometimes I think that members of the *ton* have nothing else to do.'

'I have done no harm,' Fanny sulked. 'Lady Heston did not notice, and his lordship does not know that I exist.'

'Don't be too sure of that!' Miranda warned. She knew that it was not so. Nothing that her sister did or said escaped Heston's notice. That penetrating gaze rested frequently upon her twin and she had seen speculation in his eyes. His apparently casual manner hid a mind that was razor-sharp, and it never ceased to worry her.

Fanny bridled. 'What has he been saying to you?' she demanded. 'He need not think to criticise me, for I will not have it. It seems I can do nothing right. You are all against me, except for Richard. He is the only one who does not say a word except in kindness.'

'Richard is very fond of you.' It was an incautious statement in view of the fact that Miranda had promised not to reveal his true feelings for her sister, but Fanny was unmoved.

'I know that. He is fond of both of us. When we were small I was used to wish that he were my brother, instead of Jonathan and William. He did not torment us as they liked to do.'

'He is the best of creatures,' Miranda said warmly. 'It is a pity. . .' She stopped in confusion. She had been on the verge of saying too much, but Fanny was not attending.

'I think I have behaved quite well,' she announced. 'I did not make the least fuss because Alexei cannot visit us this evening.'

'How could he possibly do so? The celebrations will go on until the early hours, and he is in attendance upon the Tsar. He did not come to London just for pleasure, as you know.'

'Well, I think it most unreasonable of his master to keep him at his duties for so long.'

'How fortunate that we are not in Russia! You would probably be beaten with a knout for that remark.'

'You may make a joke of it, but he did promise. . .at

least, he suggested a party after the Procession on the night we met, if you recall.'

'It was only a suggestion. There was nothing definite settled, and his duties must come first.'

'I suppose so. Oh dear, how dull we are this evening!'

'Well, I, for one, have had enough excitement for one day. We made such an early start this morning, then all the crowds, and the Procession. After supper I shall seek my bed.'

This suggestion met with approval from her aunt. Mrs Shere's eyes searched Miranda's face, then she nodded to herself with a strange little smile of satisfaction.

'What is it, Aunt Emma? You are looking positively conspiratorial. Have you some secret plans for us?' Fanny could not hide her curiosity.

'I have a surprise, but you are not to know of it until tomorrow.'

Not all Fanny's wheedling could persuade her to reveal her secret before the twins retired.

Fanny returned to the subject at breakfast on the following morning.

'Now do pray tell us, Aunt,' she coaxed prettily. 'I vow I have not closed my eyes all night for wondering.'

'What a story! When I looked in upon you, you were sound asleep!' Mrs Shere glanced from one twin to the other. 'Very well, then. We are to go for a drive, but I shall not tell you our destination.'

'How exciting! I love a mystery!' Fanny clapped her hands. 'What are we to wear? Must we be very fine?'

'We may be out for quite some time, so perhaps your Sardinian blue pelisses with the matching bonnets, and an extra shawl for warmth. And your parasols against the sun?'

Miranda chuckled. 'I see that this is to be a serious expedition, ma'am, if we are to go from one extreme of temperature to another.'

'There is no harm in being prepared against the weather,' her aunt reproved. 'It may be high summer, but in this climate one can never tell. . . The morning is fine, but before the day is out we may have rain, or even blazing sunshine.'

'Are we to be out all day?' Fanny's face clouded, and Miranda threw her a warning look.

Fanny must not raise objections to the outing, however much she hoped that the Count would call. Aunt Emma may have believed that Fanny's behaviour on the previous day was just high spirits, but she would not be deceived for long.

And only Fanny could believe that Alexei would offer for her. To be seen to throw herself at the young man's head would bring down Mrs Shere's severest disapproval upon her. It would be the last straw as far as their aunt was concerned. She would write at once to their mama.

And much good that would do her, Miranda thought ruefully. However unlikely the chance of such a thing occurring, her mother would be in raptures as the thought of having a Countess in the family.

Her frown quelled Fanny's objections for the moment, although she heard a few mutterings of rebellion as they tied the ribbons of their bonnets.

'I can't think why we must be out all day,' Fanny complained. 'I believe it will be too tiring, but I suppose we may come home if I am not feeling well.'

'To make an instant recovery if Count Toumanov

should happen to call? You will do no such thing! Aunt has arranged this outing for our pleasure, and you will do nothing to spoil it.'

'You always think the worst of me,' Fanny complained in an injured tone. 'You are becoming such a crosspatch.'

Miranda was tempted to inform Fanny that her behaviour would try the patience of a saint. Instead she turned the conversation to their new bonnets.

'I like these curled plumes, don't you?' she said. 'I wonder how they managed to dye these feathers to the exact shade of blue?'

Fanny looked at her reflection in the glass and gave a nod of satisfaction.

'They are pretty,' she agreed. 'Though I wonder if we should not wear the new small hats instead?'

'Aunt Emma suggested bonnets.' Miranda began to laugh. 'They are more likely to protect our faces from either snow or blazing sunshine.'

Fanny picked up her shawl. 'I wonder where we are to go? I thought we had visited almost everywhere of interest. Pray heaven it is not to be another outing to the Museum!'

'I doubt it. I did not see any parasols unfurled in there, nor gentlemen in fur hats.'

They went downstairs together to find Richard waiting for them in the salon.

'Oh, is it you?' Fanny murmured. 'We are to go out today, you know.'

'And I am to accompany you. Mrs Shere arranged it with me yesterday. . .'

That was not the full extent of Mrs Shere's arrangements. The next arrival was Lord Heston, attired in a riding coat, buckskin breeches, and gleaming Hessians. He took Miranda's hand.

'Beautiful as always!' he murmured. 'You are ready, my dear?'

'Why, yes! I did not know that you were to come with us, sir.'

'With *you*,' he corrected. 'Shall we go? I do not care to keep my horses standing.'

'But my aunt intends to travel in the family coach. . .' Miranda looked across at Mrs Shere for confirmation, and was surprised to see a conspiratorial smile again.

Still chuckling, her aunt proceeded towards her own coach and stepped inside. She was followed by Fanny and then by Richard, and the carriage set off along the cobbled street.

'I hope you know our destination, my lord, for I do not.' Miranda allowed herself to be handed up into Heston's racing curricle. She was somewhat mystified by these curious travelling arrangements. There was room and to spare for both herself and her companion in the coach. Perhaps Heston preferred to drive himself upon this strange expedition.

'I know my own, and yours.' Heston's expression was enigmatic and suddenly she felt sudden panic. Her aunt's coach had turned to the left at the far end of the street, but his lordship guided his team to the right.

'What are you about?' she cried. 'Surely we should follow them?'

'Why should we do that? They are not going in our direction.'

'You will please to stop at once. How dare you trick me in this way? I did not agree to spend the day with you. . .my aunt will be distraught.'

'I doubt it, dearest one. She knows of my intention.'

'And what is that, my lord?'

'Why, I have kidnapped you! Sadly, only for the day, but I believe that we should make the most of it.'

'And you arranged this with my aunt? How could she agree to such a plan? I can't believe it!'

'But you must. She thinks you too much in your sister's company, and so do I. It is a strain on both of you.'

Miranda's fury knew no bounds. 'My relations with my family are none of your concern,' she cried. 'You dislike Fa—my twin. You have made that clear, but you do not understand, and nor does my aunt.'

'I think we do,' he told her calmly. 'I have no wish to come between you and your sister—'

'You could not!' she burst out.

'That may be so, but confess it. Shall you not enjoy a drive to Richmond? It is peaceful there, away from the noise of the city. Both your aunt and my mother thought you in need of rest.'

Miranda was about to fly at him. Then she recalled her ladyship's sweet smile. That gentle person must have seen her inner torment. She had been about to inform Heston of her strong dislike of being discussed in her absence, but she checked the angry words.

'That was kind of her. I had not thought—'

'That you were looking "hagged"? That is your own expression, I believe? No, my love, you could not look other than ravishing, but there is an expression in your eyes. Sometimes, I have thought. . .' He left it there, and Miranda did not answer him.

No purpose could be served by either admitting or denying his words. She leaned back against the cushions as he took the road to the west.

Chapter Thirteen

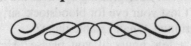

For a time he drove in silence, a fact for which Miranda was profoundly thankful. She had no wish to return to the topic of Fanny and herself, and to comment upon the weather or the charm of the countryside through which they passed held no appeal for her. It was the type of trivial conversation which Heston would find trying, though why she should care for that was puzzling.

She smiled to herself. On occasion she had noticed how his eyes would glaze with boredom when faced with a gabblemonger. At least he could not accuse her of that.

She was intensely aware of his strong hands on the reins as he sprang his team of matching chestnuts. He seemed at one with the splendid animals, never pushing them too hard, or dragging at their tender mouths, yet allowing them to cover the miles to Richmond at a spanking pace.

It was always a pleasure to watch an expert, she admitted to herself, and he was right. To escape from the city with its crowds and its fearful stench was exactly what she most needed on a day like this.

'My compliments, ma'am! You are no chatterbox!' He drew the curricle to a halt at a small inn. A groom materialised as if from nowhere, and Heston threw him the reins.

'Glad to see your lordship! It's been some time!'

'Too long, Ben! How do you like my cattle?'

The groom ran an appraising eye over the team.

'You ain't lost your eye for bloodstock, sir, and that's a fact,' he grinned. 'Shall I stable them?'

'Just for a few hours, if you please.' Heston took Miranda's arm and led her into the inn.

There he was greeted with evident pleasure by the landlord.

'Ah, Flodden, there you are. You kept your private parlour for us?'

'As if you need to ask, my lord!' The man bowed low, but there was no trace of servility in his manner. As he straightened Miranda was aware that she was the object of scrutiny from a pair of sharp blue eyes.

'My dear, this is Flodden. He is an old friend of mine.' Heston clapped their host upon the shoulder. 'Now, you old rascal, where is Annie? I must make her known to Miss Gaysford, who is to be my bride.'

Flodden was clearly startled by this news, but he made a quick recover, leading them through into an inner room where the table was already laid for two.

'You will take a glass of wine, my lord, to clear the dust?'

'Champagne, I think. The occasion calls for it. . .'

As Flodden limped away Miranda saw that he was badly crippled. One leg was bent at an awkward angle, and his left arm was almost useless. His short stature and slight build, as well as something in his walk, made her suspect that he had been a jockey.

When he returned he was accompanied by a buxom woman who was twice his size. The contrast between them was incongruous, but there was a certain dignity in Mrs Flodden's bearing that commanded respect rather than amusement.

She flushed with pleasure as Heston rose to greet her.

'Well, Annie, how do you go on? Still ruling the roost with an iron hand?'

Mrs Flodden smiled at this sally, but she shook her head in reproach. Then she made her curtsy to Miranda.

'Now, tell me, how is Mary? No further setbacks, I hope?'

'Not since your lordship sent the physician down from London. She hopes to see you, sir, to thank you herself.'

Although Miranda had never succeeded in putting Heston out of countenance, the older woman's words clearly embarrassed him.

'I'll come at once,' he said quickly. 'Perhaps Miss Gaysford will like to remove her coat and bonnet.'

Miranda's curiosity was aroused. She followed the landlord's wife to an upper room where she found all in readiness for her to wash away the dust of travel.

'Have you known Lord Heston long?' she asked.

'For many years, ma'am, and what we should have done without him I don't know.'

Miranda looked up, a question in her eyes, but Mrs Flodden would not go on.

'Ma'am, we are forbidden to speak of it. You saw how Lord Heston looked when I tried to thank him for his goodness. I fear that I disobeyed his wishes. . .' She handed a towel to Miranda. 'Will you excuse me?'

She hurried back to her kitchen, clearly preoccupied with thoughts of the meal already in preparation.

Miranda made her way downstairs. Her untouched glass of champagne stood upon a side table, the bubbles still rising to the surface. She took a sip or two, realising suddenly that she was both thirsty and hungry.

Now that she was alone she had leisure to look about her. The place was spotless in the brilliant sunshine which flooded through the windows. Horse brasses on the walls gave back reflections, as did the lovingly polished oak of a fine dresser.

She was examining a drawing of a horse race, flanked by a number of rosettes, when Heston returned.

'Was Flodden a jockey?' she asked. The connection of the oddly assorted couple with Heston had intrigued her.

'Yes.' This short reply was not an invitation for further questioning, but Miranda persisted.

'What happened? Why is he. . .?'

'A cripple? There was an accident. He was riding a young horse in its first race. Something startled the creature. . .perhaps the shouting of the crowd. . .and it ran into the rails.'

'And he was crushed?'

'No, he was thrown over the rail and into a heavy post on the other side. It was not thought that he would live.'

'My lord, I know that you do not care to speak of it, but why you? Why did you help them? I could not help but notice their gratitude.'

'Inquisitive!' He tugged at a straying curl. 'It was my horse, you see. Flodden had ridden for me for years.'

'And you set them up here?'

'What else could I do? His livelihood was gone, and the child was sick.'

Miranda was silent. Many owners would not have spared another thought for the injured man since he could be of no further use to them. Compassion was not a virtue which she had noticed much among the *ton*.

'And Mary?' she ventured.

'Their daughter is much improved since she came to live in Richmond. I have promised that she shall meet you later, if you do not object?'

'Of course not. I should like to meet her.' She eyed Heston with new respect. Perhaps it was not so strange that she should be in love with him. Behind that hard exterior lay a warm heart. If only some of that warmth might flow in her direction.

She had emptied her glass without thinking, and he refilled it for her.

'Hungry?' he asked.

'I'm starving!' Miranda smiled up at him. 'It must be the drive and the country air.'

'I'm glad to hear it. Annie is a fine cook. She will be disappointed if we don't do justice to her efforts.'

He spoke no more than the truth, and for the first time in weeks Miranda ate with a hearty appetite. She had expected the usual country fare of ham and beef and heavy meat puddings, and was surprised to be served with a feather-light omelette, followed by small strips of chicken breast in a tangy sauce. The salads were so fresh that they could only have come from the Floddens' garden that very morning.

She was lavish with her praise when Mrs Flodden appeared.

'I did not wish to overface you, miss. The day is so

warm, but if his lordship is still hungry there is a saddle of mutton. . .'

Heston shook his head and laughed. 'Annie, you would have me as fat as a flawn. I doubt if I could eat another mouthful.' There was a wicked twinkle in his eyes.

'Not my fruit pie? Oh, sir, I made it specially, knowing how you like it, and the apples are our own, stored from last year.'

'Well, if I must. . .' he said with mock reluctance. Miranda was undeceived.

'Lord Heston is joking, Mrs Flodden,' she announced. 'He tells me that your pies are famous. You should punish him by refusing to let him taste them.'

'Oh, ma'am, I couldn't do that!' Mrs Flodden was shocked. 'I'll fetch the pitcher of cream.'

She stood over him anxiously, waiting for his verdict.

'Delicious! Annie, you haven't lost your touch. I believe I might manage another morsel.' In the end he consumed a full half of the pie, much to the satisfaction of his hostess.

'You have led me astray once more,' he told her with a grin. 'Now I must walk for at least three hours or I shall fall asleep.'

'Oh, sir, you can't be meaning to keep the young lady out for all that time in the heat?'

'If she falls by the wayside, I shall sweep her into my arms and bring her back to you, I promise.' He saw her worried frown. 'Don't worry, Annie. We shall keep to the shade of the trees down by the river. I think Miss Gaysford will enjoy a stroll.'

Miranda was quick to assent. There was something about this quiet place which had done much to restore her peace of mind, and she felt at ease with these good people.

Heston took her arm and led her through the inn and down through the kitchen garden to a wicket gate. Beyond it a narrow path ran down towards the river.

He drew her arm through his and they strolled along in a companionable silence.

'Still cross with me because I brought you here?' he asked suddenly.

'No, I have enjoyed it very much. You were right. It is good to get away from the city.'

'And your worries?'

Miranda did not answer him. How could she explain that the main cause of her apprehension was standing by her side.

She pointed to the swans. 'May we not take a closer look at them? they have some cygnets.'

'Feed them if you wish. Annie sent me out prepared.' He produced a bag of broken bread from his coat pocket, and handed it to her. 'Not too close though. They can be dangerous at this time of year.'

Obediently she stood well back from the river bank and threw the bread into the water. It attracted the swans at once and they came towards her, their long, snake-like heads striking out towards the floating food. When it was gone they lost interest and swam away.

She turned to find that Heston was seated on the trunk of a fallen tree, regarding her intently. He patted the seat beside him.

'Come here,' he said gently. 'I want to talk to you.'

She wanted to refuse, but somehow she could not. She hesitated, knowing that it was folly to be alone with him like this.

'I shall not eat you, my dear love, but if you will not

come to me then I must come to you.' He rose and walked towards her. Then he took her in his arms.

'Please don't!' she murmured.

'Why not, my darling? Don't you know how much I love you?'

His words brought her to her senses. She broke away abruptly.

'Haven't you punished me enough?' she cried in a broken voice. 'On top of all else, must you pretend that you care for me?'

'You are sure that it is pretence?' He was so still that he might have been carved from stone.

'What else can it be? I admit that I was wrong, if that is what you want from me. I knew that you had no intention of offering for me, and I should not have ptetended that I did.'

'It was not a very serious pretence, my dear.' His face was calm. 'On the contrary, you gave me the impression that you wished to put me out of countenance.'

'But you. . .but you. . .'

'I decided to call your bluff.'

'Well, you certainly did so.' Miranda's voice was bitter. 'May we not end this farce here and now? I release you from your promise.'

'But I have no desire to be released. Did I not make that plain?'

'Oh, no, you cannot mean it? How can you behave so ill? You know that I have not the least desire—'

'That I must beg leave to doubt.' He bent his head and found her lips, and again the world was lost.

'Will you still tell me that you don't care for me?' he murmured. 'Your body gives you the lie.'

'You are mistaken!' Miranda struggled to free herself.

'Am I? I think not! I asked you once before to trust me. Is it so hard to do? Is there always to be this barrier between us?'

'I don't know what you mean.'

'I think you do. This secret that you guard so closely? Must it never be revealed?'

'It is not mine alone to tell,' she cried, goaded into flinging caution to the winds.

'Your sister again? Well, I had suspected it. I won't press you to reveal her confidence, but one day you will come to me in your own good time.'

'You speak in riddles, sir. Now, if you please, I should like to return to London.'

'I wonder why that should not surprise me?' His expression was imperturbable as he took her arm once more and led her towards the inn.

Miranda was desperate to get away, but she was not to be released so soon.

'I have promised to take you to see Mary,' he announced. 'I hope you will be kind to her.'

Accompanied by Mrs Flodden, he led her through to a small private parlour at the far end of the inn.

At first she did not see the child who lay among a pile of cushions on a sofa by the window. Then she was aware of being inspected by a pair of bright blue eyes. The thin little face was a perfect replica of Flodden's own.

'Here is Miss Gaysford come to see you, Mary. She is very shy. Promise that you will not frighten her as you do me?' Heston sounded solemn.

'Sir, you are teasing me,' a small voice cried merrily. 'I don't frighten you.'

'Indeed you do! Sometimes, when we have been playing spillikins, you looked so fierce that I was positively shaking in my boots.'

A peal of laughter greeted this sally. Heston was clearly a favourite with the frail little girl.

Miranda guessed that she could not have been more than eight or nine, although the traces of pain upon the child's face made her look older. She was desperately thin, with stick-like arms and legs, but her face was alive with intelligence.

Heston went across to sit beside her on the sofa.

'Well, what do you think of the lady who is to be my wife?' he said gravely.

Blue eyes and grey regarded Miranda so seriously that she began to smile.

'Mama told me that she was beautiful, and she is,' the little girl announced. 'She looks like the picture in my book.'

'You mean the wicked witch?' Heston asked mildly.

'No, sir. . . I mean the fairy princess.'

'I am relieved to hear it. I should not care to be married to a witch. She might put a spell on me.'

'And turn you into a frog?'

'I shouldn't put it past her. It would be most inconvenient to be a frog, you know. I should have to hop about the garden and eat flies.'

'Instead of Mrs Flodden's apple pies? You would not care for that, my lord,' put in Miranda.

Miranda could not hide her amusement, especially when Mary nodded her agreement.

'He would not,' she confirmed. 'Mama says that Lord Heston is a splendid trencherman. I think it means that he eats a lot. . .'

'What a reputation!' Heston rose to his feet. 'All

these agreeable compliments will turn my head. Mary, we shall come to see you soon. If you do as the doctor says and eat up all your food, you may be well enough to come for a drive.'

The child's eyes shone. 'I will!' she cried. 'Do you promise?'

'I give you my word on it. Now say your goodbyes to Miss Gaysford, for I must take her home.'

A small, claw-like hand appered from among the cushions and Miranda took it in her own.

'I hope we shall be friends,' she said with a twinkle in her eyes. 'Then you may teach me how to frighten his lordship.'

'Both of you?' Heston threw his eyes to heaven in mock dismay. 'I shall be a quivering jelly.'

Mary was still laughing when they left her.

They had covered several miles of the journey back to London before she questioned him about the child.

'Is Mary very sick?' she asked.

'She was always delicate, but she is improving. There have been setbacks, naturally, but the spirit is there. It has pulled her through on many an occasion.'

'She seems devoted to you.'

'Purely due to my expertise at spillikins.' Heston smiled down at her and her heart turned over. She turned her head, so that he should not see how her love for him betrayed her.

He drew the team to a halt in the shelter of some trees. Then a large hand reached out to cover her own.

'Can I have been mistaken? My love, we deal so well together, and in these last few days I have felt that you have changed. I think you do not dislike me as you did.

In fact, I have begun to hope that you could learn to care for me.'

Miranda did not answer him.

'You do not deny it?' he said eagerly.

She cast about wildly for some reply which would put an end to this dangerous conversation. Perhaps a half-truth would serve.

'I have misjudged you from the first,' she replied in a low tone. 'Perhaps we might be friends—'

'And that is to be all?'

Before she could protest he took her in his arms and kissed her soundly. Her mouth opened like a flower beneath his own, and he began to tease her with little flickering movements of his tongue. Her arms crept about his neck and she strained towards him, faint with longing for a fulfilment which she did not understand.

When he held her away his face was serious.

'Will you tell me now that you do not wish to marry me?' he asked.

'I can't!' Miranda did not recognise her own voice. The words had seemed to come from a stranger.

'You have not answered my question.'

When she did not reply he sat in silence for a time. Then he turned to her again.

'Promise me this at least? Do nothing hasty for the moment. Next week I shall be in Portsmouth for some days. It will give you time to consider. On my return you may give me your answer.'

When she began to speak, he stopped her.

'Don't worry, my dear. If you are still of the same mind I shall not press you further. You may put an end to our betrothal in any way you wish.'

These were the words which she had once longed to hear, but the triumph felt like ashes in her mouth.

There was nothing left to say, and indeed if she had tried to speak she must have burst into tears.

Heston picked up the reins and guided his team back on to the road. For the rest of the journey back to London both of them were silent, but in place of the easy camaraderie on the drive down to Richmond there was now an atmosphere of tension.

It was not until they reached their destination that Heston broke the awkward silence. His threw his reins to the groom, jumped down from the driving seat, and held out his arms to help Mrianda from her perch.

'Cheer up!' he murmured as his lips brushed her ear. 'Even friends are allowed to enjoy each other's company.'

She responded with the faintest of smiles, and was in no mood to listen to Fanny's strictures after he had gone.

'What a trick to play on us! I am surprised that Aunt allowed you to go jauntering off with Heston on your own, and for so long . . .'

'Haven't you enjoyed your day?'

'No, I have not. We saw no one that we knew, and if there is one thing I detest it is a picnic. There were so many creepy-crawlies, and stinging insects too. I could not eat a bite.'

'Then you must be very hungry. . .'

'Much you care when we might all have gone to Richmond.'

'Lord Heston wished to speak to me alone.'

'Are there not rooms enough in this house where you might be private with him without trailing out to Richmond on your own?'

Miranda did not reply.

'What had he to say?' her twin asked with a nervous laugh.

'He has offered to release me from my promise to him.' Something in her face warned Fanny to proceed with caution.

'And did you agree?'

'I agreed to do as he requested.'

'And that was?'

'To wait and to consider. I am to give him an answer when he returns from Portsmouth.'

'Oh, you are a darling!' Fanny threw her arms about her sister's unresponsive form. 'You did it for me, just as you promised.'

'It must come to the same thing in the end. I cannot marry him. . .'

'Well, in my opinion he would make a most disagreeable husband, always looking down his nose, and making those strange remarks which no one can understand.' She saw the pain in Miranda's eyes and stopped.

'Of course I do not know him as you do,' she continued when her sister did not speak. 'You seem to have seen something else in him, though what I can't imagine—'

'Leave it, Fanny!' Miranda begged in desperation.

'Very well,' Her sister brightened. 'You need not make a decision yet, you know. Anything may happen in the next two weeks. . .' Her face grew dreamy.

Miranda knew that she was thinking of Alexei Toumanov. Had he joined them on the infamous picnic, the stinging insects would have gone unnoticed. She could only be thankful that the handsome Russian was due to leave the capital so soon.

'I wonder that Harry Lakenham has not called upon us recently,' she said. 'You have not seen him?'

'We met him in the Park the other day,' Fanny told her in casual tones. 'He was with his friends, so we did not stop to speak.'

'He seems to have taken his dismissal very well.'

'It was you who told him that he must not try to see me.'

'Not alone and in secret, but I did not say that he should avoid your company altogether.'

'It cannot signify! I expect he feels as I do, that we were both mistaken in our hearts.'

This cool dismissal of what was to have been the love affair of the century took Miranda's breath away. Angry words rose to her lips, but she suppressed them. The same thing had happened many times before, but on previous occasions no harm had been done. She struggled for composure.

'What a pity that you did not discover it before,' she said quietly. 'Much trouble might have been avoided.'

'I can't help that, and I don't know why you should look so black at me. I thought you disapproved of Harry.'

'I think him too young and foolish to be considering marriage.'

'Well, then, you must be satisfied, and your precious Adam Heston will be delighted.'

'Not if he thinks that you have formed an attachment for the Count. . .'

The colour rose to Fanny's cheeks. 'What an idea! Pray why should he think that? Alexei has not spoken.'

'Nor will he do so, Fanny.'

'Are you so sure? He has been most particular in his attentions.'

'He likes to flirt, as do most young men, but you can't believe that he is serious?'

'You think I am beneath his notice?' Anger sparkled in Fanny's eyes.

'Of course not, but I don't want you to be hurt. You should not refine too much upon his gallantries. They may be nothing more than the usual outrageous flattery which passes for conversation in the Polite World.'

Fanny tossed her head. 'Why should you be the only one to marry well? I have a fancy to be a Countess.'

Miranda said no more. Further warnings would be useless. Her only hope that her twin would be saved from further folly lay in the fact that the Count would return to Russia within the next two weeks.

She was dismayed to find that he, together with his sister and her husband, were to be their fellow dinner-guests at Brook Street on the following evening. At Lady Heston's invitation Richard had also joined them.

He looked overawed at the prospect of visiting Lord Heston's home.

'How do I look?' he asked Miranda in an undertone. 'I expect it will be all magnificence. . .'

'You are the epitome of elegance,' she told him with a smile. She felt somewhat nervous herself, but her blonde silk gown, ornamented with cobweb-like blonde lace, was so becoming that it gave her confidence.

In the event, the evening was not the ordeal she had expected. Heston's major-domo, whilst perfectly correct in his manner, showed no trace of stiffness, and she guessed that he was an old retainer.

He announced their party to the group already gathered in the salon, and Heston came to greet them with all the easy address which was natural to him.

Miranda could not meet his eyes, but he took her

hand and kissed it, and then saluted her upon the cheek.

'Friends?' he murmured.

She gave him a look of gratitude. She had dreaded a certain awkwardness after their last meeting.

His lordship appeared to have forgotten it. To her surprise it was the Count whose manner had changed. It was imperceptible to most of the party, and through-out the meal he joined in the conversation so merrily that he kept them laughing with his stories of life at the Russian court. Yet he made no effort later to monopol-ise Fanny for himself.

Miranda looked across at the Princess Chaliapine. She, too, was speaking with her usual vivacity, but it was impossible not to wonder if she had spoken to her brother, warning him not to raise hopes which could not be fulfilled.

She prayed that Fanny would not give herself away. Her twin was incapable of dissembling, and she was already looking dissatisfied to see the Count in conver-sation with the Alderman and Mrs Shere.

Miranda threw a speaking look at Richard, and he moved at once to Fanny's side.

Accompanied by Lady Heston, Miranda went to join them.

'This has been a delightful evening, your ladyship,' Richard told his hostess warmly. 'It was kind of you to include me.'

'It was a pleasure, Mr Young. Now you three young people may advise me. I have a small gift for the Alderman. Do you think that he will like it?' She took up a small parcel from the table and unwrapped it to reveal a painting.

'How beautiful! It is one of my uncle's roses. . . He will be delighted!'

Miranda bent to examine the work more closely.

'Why, you have caught every detail,' she murmured in wonder. 'I had not realised that the petals were shaded so, and that the leaves are not all a solid green. . .'

Even Fanny was intrigued. 'Ma'am, it is hard to believe that you have made the painting so quickly. Why, it is not more than a day or two since you took the flowers.'

'That is experience, my dear, and a sad habit of ignoring all else in order to paint.'

'How better could you spend your time, my dearest?' Heston had joined their little group. 'We are all waiting for your *magnum opus*.'

'Now, Adam, I beg of you. . .' Lady Heston shook her head in reproach.

'Please tell us what it is, ma'am, if you do not object.'

Richard was so clearly interested that her ladyship did not refuse.

'I am trying to record the flora and fauna in our part of Warwickshire,' she admitted shyly. 'It is a lengthy task.'

'But well worth doing, Lady Heston. It will be a wonderful record for the future.' Richard quite forgot his own diffidence as he began to tell her about the countryside in Yorkshire.

Heston took Miranda's arm. 'We are *de trop*,' he told her with a smile. 'If you ladies do not rescue me, I shall be forced to display my ignorance. Do you care for cards, or a game of billiards?'

'Billiards, my lord? I have never played, but I should like to try.' Fanny's expression brightened in an instant.

'Then you shall do so.' He led them through the hall and into a massive billiard-room, complete with baize-covered table and cues in racks upon the walls.

Fanny showed a surprising aptitude for the game.

'What fun it is!' she cried. 'I had thought it only a game for gentlemen.' She grew excited as her score increased, and her face was vivid with enjoyment. For the moment she had forgotten the Count's defection.

Miranda sighed with relief. 'When do you go to Portsmouth?' she asked Heston.

'In a day or two. Alexei is to go ahead of the main party, to make sure that all is in readiness for the Tsar's suite.' The penetrating eyes held amusement in their depths. 'You have no need to worry, I assure you.'

'No. . .no, of course not. It is just that. . .'

'You need say no more. I am not blind. Now will you not try your hand at this absorbing game? If you allow your sister to outshine you, she will be insufferable.'

A smile took the sting out of his words and Fanny laughed at him as she relinquished her cue.

'You shall both try to beat me,' she announced.

'Not I!' his lordship shuddered. 'I have too much regard for the surface of this table.'

'Lord Heston, you are joking!' Fanny reproached. 'I suspect that you are an expert at this game.'

'This. . .and others. . .' he murmured in Miranda's ear. 'Now let me show you how to hold the cue.'

He stood behind her, long arms stretched out, and his hands covering her own. 'Don't rush at it,' he advised. 'Take it gently, and keep your eye upon the ball.'

His nearness made Miranda feel faint with longing. She tried to pot the ball, and missed completely.

Fanny's laughter echoed round the room. 'That is not the way,' she cried. 'Here, let me show you.'

Miranda dropped the cue and turned, only to find herself still enclosed within his lordship's arms. Beneath the fine cambric of his shirt, she sensed the beating of his heart, and the pounding in her own breast threatened to overcome her.

Then Heston moved away. 'We shall be missed,' he said lightly. 'Shall we join the others?'

They returned to the salon to find the Alderman lost in admiration of his painting. 'I have just the place for it,' he said with pride. 'I'll have it framed to match the gilding in the drawing-room. Then I shall see it every day.'

He was still gloating as they returned to Bloomsbury.

Chapter Fourteen

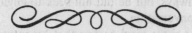

Fanny was unusually quiet on the following day. The reason was not far to seek, but Miranda did not question her.

'I thought Alexei seemed a little strange last night, did not you?' Fanny asked at last.

'He was pleasant, as he always is.'

'Yes, but. . .well. . .he is used to be more loverly.'

'You could not expect him to flirt openly in company.'

'You mean in the company of his sister, I suppose?'

'Among others.'

'No, it is she who does not like me. I knew it from the first. A Princess, indeed! Why, her husband is old enough to be her father.'

'That is not our concern.'

'Not yours, perhaps, but it is mine. She is so puffed up with family pride—'

'Oh, Fanny, that isn't true! I find her charming.'

'That is because she doesn't try to interfere in your affairs.' Fanny's laugh was angry. 'It is to be hoped that she does not intend to join us for our visit to the Pantheon. Without her, Alexei is so different.'

* * *

Her hopes were realised on the following evening, and Fanny was so delighted by the absence of the Princess that she failed to notice Alexei's continued reserve.

As always, his manners were delightful, but there was certainly a change in him.

It was obvious to Miranda. Alexei was his usual charming self, solicitous for their comfort and as entertaining as always, but he did not seek to engage Fanny in private conversation.

Surely her sister must realise that his interest in her went no further than the lightest of flirtations. A look at Fanny's expression convinced her otherwise. Her twin was gazing up at the Count with adoration in her eyes. She could not have made her feelings clearer if she had spoken them aloud.

'Out of the frying pan and into the fire?' Heston murmured wickedly. His words were for Miranda's ear alone, and she threw him a look of reproach.

'My sister is too susceptible,' she admitted with an uneasy laugh.

'Unlike yourself?' There was something in his eyes which challenged her to deny it.

'We. . . we are very different, she and I,' she said hastily.

'Indeed you are! It would be difficult to find two women less alike in temperament. I confess that your previous attachment to Harry Lakenham and his to you has often puzzled me.'

His remark was so unexpected that it caught Miranda unawares. Her head went up and she looked at him in panic. Then she made a valiant effort to cover her confusion.

'Why should you find it strange, my lord? I explained my reasons well enough. . .'

'So you did! It was a splendid explanation, but I was thinking more of Harry. . .'

'I don't know why you should feel his wish to marry me outrageous.'

'Not outrageous. . .just astonishing! Did he not quail at times?'

'That remark is unworthy of a gentleman, sir. You make me out to be some kind of dragon.'

'Not a dragon, my love, although I have seen you breathing fire upon occasion.' He looked down at her and she heard the laughter in his voice. 'Now how shall I find the words to describe you when you are upon your high ropes. . .perhaps a pretty little hissing kitten, out to defy the world?'

'That is nonsense!' she said coldly. 'Now, if you please, I should like to listen to the play.'

'Of course. I, too, shall enjoy it. It is such a comfort to know that both your own undying passion and that of Lakenham is unlikely to survive into old age.'

Miranda did not reply, although she herself had wondered why Harry no longer called upon them. After all, in the first hot throes of love he had been prepared to defy his grandfather. Yet that devotion had not survived an enforced separation. She realised that it was for the best, but it said much for the fickleness of a man's affection. Most probably they were all the same with their honeyed words at one moment, and indifference in the next. It was a lowering thought.

'Cheer up!' Heston teased. 'I shall not change.'

'No, I don't suppose you will,' she snapped. 'And that, my lord, is not a source of comfort to me!'

'Milling me down again?' His shoulders began to shake. 'I shall advise my friends that they need not visit the great Jackson for lessons in the art of self-defence. They should come to you instead.'

Miranda gave him an unwilling smile. Such a notion was so ridiculous that it appealed to her sense of humour.

'That's better!' he approved, and relapsed into silence until the interval. The one-act play which opened the evening's entertainment had not been received with much acclaim, but before the main performance could begin a buzz of excitement ran around the theatre.

Then the audience rose and began to clap and cheer. A woman had entered the opposite box, and now she came forward, bowing to the crowd.

Miranda knew at once that it was the Prince Regent's estranged wife, Caroline of Brunswick. Rumour had not lied, she decided. The Princess was heavily built, with rather coarse features. Her colouring was difficult to distinguish beneath the garish layers of paint and powder. Against the thick white coating blotches of scarlet rouge stood out in such startling contrast that they gave her the appearance of a clown.

The plunging neckline of her gown revealed a magnificent bosom, but it was cut even lower than those of the demi-reps who plied their trade on such occasions.

As Miranda watched the Princess threw back her head and laughed, displaying broken and discoloured teeth.

The vulgarity of her manner did not dismay the crowd. They cheered her to the echo.

'I did not know that the Princess was so popular,' Mrs Shere announced.

'We are about to find out just how popular,' Heston said with a significant glance at the adjoining box.

It was unfortunate that the Regent himself had chosen that particular moment to arrive at the theatre. He went unnoticed for a moment or two, and was forced to content himself with a back view of those of his fellow countrymen who had chosen to welcome the Princess Caroline. Then a murmur ran through the crowd. They turned and stood in silence as the heir to the throne took his seat.

The audience could not have made their opposition clearer, but the Prince's manner remained unchanged. He did not betray by the flicker of an eyelid that he was acquainted with the woman in the opposite box.

'Why, this is more exciting than the play,' Fanny whispered to Miranda. 'The Prince and his wife are looking through each other.'

'I think it sad,' Mrs Shere said quietly. 'Sometimes men and women are ill suited to each other. They cannot be blamed for that.'

'The blame is laid at the Prince's door,' Heston told her. 'He is considered to have treated both his wife and his daughter in a shabby way. The people will not stand for it. They have a love of justice, as you know.'

'Perhaps they do not know the whole,' Mrs Shere said kindly.

'You are generous, ma'am, and you are right. The Prince believes his wife to have an unfortunate influence on his daughter.'

Mrs Shere was silent. She, like everyone else in the capital, had heard rumours that the Princess Charlotte had been actively encouraged by her mother into conduct which lacked propriety. On one occasion, Caroline of Brunswick had locked her into a bedroom with a handsome aide-de-camp, telling the couple to enjoy themselves.

'That will be ended when the Princess Charlotte is wed,' Mrs Shere assured him.

'Let us hope so, ma'am, but she has just cried off from her engagement to the Prince of Orange, believing it to be a trick to get her out of the country.'

'Oh, no, I don't believe it! Whatever his faults, the Regent has always loved his daughter.' Mrs Shere spoke with conviction. From his early days, when the Prince was known and loved by all as the handsome Prince Florizel and the hope of the country, Mrs Shere had been his staunch supporter.

Heston smiled down at her. 'Ma'am, the Prince stands in need of more friends like you,' he said. 'It is too easy to think the worst of him.'

Miranda threw him a warm glance of approval. She was unsurprised to find him ready to defend his friend. Extravagant the Prince might be, changeable in his politics, easily swayed by the termagants who took his fancy, and emotional to a fault, but beneath the surface Heston had found a warm-hearted, cultivated man who believed in a civilised way of life, and would settle for nothing but the best in any field of the arts.

During the next interval she was able to study the Royal Party more closely. The Prince's appearance was as artificial as that of his wife. The paint and powder failed to disguise the fact that he had paled at the sight of her, and now looked morose.

Against the brilliant splendour of the satin coat and breeches which clothed his massive form, the dress of his Allies appeared simple and unostentatious. But it was for them that the cheering had begun again as they entered his box. The Regent had joined them in bowing to acknowledge the plaudits of the crowd, but there was a bitterness about his expression which Miranda could not fail to mark. He had suffered a public humiliation and she pitied him.

'Will the Princess Caroline be invited to attend the Proclamation of Peace with France tomorrow?' Mrs Shere enquired.

'No, ma'am. She does not attend official occasions.' Heston frowned. 'It is to be hoped that she won't invite herself and cause a disturbance.'

'Shall you go with the Prince, my lord?' Miranda asked.

'No, I think not. You know my views upon this so-called peace, my dear. In my opinion it is but a temporary cessation of hostilities. We haven't crushed Napoleon yet.'

He spoke in a low tone, for which Miranda was profoundly grateful. Mrs Shere had suffered enough as her eldest son had fought his way through the Peninsula with Wellington.

Miranda looked at the Prince again. 'If you are right, will the Regent lead his troops in battle? I heard that he had always longed to do so.'

'The King would never permit it.'

'But why? His royal brothers hold the highest ranks in the army.'

'That was one cause of the estrangement between Prince George and his father. He does not lack personal courage, but he was made to appear a coward through no fault of his own. It was in part a desire not to risk the life of the heir to the throne, but the main reason was the old king's dislike of his eldest son. Any request was met with a refusal as a matter of course.'

'They are an unfortunate family,' Miranda sighed.

'Indeed they are, but let us drop this depressing subject. Tomorrow I intend to leave for Portsmouth.'

'So soon? The Review of the Fleet is a full five days away. . .'

'Would you keep me by your side?' he teased.

Miranda looked up to see a twinkle in his eyes.

'Your private arrangements are none of my concern, my lord. . .' She turned away, but not before the tell-tale colour had risen to her cheeks.

'Crushed again, and just as I was beginning to hope.' He took her hand and raised it to his lips. 'I intend to call upon Lord Rudyard,' he told her. 'He is not in the best of health, and as he lives near Midhurst, it seemed an excellent opportunity. . .'

'To report upon myself and Harry?' Miranda's tone was sharp.

'Why, no!' He looked at her in mock surprise. 'I see no need for that.'

'He is sure to ask.' She felt uncomfortable.

'I don't intend to worry him with details of a matter which is now in the past. And Harry is behaving better than we might have hoped. I haven't seen him at the gaming tables, and to my knowledge he hasn't attempted any more balloon ascents.'

Miranda could not take so sanguine a view of Harry as a reformed character. In the past few months she had come to know him well, and his absence from his usual haunts had worried her.

For a time she had suspected that he and Fanny might be meeting in secret, but since her sister had transferred her affections to Alexei Toumanov she had dismissed the idea. Fanny was transparent and, apart from the fact that she had had no opportunity to make furtive assignations, it was clear that she no longer had any wish to revive her former love affair.

'Will Count Toumanov go with you?' she asked.

Heston shook his head. 'Tomorrow he is on duty. He will follow later.'

Fanny looked across at her twin with a radiant smile. Without Heston by his side this would be an opportunity for Alexei to declare his love. She was in the highest of spirits for the rest of the evening.

Throughout the following day her air of suppressed excitement did not go unnoticed by the Alderman and his wife.

'What a child you are!' her aunt said fondly. 'Such enthusiasm for our trip into the city! I hope it will be all that you expect, my dear.'

They were not to be disappointed. As the family coach turned into the Strand, the crowd slowed them to a halt. The city was in gala mood and there was dancing in the streets. Every building was decked with flags and banners, and the fountains ran with wine.

'What a sight!' Tears sparkled in Mrs Shere's eyes as she turned to her husband. 'May we not go into St Paul's Cathedral, my love? I should like to give thanks that our boy will now be safe. . .'

'Perhaps another day, my dear Emma. I think we should not leave the coach, or there is every likelihood of our being either separated or trampled underfoot.'

The press of people was so great, and the shouting so loud, that the horses grew uneasy. The Alderman was quick to see the danger, and he ordered his coachman to turn for home. It as not easily accomplished, and it was late afternoon before they reached Bloomsbury again.

Mrs Shere sank into a chair. 'What an exhausting day! I am glad to have seen the celebrations, but what a blessing it will be when all these foreigners leave the city. . .'

Miranda smiled at her. 'You will like to have a quiet evening, ma'am, with perhaps a little music?'

'More than anything, my dear, if you are not too tired to play.'

After their evening meal Miranda took her place at the spinet, signing to Fanny to turn the music for her. It soon became apparent that her sister's attention was elsewhere.

'Do pay attention, Fanny. You have missed the place three times.'

Fanny's eyes were upon the clock, and her face grew longer as the hours ticked by.

'It is so late,' she whispered. 'He won't come now.'

'Of course not!' Miranda did not pretend to misunderstand. 'Tonight there is a dinner at Carlton House.'

'A dinner at Carlton House, do you say?' The Alderman settled himself more comfortably in his chair. 'The Prince will be hard put to beat the dinner we gave him at the Guildhall. Did I tell you that we had the first turtle soup of the season?'

'Many times,' his wife assured him with a smile. 'My dear, would you not be more comfortable in your bed instead of dozing in your chair? These girls must be tired to death.'

It was a disconsolate Fanny who sought her bed-chamber that evening.

'I quite thought that Alexei would have come tonight,' she told Miranda.

'But I explained. The dinner will go on until the early hours.'

'Yes, that must be it, but pray do not suggest that we go out tomorrow. He is sure to call...'

* * *

Her hopes were to be dashed. They had a number of visitors on the following day, but the Count was not among them.

'Do you think that he is ill?' she asked Miranda anxiously. 'There must be a reason why he does not come to see us.'

'We have no way of finding out.' Miranda did not have the heart to voice her own interpretation of the reasons for the Count's absence. Fanny had been unable to hide her feelings for him, and he was too much of a gentleman to encourage her in a hopeless passion.

As the days passed Fanny grew more and more distraught. When Richard arrived she could not wait to question him.

'We have been worried about Count Toumanov,' she said. 'Have you heard that he is ill?'

'He was looking well when I saw him yesterday. He was on his way to Portsmouth.'

This apparently innocuous remark brought a gasp from Fanny. She fled the room with her handkerchief to her eyes, and Miranda could only be thankful that she and Richard were the only witnesses of her distress.

His face fell. 'Miranda, I know that you told me not to give up hope, but I can't believe that Fanny does not love the Count.'

'Another infatuation!' Miranda told him calmly. 'By next week he will be gone. Richard, if you are still of a mind to wed my foolish sister, I suggest that you seize the opportunity to offer for her. The love of a dear friend cannot but help to mend a broken heart.'

'She won't look at me.' His face was sad. 'She thinks of me as a brother.'

'Then you must change her mind.' She gave him a rueful look. 'But who am I to advise you? I cannot manage my own affairs.'

'How do you go on with Heston? Don't tell me if you don't wish it. I have no right to ask, but I should like to see you happy.'

Miranda hesitated for a moment. 'He says he loves me,' she replied. 'But I can't believe it.'

'I believe it. I have thought so for some time, as I once told you.'

'Even supposing it were true, I cannot marry him. In the first place, I should be forced to tell him of the way I have deceived him. What man could hear of it without disgust?'

'You are convinced that he has no suspicion of what has happened?'

'I am. I know well enough what his reaction would be.' She shuddered. 'I could not bear to hear what he would say. . .'

'Miranda, you misjudge him. He is one of the wisest men I know. His pride might be hurt, but he would soon forgive you.'

'You sound like Aunt Emma. I know you mean to comfort me, but it is to late for that. He offered to release me from my promise to him. . .did Fanny tell you?'

'No, but I must hope that you didn't accept.'

'I can do nothing else. When he returns from Portsmouth, I shall give him my decision.'

'If he accepts it, he is not the man I think him.' With those enigmatic words he prepared to take his leave.

'Will Fanny care to see the battle on the Serpentine?' he asked. 'It is not until next week, but. . .'

'By then the Count will be gone. No doubt she will welcome the diversion.' Miranda gave him her hand.

'What a staunch friend you are!' He bowed and left her.

Miranda went in search of Fanny, only to find her sister weeping in their room.

'How could Alexei do this to me?' her sister moaned. 'He must have known how much I longed to see him.'

'You certainly made it obvious. Fanny, I wish you will listen to me. . .'

'I won't! I won't! You don't understand! You have never cared for anyone as I care for him.'

'Perhaps not!' Miranda lied. 'But must you advertise it to the world? Richard was distressed to see you so upset.'

'Richard understands. He is the only person in the world who does not criticise me.'

'Then I am surprised that you are not kinder to him.'

Fanny ignored this last remark. 'When does the Court return from Portsmouth?' she asked. 'There is so little time left to us. Perhaps Alexei does not know of my feelings for him.'

'Then he must be blind. Fanny, I beg of you. . .please try for a little conduct. You lay yourself open to gossip.'

Fanny was not attending. 'That must be the reason. He thinks that I don't care for him. What a fool I have been! When he returns, I shall make my feelings clear.'

'Oh, love, please don't! Think how mortifying it would be to discover that he does not feel the same.'

Fanny glared at her. 'Why should he not? The most mortifying thing to me is to discover that you are eaten up with jealousy. Do you want him for yourself?'

The gibe was unworthy of a reply and Miranda changed the subject.

'Richard has asked if you would like to see the mock battle on the Serpentine next week. Shall you care to go? It is to be a re-creation of the battle of Trafalgar.'

'I suppose so. Anything would be preferable to this dreadful boredom. How dull we are without Alexei!'

Miranda held her tongue. She, too, was finding that life had lost much of its savour. It came as a surprise to realise just how much she had grown to enjoy her daily battle of wits with Adam Heston.

She missed the stimulation of his company, the laughter, the teasing, and above all the excitement when he held her in his arms.

She could not deny that she loved him with all her heart and she longed for the sight of his tall figure, the warmth of his smile, and his passionate caresses.

Without him the future would be bleak indeed. More than anything in the world she wanted to become his wife. It was cruel to think that she had found her love at last, only to be forced to give him up.

Yet their next meeting must be their last. The Review of the Fleet was to take place on the following day and then he would return from Portsmouth to seek her answer.

The thought of refusing him was agony, but she must be strong. To see him just once more was all she could hope for now. She looked so sad that Fanny was moved to question her.

'Are you ill?' she asked. 'You don't look at all the thing.'

'I have the headache, that is all.'

'So have I,' Fanny sighed. 'This waiting is enough to give anyone the megrims. I believe we should go shopping. That will cheer us up, and Aunt Emma will enjoy it.'

She hurried away to find their aunt and returned with the news that the carriage would be at the door in half an hour.

Miranda as too preoccupied to take much interest in their expedition, though she did her best to hide her worries. Perhaps the Tsar and his retinue would sail back to Russia direct from Portsmouth after the Review. There had been some talk of it. That would prevent Fanny from carrying out her plan to tell Alexei of her love.

Three days later her hopes were dashed when the Count was shown into their drawing-room.

Chapter Fifteen

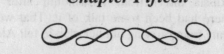

Fanny jumped up at once, oversetting her embroidery frame and scattering the brightly coloured silks across the carpet.

'At last!' she cried. 'Oh, how I have missed you!'

Miranda was ready to sink with embarrassment at this open declaration and a glance at Mrs Shere told her that her feelings were shared. She tried to retrieve the situation.

'We have all missed your company, Count Toumanov. Is that not so, Aunt Emma?'

'Indeed it is! The Review went well, I hope?' Mrs Shere tried to hide her anger at Fanny's shocking lack of decorum.

'It was a great success, ma'am, but now, alas, I am come to take my leave of you.' He did not look at Fanny as he spoke.

An audible gasp drew all eyes to her. Her colour rose and then receded, leaving her very pale.

'No, not yet!' she pleaded. 'Oh, I cannot breathe! Sir, will you help me into the garden?'

'I will take you to your room.' Mrs Shere rose to her

feet. 'Count Toumanov, will you excuse us? My niece has not been well.'

'I am sorry to hear it, and I must hope that Miss Gaysford will make a quick recovery. . .' He opened the door and stood aside as Mrs Shere thrust Fanny from the room.

An awkward silence followed their departure.

Then the Count walked over to the window. For some moments he was lost in thought.

'Have I been at fault?' he said at last. 'I would not willingly give pain.'

'The fault is not yours, sir.' Miranda felt unable to discuss her sister further. It had been an appalling scene, and she wished to spare the young man further embarrassment.

'Adam did not return to London with you?' she asked.

'Forgive me, Miss Gaysford, I had quite forgot. I am charged with messages for you. Adam sends his duty to Alderman and Mrs Shere, and rather more than that to you, I fancy.' He managed a faint smile. 'He is gone to see his godfather.'

'I thought he had intended to call upon Lord Rudyard on his way down to Portsmouth.'

'He did so, and found the old man sadly pulled down. Adam was so worried that he decided to return.'

'I see. Then we must expect him when we see him.'

'That won't be too long, I imagine. He is anxious to return to you, as I'm sure you know.' The Count pulled on his gloves. 'This has not been the happiest of leave-takings, Miss Gaysford, and for that I must blame myself. I should not have come today.'

'After all our happy times together? We should have taken it amiss if you had not called to say farewell.'

Miranda hoped that her words would reassure him, but his face was troubled as he took his leave of her.

She was given no time to worry about it, for at that moment the door burst open and Ellen rushed into the room.

'Miss, will you come at once? Your sister is in strong hysterics, and Mrs Shere can do no good with her. . .'

Miranda hurried up the stairs. She could hear Fanny's screams from the first landing. Fanny was lying on her bed, laughing and crying by turns.

'Shall I send for the doctor?' Mrs Shere turned an anxious face towards her.

'Leave her with me.' Miranda walked over to the bed and slapped her twin across the face. The laughing and screaming stopped as Fanny subsided into hiccuping sobs.

'My dear child, I had not the least idea that your sister had formed an attachment for the Count.' For once Mrs Shere looked every year of her age.

'Infatuation, ma'am,' Miranda told her crisply. 'It has happened before.'

'But Count Toumanov? Has he led her to believe. . .?'

'No, that is all in my sister's mind.'

'Then I must wonder how your mama puts up with all this nonsense. I would suggest that she goes home, but your marriage is so close, and she must return for that.'

'Aunt, if you will allow me, I will speak to her alone.'

'Very well, my dear. You may succeed in bringing her to her senses where I could not.' Her manner was unusually stern as she left the twins together.

Miranda walked over to the bed and looked at the weeping figure of her twin.

'You may stop that!' she said coldly. 'It will not wear with me.'

'How could it? You can have no idea of how I feel. Oh, how could he be so cold? I tried to see him alone, but he did not support me.'

'Fanny, your behaviour was the outside of enough. That blatant attempt to persuade the Count into the garden! I thought I must have died of shame.'

Fanny's sobs ceased. 'That is all you care about,' she accused. 'I declare you are become as stuffy as Heston himself. You should deal well together.'

'Don't try to change the subject. We are not discussing Heston. Surely you must realise now that Count Toumanov had no intention of offering for you?'

Fanny began to wail again. 'I shall become a dried-up spinster,' she declared. 'Lakenham has deserted me, and now the Count. I hope you are satisfied.'

'None of it was of my doing,' Miranda declared with some asperity. 'Now wash your face. You must apologise to Aunt Emma. She had almost decided to send you home.'

'I should not care,' her twin said in a sullen tone. 'I am beginning to hate London. Nothing pleasant ever happens here.' She turned her head away and buried her face in the pillow.

Miranda left her to her sulks.

By the evening of the following day she was growing worried. No food had passed he sister's lips, and Fanny replied to questions only in monosyllables.

'Perhaps we were too hard on her. You do not think that she will fall into a decline?' Mrs Shere was clearly anxious.

'No, I don't.' Miranda gave her aunt a reassuring smile. 'I'll speak to her. She may be feeling better now.'

As she made her way upstairs she felt perplexed. It was difficult to know exactly what to do. Fanny might be genuinely ill, in which case they should summon the doctor without delay. On the other hand, this refusal to eat could be her way of punishing her sister and her aunt for the lectures which she had suffered.

She opened the door to the bedchamber as quietly as possible, in case her twin was sleeping. The blinds were drawn against the evening sunlight, but Fanny was sitting up in bed. She looked up startled as Miranda entered and pulled the bedcover up to her chin.

'Are you cold? Will you have a hot brick for your feet?'

'No!' Fanny mumbled. Her guilty expression aroused Miranda's suspicions. She crossed over to the bed and threw back the coverlet to reveal a plate of cakes.

'I see! Ellen has been smuggling food to you. You have not been starving, have you?' The contempt in her voice made her sister blush. She did not reply.

'How could you, Fanny? Aunt has been so worried and so have I.'

There was still no answer.

'You can't hide up here for ever,' Miranda continued. 'You must come downstairs and speak to Aunt.'

'I won't! I'm tired of being scolded. I wish we had never come here. . .' Fanny scowled at her.

'It's too late to think of that. We are here and you must make the best of it. Now pray get dressed and do as I ask. . .'

'Not tonight. I'll come down in the morning. You may tell Aunt Emma that I feel a little better.'

Miranda felt dispirited as she returned to the salon,

but her anger was mingled with relief. If Fanny might be persuaded into an apology, Mrs Shere would readily accept it. Count Toumanov was gone, so there could be no repetition of Fanny's ill behaviour as far as he was concerned.

'I think we have no further cause to worry, ma'am,' she said. 'My sister is much recovered and will come down in the morning. She is distressed to think that she has worried you. . .'

'That she did!' Mrs Shere replied with feeling. 'I cannot like the way that she goes on. If it were not for your wedding, I should send her home.'

'Ma'am, pray try to understand. . .she is so impressionable and she does not always consider. . .'

Mrs Shere gave Miranda a reluctant smile. 'You will always defend her, my dear girl, and I admire your loyalty, but I could wish that she were wed to some sensible man such as Mr Young. With her children about her she might settle down.'

'Aunt, I share your hopes, and so does Richard. He is devoted to her.'

'Heaven protect him!' Mrs Shere threw her eyes to heaven. 'He cannot wish for a quiet life.'

'He knows her very well, Aunt Emma, and he does not mind her fits of temperament. When we were children he could always coax her out of them, and was happy to do so.'

'He must be a saint.'

'I have often thought much the same myself, but she must be loved, you know, and he would give her all the love she needs.'

'Your twin is spoilt, my dear, but there, I shall say no more to distress you.'

'Or her?' Miranda begged.

'I suppose not. My only comfort is the thought that you are to be wed so soon, and will no longer bear responsibility for her. When does Lord Heston return?'

'I'm not quite sure. He is staying with his godfather. The Count told me that Lord Rudyard is not well.'

'Doubtless reports about Harry Lakenham have reached him. I do not understand the young these days. It makes me wonder what the world is coming to.'

On this sombre note both ladies retired.

Fanny was on her best behaviour for the next few days. Her apologies were given and received with good grace. Then she exerted all her charm in an effort to restore Mrs Shere's kind opinion.

This was the calm before the storm, Miranda thought with a shudder. When Heston returned and she refused him, they would be plunged into further scenes involving herself.

And with each day that passed she missed him more. Even to endure his anger would be preferable to not seeing him at all. Perhaps if she threw herself upon his mercy he might forgive her? Then the memory of that harsh dark face rose before her eyes. No, he would not forgive deception followed by humiliation. It was alien to his nature, and an offence to any man of honour.

It was in no happy frame of mind that she joined the others in the carriage as they set off to see the mock battle on the Serpentine.

The Park was crowded, but Richard found a place for them beside the water's edge. Fanny was in the highest of spirits, Count Toumanov apparently forgotten. She chattered gaily, begging to be told the names of all the miniature ships upon the lake.

'They are larger than I had expected. . . I thought they would be toys.'

'Not if they are to hold the crews. It is all to be as realistic as possible, you know. The Prince has spared no expense.' Richard was eager to explain. 'He wished to mark the centenary of the House of Hanover in appropriate style. What better than a re-creation of the Battle of Trafalgar?'

Miranda looked about her. 'I wonder if we should not move further back?' she said. 'The crowd is pushing from behind and we are so close to the lake. . .'

'No, no!' Fanny clapped her hands. 'We have a splendid view. I won't give up my place.'

The Alderman had seen the danger. He took his wife's arm and moved back a pace or two, pushing the jostling mob aside. Others took their place at once, and soon they were lost to sight.

Miranda heard him call to her to come away. Then his words were drowned in a cannonade of gunfire.

Startled, Fanny screamed and lost her footing as he turned. Then she plunged headlong into the lake.

A roar of laughter ran through the crowd as Richard waded after her.

'Oh, she will drown!' Miranda cried in anguish.

'No, ma'am, it ain't deep enough just here,' the man beside her comforted. 'See, the young man is only in the water up to his waist.'

At that moment Fanny found her footing and flung her arms in a stranglehold about Richard's neck. It took him by surprise and they fell together into deeper water. The crowd grew silent.

'She will drown the pair of them,' Miranda's companion murmured. He sat down and began to struggle out of his boots.

Miranda was frozen into silence as she watched the struggling pair. Then Richard brought both arms up through her sister's grip and broke it. He cupped one hand beneath her chin and forced her head back. Then he slipped behind her and began to tow her to the shore.

A circle formed about them as he lifted Fanny's unconscious figure up onto the bank. Then he turned her over and pressed upon her back. Streams of water flowed from her mouth and then her eyelids fluttered.

Alderman Shere was on his knees beside them. 'Well done!' he said in a low voice. 'Is she conscious?'

Richard nodded. 'It is all my fault, sir. I should not have let her stand so close to the edge.'

'You are not to blame. Let us take her home.'

Miranda slipped an arm about her aunt's shoulders. The older woman was badly shaken, but with commendable restraint she refrained from any comment upon the accident.

It was only later, when Fanny had been taken to her room and the doctor summoned, that she began to cry.

'Now, Emma, don't give way,' the Alderman admonished. 'You ladies have held up well in spite of the shock, and there is no harm done.' He looked across at Richard. 'My dear sir, you showed great presence of mind, for which I thank you.'

Clad in the Alderman's coat and breeches, which were too big for him, Richard was a comic figure, but no one smiled.

'She might have drowned!' He buried his face in his hands. 'I shall never forgive myself.'

'Nonsense!' Miranda told him briskly. 'The lake is shallow. She might have walked out of it herself if she had not panicked.'

'But she did, and she can't swim.'

It took some time to comfort him, but reassured at last by the doctor's hopeful diagnosis he took his leave of them.

Fanny was unharmed, and the ducking had not resulted in an inflammation of the lungs as Mrs Shere had predicted. Once recovered from the shock she took full advantage of the near-tragedy, happy to be the centre of attention.

Richard was now her hero, though he disclaimed the honour.

'The lake was not deep, you know. We might have walked out if. . .'

'If I had not been so foolish?' Fanny smiled up at him. She was lying upon a sofa in the salon, dressed in one of her most becoming gowns. 'Oh, Richard, you saved me from a watery grave. I never was so frightened in my life. . .'

'It is all over. You must forget it.' He took her hand and held it in his own.

'How can I? What should I have done without you?'

He was spared the need to reply when Charlotte Fairfax was announced, and his gaze was rueful as he looked up at Miranda.

She smiled and shook her head. 'There will be other opportunities,' she assured him. 'I believe you have slain the dragon.'

After that, Charlotte was a frequent visitor, somewhat to Fanny's surprise.

'I thought her more your friend than mine,' she said one day. 'Yet she has asked if I will go to stay with her.'

'An excellent plan!' Mrs Shere intervened. 'It will give you a change of scene.'

'But shall you wish to go?' Miranda asked. 'It seems a little strange when she does not live above a mile away.'

'Oh, I think so.' Fanny dismissed the objection. 'It will be only for a day or two, and Aunt is right. It will suit both of us. Charlotte is lonely, so she tells me. . .'

Miranda suspected that Fanny's main reason for agreeing to this plan was to avoid the stricter supervision which her aunt had threatened after the contretemps with Count Toumanov, but she made no comment.

When Fanny had gone, Mrs Shere did not mince her words.

'I cannot but be glad that you are separated for a time,' she said. 'Sometimes you look positively hagged, my love. Don't tell me that your sister is not a worry to you, for I won't believe it.'

'She did not mean to fall into the lake,' Miranda murmured.

'I was not referring to that, although the accident was due more to her own folly than to a lack of care upon the part of Mr Young.'

'It may be no bad thing,' Miranda chuckled. 'He is now her hero.'

'I know it. That was the only reason why I agreed to let her go to Charlotte. And Sir William Fairfax is a stern papa, you know. The girls will be carefully supervised.'

Miranda grew thoughtful. Sir William's reputation as a disciplinarian was well known. She doubted if Fanny would care to stay for long in such a household, but in the meantime it was a relief to be spared the need to fret about her.

In the next few days her life took on an almost dream-like quality. She wandered about the garden, helping the Alderman where she could, between intervals of playing on the spinet, much to her aunt's delight. Her book was long since finished, but she had managed to obtain a recently published copy of *Waverley*, which had taken the town by storm. It kept her occupied for many hours.

Even an invitation to take tea with Lady Heston did not trouble her as it might have done. The visit passed off without incident, and if she seemed preoccupied neither her aunt nor Lady Heston mentioned it.

Time seemed to have stopped. She was waiting in limbo as the dark cloud at the back of her mind grew ever larger. Heston must soon return and then. . .? Her face grew sombre. She dreaded the thought of that last interview with him, but it must be final. She would make sure of that.

'My dear, won't you take up your embroidery again? You have neglected it for so long, and it will help to pass the time,' Mrs Shere said kindly. 'His lordship cannot be long delayed, and then you will be happy once more.'

'I beg your pardon, aunt Emma. I did not mean to be so gloomy.'

'Not gloomy, dearest, just a little sad. It is under-standable when Lord Heston has been gone for all this time. I'm sure he would not wish you to give up all your pleasures. We might drive out, you know, or visit the shops in Bond Street. . .'

Miranda excused herself from the proposed expedition, and Mrs Shere did not argue.

'You fear that he might call when we are out? Very well, but I must go. I shall not be away for long.'

Miranda settled herself at her embroidery frame, and began to look through the coloured silks. She threaded her needle, but it was only the striking of the clock which told her that she had not set a stitch for the past hour.

Lost in a reverie, she did not at first attend when the door opened.

'Lord Heston, ma'am,' the servant announced.

Miranda looked up to find his lordship advancing towards her. Her smile of welcome vanished when she saw the expression on his face. His eyes were stony with contempt and his jaw was rigid. At that moment he looked capable of murder.

'Where is Fanny?' he said without preamble.

Miranda froze. 'My lord, are you not mistaken?' she faltered. Then she heard an ugly laugh.

'Come, madam, let us have done with this charade. It has gone on for long enough.'

Miranda made a last attempt to save herself. 'I. . . I don't understand you.'

He caught her wrist in an iron grip which made her wince and dragged her to her feet.

'Don't you? Will you deny that you have tricked me from the first? You shall not take me for a fool. Did you think it amusing to take your sister's place?'

Miranda knew that all was over. It would be useless to prevaricate further.

'How long have you known?' she asked in a low tone.

'Does that matter? It did not take long, I assure you.

You made a number of mistakes, although I did not need them to convince me. You and Harry Lakenham? It wasn't possible.'

'Not even for the money and the title?' Miranda flared. He was entitled to be furious, but his icy disdain was not to be borne.

'Don't trifle with me! There is no time! I ask you again. . .where is your sister?'

'What concern is that of yours? If you must know, she is staying with Charlotte Fairfax. . .'

'Is she? You had best read this.' He produced a letter from his pocket and thrust it into her hand.

Miranda opened it with shaking fingers. The characters seemed to dance across the page, blurring as she tried to make them out. They began to swim before her eyes.

'Here, let me!' Heston said roughly. As he read the note to her, Miranda's worst fears were realised.

It was from Harry Lakenham, informing Heston that he had eloped. By the time the letter was received, he would be married.

Miranda swayed as the room seemed to spin about her. She sat down suddenly, feeling that her legs would no longer support her.

'I don't believe it!' she whispered. 'Fanny would not. . .she could not. . .'

'On the contrary, I believe her capable of anything. Was this your idea?'

Miranda felt dumb with misery. She could not answer him.

'Don't play the innocent with me, my dear. It was a clever plan, I'll give you that. Were you to keep me occupied and throw me off the scent until Lakenham and your sister found a suitable opportunity to disappear?'

'No! I thought she had changed her mind in favour of Count Toumanov.'

'Another clever ploy? It will not serve. Both you and she would know that Toumanov would never offer for her.'

'I knew it, but she did not, and you yourself threw them together.'

'I admit it. I have never trusted her. She was meeting Lakenham after you were supposedly betrothed to me. Don't trouble to deny it, for I have proof.'

'Please listen to me,' Miranda cried in despair. 'Let me explain. I owe you that at least.'

'Pray go on,' he said in an ironic tone. 'It should make an interesting story.'

'It is the truth,' she said brokenly. 'When you first came here, Fanny would not see you. We thought that you had come to offer for her. I was simply to refuse you, and that was to be an end of it.'

Heston said nothing, but his eyes never left her face.

'And then. . .and then you were so insulting that I lost my temper. I said more than I intended. You shall not blame Fanny for that. It was all my fault.'

'I lost my temper, too,' he admitted in a kinder tone. 'I had no right to force you into a betrothal.'

'I could not believe that you would go on with it. Each day I hoped that you would release me from my promise. I knew that you wished to punish me, but when everything went so far I could see no way of escape. . .'

'And did you wish to escape?' There was something in his voice which brought the colour to her cheeks.

She turned her head away. 'I had to. I tried to cry off, if you recall, on the day we went to Richmond.'

'I remember it well.'

'Then why didn't you agree? By then you knew of the deception. . .'

'By then I had changed my mind.'

Miranda did not speak, but a tiny flicker of hope stirred in her heart. She stifled it at once. It would be too cruel to raise expectations which could never be fulfilled.

'Have you nothing more to say to me?' Heston enquired softly.

'I can only apologise, my lord. What you must think of us. . .of me. . . I can't imagine.'

'Then I must tell you some time.'

Miranda looked up at that, and was surprised to see a twinkle in his eyes. She felt confused.

'I wanted to tell you the truth. I was ashamed to do so, especially when I thought about my aunt and uncle, and Lady Heston too. They were all so kind. Oh, sir, if only a scandal might be avoided. . .!'

'It might be possible.' Before she could protest, he took her in his arms. 'My love, you are a goose! Can it be that you don't know how much I love you?' He dropped a tender kiss upon her brow.

'But you can't! Not after the way. . .'

'After the way you have stolen my heart? I have deceived you too, you know, in pretending that I thought that you were Fanny. It is I who should beg for your forgiveness. Will you dash my hopes?'

Miranda found that she hadn't the least desire to release herself from his embrace. She buried her face in his shoulder.

'Why did you go on with it?' she asked in muffled tones.

'Well, you know, I hoped that you had learned to trust me enough to tell me the truth.'

'I couldn't. I loved you so, and—' She could not go on as he caught her to him, and his mouth found hers. Miranda clung to him in ecstasy, lost in the wonder of his love. Then the door opened.

'I thought I should find you here,' said Fanny.

Chapter Sixteen

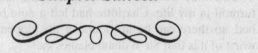

Two pairs of startled eyes regarded her, and then Miranda sat down suddenly.

'What are you doing here?' she asked in a faint voice.

'I live here, in case you had forgotten.' Fanny was clearly in the grip of some powerful emotion. 'You won't believe what I have to tell you.' She threw herself upon the sofa in a dramatic attitude. 'I have been tricked in the most shameful way.'

'Who has tricked you?' Miranda feared the worst.

'Why, Charlotte and Harry Lakenham. It is the most deceitful thing. They have eloped!'

Her injured expression was too much for Miranda's composure, but she tried to keep her voice steady.

'Are you quite sure?'

'Of course I am. I suppose I may believe the evidence of my own eyes. We were shopping in the Emporium in Bond Street when I missed her. I looked about and then I saw her disappearing through the door at the back of the shop. When I followed, Harry was helping her into a closed carriage. . . I called to them, but they did not answer me.'

'And then?'

'Well, I could not make it out. It seemed so strange of them to go for a drive without inviting me, and in a chaise with the blinds pulled down. I could not follow them, so I went back to Charlotte's home to see if they had returned, but they weren't there.'

'Oh, Fanny, what a worry for you!'

'You may believe it! I never walked into such a turmoil in my life. Charlotte had left a note beside her bed, so there be no doubt of the elopement. The worst of it is that Sir William blames me!'

'Astonishing!' Heston murmured. 'What could have given him the idea that you would be party to such a plan, I wonder?'

Miranda threw him a reproachful look. 'You knew nothing of it?'

'No, I did not. Charlotte may not think herself my friend in future. I shall not speak to her again. To steal off with Harry in that way. . .? It is beyond anything!'

'But you no longer care for him, I think?'

'No, I don't. He is a fribble. I have had a lucky escape, but that is not the point. I might have eloped with him myself. . .'

There seemed to be no immediate answer to this remark, but Fanny's expression tried Miranda sorely. Her sister resembled no one so much as a child who had been robbed of a favourite toy. She dared not look at Heston, but she guessed that his feelings were much the same as her own.

Fanny's glance was suspicious as she looked at the faces of her companions.

'You seem to find the situation amusing,' she said sharply. 'Had you not best go after them, my lord?'

'I think not, my dear Miss Gaysford. I believe I must leave that task to Sir William Fairfax.' Heston took

Miranda's arm. 'Will you not take a turn about the garden with me, dearest, that is, if your sister will excuse us. . .?'

Fanny flounced out of the room, a thunderous expression on her face.

'Oh dear, I should not laugh,' Miranda choked.

'Certainly not in here. Let me beg you to restrain yourself until we reach the summer-house. . .'

There Miranda laughed until she cried.

'What a wretch I am!' she gasped as she wiped her streaming eyes. 'It is not kind to be so unfeeling, but Fanny looked so. . .so. . .'

'Injured?' Heston's own shoulders were shaking. 'I thought I had best rescue you before you disgraced yourself in your sister's eyes.'

'She must be so hurt.'

'Not at all! Your beloved twin is mortified to find that she is not the central figure in this elopement. The injury is to her pride, and I have no doubt that Sir William Fairfax further injured it.'

'Fanny was right in one respect, my lord. This elopement will be a sad blow to Harry's grandfather, as well as to Charlotte's parents. Can you do nothing?'

'I wouldn't, even if I could. Sir William is a martinet, as Harry will discover to his cost. He may forget his previous ways. Sir William will have none of them.'

'Then you think it may be for the best?'

'I do. I can think of nothing better to bring Harry to his senses.'

'If they are already married. . .'

'Harry won't waste time. He is still under age and would fear pursuit. I imagine he would make for Doctors Commons with a licence in his pocket.'

'But Sir William may annul the match.'

'I doubt it. Harry bears an ancient name, and he will soon be in possession of his fortune.'

'But Lord Rudyard? Oh, dear, he is not well. . . The shock may be too much for him.'

'He knows Sir William, and that will be enough for him.'

'You seem so sure?'

'I am, my dearest one. Besides which, I am ready at this moment to consign Charlotte, Harry and even your sister to perdition. We have been parted for a full two weeks, and I have missed you so.' He looked down at her with such a tender expression that her heart began to pound.

She lifted her face to his. 'I felt the same,' she said simply. 'Without you, the days seemed endless. . .'

He bent his head and she surrendered her lips to his. With that kiss the world was lost to both of them. All the heartache of the past few weeks vanished in a rising tide of passion, and Miranda felt a joy which she had not known before. He loved her. Now she could be sure of it, and the knowledge sent her spirit soaring.

When he released her she was breathless. She rested her head against his shoulder and took his hand in hers, absently stroking his fingers.

'My lord. . .' she began.

'Adam,' he corrected. 'Or are we not yet well enough acquainted for you to give me my name?'

Miranda blushed as she saw the laughter in his eyes. She could not mistake his meaning. Her overwhelming delight in that kiss had been equal to his own.

'Adam. . .when did you first know? I mean, when did you decide that I was not the termagant you thought me?'

'It was difficult,' he told her gravely. 'Those dagger

looks quite sunk me. They did serious damage to my self-esteem. At times I considered putting a period to my existence.'

'I wish you will be serious,' she reproached him. 'I asked you a sensible question.'

'There was nothing sensible about my feelings, I assure you. I think I must have loved you from the first time that we met.'

'Oh, what a fib! You called me a doxy.'

'Did I say that? You caught me off balance, my beloved. I had not expected to receive such a severe setdown, though I deserved it.'

'You did indeed!' she scolded with a loving smile. 'I may tell you that I have never disliked anyone so much. You were a perfect monster, and I wanted to crush you into very small pieces.'

Adam began to nibble her ear. 'What a fate! When did you change your mind?'

'I don't quite know,' she told him in a serious tone. 'As I grew to understand you better, I felt that I must have been mistaken in your character and your motives for behaving as you did.'

'They were always dastardly,' he assured her with a wicked grin. 'You have no fear that I shall beat you daily, and lock you in your room for weeks?'

'No!' she said demurely. 'I doubt if you would wish to lock me away.'

'Minx! What a dance you will lead me!' The prospect did not appear to worry him, for he kissed her again until her head began to spin. 'My dearest, I love everything about you, from the tip of your head to those charming little toes. How well I know that enchanting face! It is the mirror of your soul.'

'Even when I am looking cross?'

'Especially when you are looking cross. Your chin goes up and your eyes begin to sparkle. . .'

'At least I do not arch my back and hiss, you will admit. You told me once that I looked like an angry kitten.'

'Ah, you remembered that?'

'I think I remember every word you've ever spoken to me.' She pressed her lips against his hand.

'Oh, dear, not all of them, I hope? Remember only that I love you more than life, my darling. . . Will you do that?'

Her answer was in her eyes. He held her to him and then they heard the sound of approaching footsteps.

Alderman Shere was hurrying down the path towards them.

'Ah, there you are, my dear. Your aunt is returned and wishes to speak to you.' He bowed to Heston. 'There is no immediate hurry, my lord.'

'I will come at once.' Miranda rose to her feet. 'Will you join us, Uncle? We have something to say to you.'

'Nothing is amiss, I hope?' He looked at their faces and was satisfied. 'No, I see that there is not. . .but this is a bad business about Charlotte Fairfax.'

He turned back to the house, leaving them to follow him.

'I shall have to tell them,' Miranda said in a low voice. 'I can't go on with this deception, but what on earth am I to say?'

'Will you leave it to me?' Adam slipped an arm about her waist and hugged her. 'Don't worry, my dearest. I promise you that all will be well. You must learn to rely on my support, you know.'

Miranda threw him a speaking look of gratitude. It

was a comfort to think that she need no longer carry her burdens alone.

They found Mrs Shere alone in the salon and she was looking stern.

'My lord, you will forgive me for speaking out in front of you, but I must know. My dear, did your sister play any part in helping Charlotte to elope? She denies it, but there is no speaking to her. . .'

'No, ma'am, she did not. Fanny was as shocked as we were ourselves.'

'Fanny? But you are Fanny. It was Miranda who went to stay with Charlotte. . .'

'No, ma'am.' Adam sat down beside her and took her hands. 'We must beg your forgiveness, Mrs Shere, and yours too, my dear sir. When I first came to you, I asked if I might pay my addresses to Miss Gaysford. I should have asked for Miss Miranda Gaysford. It was she who had my heart. The fault is mine. It was a foolish mistake, but I had thought Miranda the elder of the two.'

'But, Lord Heston, you should have spoken when you found out your mistake. We should have understood. . .'

'You are too kind, ma'am, but I felt an utter fool. My pride was at stake. It is a sad failing in me, I fear. The trouble was that I did not at first realise. . .fond though I was, I did not know your nieces well.'

'Perfectly understandable.' The Alderman laughed aloud. 'Emma, have I not always wondered how Lord Heston knew one twin from the other?'

Mrs Shere was not so easily satisfied. 'The girls are not in the least alike in temperament,' she said doubtfully. 'I confess that it was a puzzle to me to learn that my sister relied so heavily upon Miranda when I found her such a scatterbrain. . .'

'That was Fanny, ma'am. I feel a perfect wretch. I should have thrown myself upon your mercy long ago.'

He was smiling as he spoke and Mrs Shere could not resist his charm. He had always been a favourite with her.

'I should give you a cruel scolding, and Miranda too,' she said with mock severity.

'And I should deserve it, ma'am.' He bent his head and looked so meek that Mrs Shere began to smile.

'Pray do not add play-acting to your other misdeeds, my lord. . . Just tell me one thing. Are you convinced that the lady by your side is indeed Miranda?'

'I'm certain of it, ma'am. Aren't you?' He stretched out a hand and drew Miranda to his side.

'Yes, I am, and I wish you happy, sir. You will not find a better wife.'

Miranda threw her arms about her aunt and kissed her. Then she went to hug her uncle.

'May I tell Fanny that you know the truth?' she asked.

Mrs Shere reached out for the bell-pull and sent her servant to summon Fanny to the drawing-room.

She entered, looking subdued and in the expectation of another scolding, but Miranda set her mind at rest.

When Heston's apparent folly was explained to her, she looked at him with awe. Then she began to laugh.

Mrs Shere took her to task at once. 'This is no laughing matter, Fanny. I am surprised that you should find it so amusing. Pray do not try to convince me that you knew nothing of it.'

'No, ma'am, but you see. . . I was trying to protect Lord Heston's reputation.'

'Lord Heston has no need of your protection. He would do nothing dishonourable.'

It was clear that Adam was now to be absolved of all blame for his part in the charade.

'Don't look so smug!' Miranda hissed at him. 'We have still to face your mother.'

'She knows all about it, my love. I had to tell her. She was so worried about you.'

'Deceiver!' Miranda threw him a fulminating glance. She might have said more but at that moment Richard was announced.

He seemed unsurprised to discover that a change had taken place and that he might now address his love by her own name.

The conversation now centred upon the arrangements for Miranda's wedding, and for the first time she was able to take part in the discussion with a happy heart.

'And your honeymoon, my lord. Where will you go for that?' Mrs Shere asked.

'Paris, I think, if Miranda agrees.' Adam looked a question at her, but before she could reply Fanny intervened.

'Famous!' she cried. 'I shall enjoy that above anything. . .'

Miranda stared at her in stupefaction. Beside her, she sensed that Adam was about to speak, but before he could do so Richard walked over to her sister and took her hand.

'You cannot go with Miranda,' he said gently.

'Why not? It is quite the thing, you know, for a bride to have a friend or a relative with her for companionship.'

Adam stirred again, but Miranda stilled him with a hand upon his arm.

'I thought you might prefer to go there as a bride yourself, Fanny.' Richard stood quite still, but his face was alight with hope.

'How can I? I have no husband.'

'You might have, if you will take me?'

He had Fanny's attention then. She stared at him.

'You can't mean it! Are you making me an offer?'

'Hand and heart, dear Fanny. Will you disappoint me?'

Fanny looked about her. The Alderman and Mrs Shere were speechless with astonishment, but Adam and her twin were smiling. It was a most public declaration, and she was certainly the focus of all eyes.

'I'd like to marry you,' she announced. 'But, Richard, I always wanted to elope. . .'

'Then, of course, we shall elope, but there are arrangements to be made. Your aunt and uncle will wish to know where we are going.'

'Is that usual?' she asked doubtfully. 'I thought it was always meant to be a secret?'

'Not always!' Richard's face was grave. 'I thought we might elope to Yorkshire, and go to Paris later. Then your mother and my father will be able to attend the ceremony. . .'

Beside her, Miranda felt Adam's shoulders begin to shake. 'Hush!' she whispered. 'Will you spoil everything?'

'I couldn't if I tried,' he moaned in anguish.

Miranda dug her elbow into his ribs. Thankfully, Fanny had not noticed his paroxysms. She bestowed an enchanting smile upon her suitor and allowed him to clasp her in his arms.

Over her head Richard sought Miranda's eyes. His own held a curious mixture of love and rueful amusement but she nodded, happy to think that he had won his heart's desire. Life with Fanny would not be easy, but he loved her dearly and he knew her well. She need have no fears for her sister's future happiness.

'I am about to collapse,' Adam whispered in a voice intended only for Miranda's ears. 'In a moment I shall disgrace myself. . .'

He was rewarded with a stern look.

'Don't torture me,' he begged. 'I rescued you. Won't you do the same for me?'

Her own composure was sorely tried, but she made her excuses after offering the happy pair her good wishes for their future life together. Then she allowed Adam to lead her back into the garden.

This time they did not reach the summer-house. Adam clung to one of the supports of the pergola, unable to speak.

'My lord, I do not take this kindly,' she told him with quivering lips. 'Richard meant well. . .'

'I know it,' he choked out at last. 'The man is braver than Wellington himself. It was the elopement that was too much for me.'

'You have a sadly frivolous side to your nature, sir.'

'No, you are mistaken. I am the dullest dog in all the world. It did not occur to me to offer you an elopement, although you must have wished it.'

'You are behaving very ill, my lord.' Her own voice was not quite under her control. 'If you go on like this, I shall begin to doubt your sanity.'

'Only mine?' The look he gave her destroyed the last vestiges of her self-control, and her peals of laughter rang around the garden.

'Pray don't go on!' she gasped at last. 'I feel quite weak. . .'

'Not weak enough to invite a companion to join us on our honeymoon journey, I hope?'

Miranda studied her fingers. 'I had considered it,' she announced.

'Really? You do not feel that I shall provide enough companionship for you, both day and night?'

'I don't know,' she murmured wickedly.

'I think we had best continue this conversation in the privacy of the summer-house, my love. . .' He slipped an arm about her waist and led her along the path. Once inside the little wooden building he gripped her shoulders and looked down, still laughing, into her eyes. Then he shook her gently.

'Exasperating creature!' he said fondly. 'Haven't I been punished enough? Must you continue to tease me?'

'Why, sir, I can't think what you mean.'

'Can't you? Then I had best show you.' He sat down and drew her on to his knee.

'Now, fair maiden,' he uttered in melodramatic tones. 'I have you in my power. To struggle will avail you nothing.' He twirled an imaginary moustache.

Miranda found that she had no desire to struggle. Instead she slid her arms about his neck.

'You are behaving very foolishly,' she whispered.

'I expect to behave foolishly for the rest of my life, my darling.' He pressed his lips into the hollow of her throat. 'Shall you mind?'

'I think I shall like it very much.' She kissed his cheek, aware only that his lips were teasing as they travelled upwards. Then his mouth found hers, and all else was forgotten in the wonder of his love.

$\mathcal{H}istorical\ \mathcal{R}omance^{™}$

Coming next month

THE EARL OF RAYNE'S WARD
Anne Ashley

Rebecca Standish *refused* to comply with Drum Thornville's outrageous demand... Since she was twelve years old her best friend Drum had tried to curb her wild ways. When he'd left to join the army she had been freed from his domination, but seven years later he was back! He was still as overbearing, arrogant and authoritarian as ever—and very handsome! She vowed to ignore him, but that proved impossible when she was forced to stay at Rayne Park, Drum's residence, while her grandfather travelled! She soon discovered that he had *every* right to boss her around, but he had *no* right to let her fall in love—with him!

GABRIELLA
Brenda Hiatt

Gabriella Gordon knew that she would have to agree to a London Season sooner or later or her Society sister would plague her to death. So when the celebrated Duke of Ravenham came to call, supposedly owing to the outcome of a wager, the duke was obliged to lend Gabriella his escort and consequence. Gabriella's sister was in raptures, but Gabriella most definitely was not. She was determined to be as difficult as possible but found that was easier said than done...

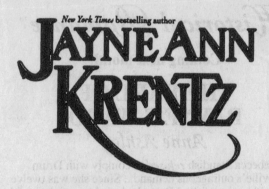

New York Times bestselling author

JAYNE ANN KRENTZ

Full Bloom

Part bodyguard, part troubleshooter, Jacob Stone
had, over the years, pulled Emily out of countless
acts of rebellion against her domineering family.
Now he'd been summoned to rescue her from a
disastrous marriage. Emily didn't want his
protection—she needed his love. But did Jacob
need this new kind of trouble?

"A master of the genre...nobody does it better!"

—Romantic Times

**AVAILABLE IN PAPERBACK
FROM MAY 1997**

FOUR FREE
specially selected
Historical Romance™ novels
PLUS a FREE Mystery Gift
when you return this page...

Return this coupon and we'll send you 4 Historical Romance novels and a mystery gift absolutely FREE! We'll even pay the postage and packing for you.

We're making you this offer to introduce you to the benefits of the Reader Service™– FREE home delivery of brand-new Historical Romance novels, at least a month before they are available in the shops, FREE gifts and a monthly Newsletter packed with information, competitions, author profiles and lots more...

Accepting these FREE books and gift places you under no obligation to buy, you may cancel at any time, even after receiving just your free shipment. Simply complete the coupon below and send it to:

MILLS & BOON READER SERVICE, FREEPOST, CROYDON, SURREY, CR9 3WZ.

READERS IN EIRE PLEASE SEND COUPON TO PO BOX 4546, DUBLIN 24

NO STAMP NEEDED

Yes, please send me 4 free Historical Romance novels and a mystery gift. I understand that unless you hear from me, I will receive 4 superb new titles every month for just £2.99* each, postage and packing free. I am under no obligation to purchase any books and I may cancel or suspend my subscription at any time, but the free books and gift will be mine to keep in any case. (I am over 18 years of age)

H7XE

Ms/Mrs/Miss/Mr_____

BLOCK CAPS PLEASE

Address_____

_____

_____ Postcode _____

Offer closes 30th November 1997. We reserve the right to refuse an application. *Prices and terms subject to change without notice. Offer only valid in UK and Ireland and is not available to current subscribers to this series. Overseas readers please write for details.

You may be mailed with offers from other reputable companies as a result of this application. Please tick box if you would prefer not to receive such offers. ☐

Mills & Boon® is a registered trademark of Harlequin Mills & Boon Limited.

NEW YORK TIMES
BESTSELING AUTHOR

Anne Mather

Dangerous Temptation

He was desperate to remember... Jake wasn't
sure why he'd agreed to take his twin brother's
place on the flight to London. But when he
awakens in hospital after the crash, he can't even
remember his own name or the beautiful woman
who watches him so guardedly. Caitlin. His wife.

She was desperate to forget... Her husband
seems like a stranger to Caitlin—a man who
assumes there is love when none exists. He is
totally different—like the man she'd thought
she had married. Until his memory returns.
And with it, a danger that threatens them all.

"Ms. Mather has penned a wonderful romance."
—Romantic Times

**AVAILABLE IN PAPERBACK
FROM MAY 1997**